Aging Facial Skin: Lasers and Related Spectrum Technologies

Guest Editor

DAVID A.F. ELLIS, MD, FRCSC

FACIAL PLASTIC SURGERY CLINICS OF NORTH AMERICA

www.facialplastic.theclinics.com

May 2011 • Volume 19 • Number 2

SAUNDERS an imprint of ELSEVIER, Inc.

W.B. SAUNDERS COMPANY
A Division of Elsevier Inc.

1600 John F. Kennedy Blvd., Suite 1800, Philadelphia, PA 19103-2899

http://www.theclinics.com

FACIAL PLASTIC SURGERY CLINICS OF NORTH AMERICA Volume 19, Number 2
May 2011 ISSN 1064-7406, ISBN 978-1-4557-0649-5

Editor: Joanne Husovski
Developmental Editor: Donald Mumford

Facial Plastic Surgery Clinics of North America (ISSN 1064-7406) is published quarterly by Elsevier Inc., 360 Park Avenue South, New York, NY 10010-1710. Months of issue are February, May, August, and November. Business and Editorial Offices: 1600 John F. Kennedy Blvd., Suite 1800, Philadelphia, PA 19103-2899. Periodicals postage paid at New York, NY, and additional mailing offices. Subscription prices are $329.00 per year (US individuals), $459.00 per year (US institutions), $375.00 per year (Canadian individuals), $550.00 per year (Canadian institutions), $449.00 per year (foreign individuals), $550.00 per year (foreign institutions), $156.00 per year (US students), and $217.00 per year (foreign students). Foreign air speed delivery is included in all *Clinics* subscription prices. All prices are subject to change without notice. POSTMASTER: Send address changes to *Facial Plastic Surgery Clinics*, Elsevier Health Sciences Division, Subscription Customer Service, 3251 Riverport Lane, Maryland Heights, MO 63043. **Customer service: 1-800-654-2452 (US and Canada); 1-314-447-8871 (outside US and Canada); Fax: 314-447-8029; E-mail:journalscustomerservice-usa@elsevier.com (for print support); journalsonline support-usa@elsevier.com (for online support).**

Reprints. For copies of 100 or more of articles in this publication, please contact the Commercial Reprints Department, Elsevier Inc., 360 Park Avenue South, New York, NY 10010-1710. Tel.: 212-633-3812; Fax: 212-462-1935; E-mail: reprints@elsevier.com.

Facial Plastic Surgery Clinics of North America is covered in *MEDLINE/PubMed* (*Index Medicus*).

Contributors

CONSULTING EDITOR

J. REGAN THOMAS, MD, FACS
Professor and Chairman, Department
of Otolaryngology, University of Illinois
at Chicago, Chicago, Illinois

EDITORIAL BOARD

SHAN R. BAKER, MD
Professor and Chief, Section of Plastic
and Reconstructive Surgery, University
of Michigan, Ann Arbor, Michigan

ROBERT KELLMAN, MD
Professor and Chairman, Department
of Otolaryngology, State University of
New York Upstate Medical University,
Syracuse, New York

RUSSELL W.H. KRIDEL, MD
Clinical Associate Professor, Department
of Otolaryngology–Head and Neck Surgery,
Division of Facial Plastic Surgery,
University of Texas Health Science Center,
Houston, Texas

STEPHEN W. PERKINS, MD
Private Practitioner, Perkins Facial Plastic
Surgery, Indianapolis, Indiana

ANTHONY P. SCLAFANI, MD, FACS
Director of Facial Plastic Surgery,
The New York Eye and Ear Infirmary,
New York, New York; and Professor of
Otolaryngology–Head and Neck Surgery,
New York Medical College, Valhalla,
New York

GUEST EDITOR

DAVID A.F. ELLIS, MD, FRCSC
Professor, Division of Facial Plastic Surgery,
Department of Otolaryngology–Head and Neck
Surgery, University of Toronto; Medical
Director, Art of Facial Surgery, Toronto,
Ontario, Canada

AUTHORS

**MACRENE ALEXIADES-ARMENAKAS,
MD, PhD**
Assistant Clinical Professor, Department of
Dermatology; Director, Dermatology and Laser
Surgery Center, Yale University School of
Medicine, New York, New York

S.M. ATHAVALE, MD
Resident in Otolaryngology, Department of
Otolaryngology, Vanderbilt University Medical
Center, Nashville, Tennessee

SUZANNE BRUCE, MD
Suzanne Bruce and Associates, The Center for Cosmetic Dermatology, Houston, Texas

PAUL J. CARNIOL, MD
Clinical Professor, Department of Otolaryngology Head and Neck Surgery, New Jersey Medical School-UMDNJ, Newark, New Jersey

JOHN DESPAIN, MD
DeSpain Cayce Dermatology Center, Columbia, Missouri

DAVID A.F. ELLIS, MD, FRCSC
Professor, Division of Facial Plastic Surgery, Department of Otolaryngology–Head and Neck Surgery, University of Toronto; Medical Director, Art of Facial Surgery, Toronto, Ontario, Canada

RICHARD D. GENTILE, MD, MBA
Medical Director, Associate Professor, Facial Plastic and Aesthetic Laser Center, Northeastern Ohio College of Medicine, Youngstown, Ohio

LISA DANIELLE GRUNEBAUM, MD
Assistant Professor of Facial Plastic and Reconstructive Surgery and Dermatology, University of Miami Miller School of Medicine, Miami, Florida

SANAZ HARIRCHIAN, MD
Resident in Otolaryngology, Department of Otolaryngology Head and Neck Surgery, New Jersey Medical School-UMDNJ, Newark, New Jersey

RYAN N. HEFFELFINGER, MD
Assistant Professor, Director, Division of Facial Plastic and Reconstructive Surgery, Thomas Jefferson University Hospital, Philadelphia, Pennsylvania

J. DAVID HOLCOMB, MD
Holcomb Facial Plastic Surgery and Institute for Integrated Aesthetics, Sarasota, Florida

GIA E. HOOSIEN, MD
Resident, Department of Otolaryngology–Head and Neck Surgery, University of Miami Miller School of Medicine, Miami, Florida

WHITNEY HOVENIC, MD
Chief Resident, Department of Dermatology, University of Missouri, Columbia, Missouri

ERIN KELLY
Student, Wake Forest University, Winston-Salem, North Carolina

JEANNIE KHAVKIN, MD
Previous Fellow, Division of Facial Plastic Surgery, Department of Otolaryngology–Head and Neck Surgery, University of Toronto, Toronto, Ontario, Canada

WENDY W. LEE, MD
Assistant Professor of Clinical Ophthalmology/Oculofacial Plastic and Reconstructive Surgery, Bascom Palmer Eye Institute, University of Miami Miller School of Medicine, Miami, Florida

JENNIFER MURDOCK, BS
University of Miami Miller School of Medicine, Miami, Florida

MARITZA I. PEREZ, MD
St Luke's Roosevelt Hospital Center, New York, New York

KRISTEL D. POLDER, MD
Clinical Assistant Professor, Department of Dermatology, University of Texas at Houston; Suzanne Bruce and Associates, The Center for Cosmetic Dermatology, Houston, Texas

JAGGI RAO, MD, FRCPC
Associate Clinical Professor of Medicine; Director, Dermatology Residency Program, Division of Dermatology and Cutaneous Sciences, University of Alberta, Edmonton, Alberta, Canada

W.R. RIES, MD
Professor, Division of Facial Plastic Surgery, Department of Otolaryngology, Vanderbilt University Medical Center, Nashville, Tennessee

ANTHONY M. ROSSI, MD
St Luke's Roosevelt Hospital Center, New York, New York

G. DANIEL SCHACHTER, MD, FRCPC (Dermatology), FAAD
Department of Dermatology, Women's College Hospital; Lecturer, Department of Dermatology, University of Toronto Medical School, Toronto, Ontario, Canada

KEVIN C. SMITH, MD, FRCPC (Dermatology), FAAD
Niagara Falls Dermatology and Skin Care Centre Ltd, Niagara Falls, Ontario, Canada

MICHAEL STAMPAR, DO
Private Practice, Punta Gorda, Florida

WHITNEY VALINS, MD
University of Miami School of Medicine,
Miami, Florida

MARTHA H. VIERA, MD
Resident of General Surgery PYG1,
Department of General Surgery, University
of Miami, Miami, Florida

JOSEPH K. WONG, MD, FRCS(C)
Department of Otolaryngology–Head and Neck
Surgery, Credit Valley Hospital-Peel Regional
Cancer Centre, Mississauga; Director,
Advanced Aesthetic Surgical Centre,
Toronto, Ontario, Canada

HEATHER WOOLERY-LLOYD, MD
Voluntary Assistant Professor, Director
of Ethnic Skin Care, Department of
Dermatology and Cutaneous Surgery,
University of Miami, Miami, Florida

Contents

> Skin is a complex organ covering the entire surface of the body. Aged skin is characterized by appearance of wrinkles, laxity, and pigmentary irregularities. These changes occur under the influence of intrinsic and extrinsic factors, with sun exposure being the most deleterious to the skin. Skin changes associated with aging are the focus of many surgical and nonsurgical procedures aimed to improve the appearance of skin. Knowledge of skin histology and physiology will deepen the understanding of cutaneous changes associated with aging and will promote optimal cosmetic and functional patient outcomes.

> This article deals with the technical characteristics of fractional light devices, fractional lasers, and light sources that cause their biologic effects by increasing the temperature of the target tissues to the point where the target is either killed, or in other cases where the temperature of the target tissue is increased to the point where repair and remodeling systems are turned on but tissue is not killed. Resurfacing devices act by causing ablation and/or coagulation.

> Photographic documentation is an essential part of facial plastic surgery practice. Standardization of photographic technique is critical to achieve accurate and consistent images to be used for medicolegal, surgical planning, outcome review, research, and teaching purposes. Standardized, high-quality images can be obtained by using proper equipment, lighting, and patient positioning. Standardized photography is especially important for facial resurfacing procedures when fine details, such as pore size, skin texture, pigmentation, and rhytids, need to be captured and accurately assessed. The purpose of this review is to discuss how to obtain standardized, high-quality images of skin surface.

ABLATIVE

> Fractionated CO$_2$ lasers are a new treatment modality for skin resurfacing. These lasers have been shown efficacious in treating facial photoaging changes and scars. These lasers have an improved safety and recovery profile compared with traditional CO$_2$ laser resurfacing. Precise treatment parameters vary between patients, the pathology treated, and the details of the particular laser.

The 2790-nm wavelength YSGG laser was introduced for aesthetic purposes under the trade name Pearl by Cutera in 2007. In clinical use, the Pearl superficial resurfacing laser has proved effective and well tolerated for the correction of superficial brown epidermal dyschromia and superficial fine lines and scars, and the Pearl Fractional laser produces excellent improvement in both dyschromia and improvement of deeper lines and moderately deep acne scarring. The two laser treatments can be combined in a single treatment session on different parts of the face or on the entire face, depending on patient needs and priorities.

For the laser surgeon, the Er-YAG laser is an invaluable tool that delivers unsurpassed ablation efficiency, and with appropriate functionality (quasi long-pulse feature) provides sufficient tissue coagulation to remodel deep rhytids. As such, the 2940-nm wavelength is well suited for routine laser skin rejuvenation in full-field, fractional, and point-beam modes with additional benefits, including applicability to diverse skin types, short healing times, and a low likelihood of energy-related complications. The author presents a technique video at www.facialplastic.theclinics.com.

Acne scarring is a common and expected result of moderate to severe acne vulgaris. Given the clinical variety of acne scars and the plethora of treatment options available, management of cutaneous scarring from acne can be challenging and confusing. This article discusses the pathophysiology of acne and acne scarring to better understand its biologic and structural nature. A simple, yet practical classification schema is presented, allowing caregivers to better organize their assessment of acne scarring and develop useful management strategies from this model. This article highlights the various useful laser options that are available for the treatment of acne scarring.

Modern cosmetic medicine requires accurate recognition of all types of rhytids and their molecular causes such that treatments may be tailored for improving skin appearance for each unique patient. This article examines the causes and treatment of fine rhytids. Laser rejuvenation therapies that affect the epidermis, dermis or both and induce neocollagenesis and dermal remodeling can be effective against the stigmata of mature skin.

NON-ABLATIVE LASERS

Cutaneous vascular lesions are common in both children and adults. The vast majority of these lesions respond well to laser treatment. A select few lesions may require surgical intervention. In order to choose the optimal laser treatment for a given lesion, it is important to have a thorough understanding of the available technology. This understanding includes the characteristics of each laser wavelength, pulse duration, and possible associated epidermal cooling. Furthermore, it is important to understand the specific characteristics of each individual vascular lesion. Together, laser treatment of cutaneous vascular lesions of the head and neck region can be optimized.

coupled radiofrequency (MRF). The authors discuss clinical studies using MRF. The authors also discuss their clinical experiences as well as recommendations for optimal results. MRF using the Thermage CPT system (Solta Medical, Hayward, California) offers minimal downtime with a favorable side-effect profile. Although there are many radiofrequency devices on the market for aesthetic use, MRF has the most clinical trials to date to support its use as an effective, evidence-based modality to improve rhytids and tighten the skin.

The application of infrared broadband light is the more recent addition of nonsurgical laser and light-based treatment for skin laxity and rhytids. Infrared broadband light, when used with the mobile technique, offers a painless, safe, nonsurgical alternative treatment option for treatment of skin laxity on the face and neck. Multiple clinical studies have demonstrated improvements in skin laxity correlated histologically with neocollagenesis and neoelastogenesis over a 6–12 month period. The consistency of clinical improvement in skin laxity supports the use of this approach for moderate skin laxity. The author presents a technique video at www.facialplastic.theclinics.com.

The greatest fear of using lasers subcutaneously in the face is that facial motor nerve injury will occur. With SmartLifting procedures, this is not a complication that occurs provided the laser and surgical guidelines are followed. We have seen several short-term, marginal mandibular neuropraxias in several patients, all of which resolved within weeks. There have been no permanent nerve injuries in any patient undergoing SmartLifting procedures. There is temporary interruption of cutaneous sensory nerves during the rhytidectomy, and the resolution of the temporary sensory deficits is identical to the resolution of non–laser-elevated rhytidectomies.

USING LASERS FOR SPECIFIC SKIN TYPES

Because the Latino/Hispanic ethnic group is made up of various skin phototypes there is no one particular laser parameter applied to all Latinos. This review examines specific laser therapies and tailors them for usage in the Latino population. Particular emphasis is placed on the selection of laser parameters, wavelengths, and pulse durations that are suitable and safe to use in Latino subtypes. Limitations are noted in the availability of certain lasers and the cost of such treatments as well as how the phototype of the patient limits what parameters can be used.

This article provides a systematic overview of laser, light, and other energy devices for patients of African descent. It also reviews complications in skin of color and some treatment options for these adverse events.

The term Asian refers to East Asians of the Pacific Rim who share not only a common heritage and skin type but also the same set of clinical skin problems. Pigmentation of the skin is often considered the number one esthetic skin concern in Asians. Asians idealize unblemished complexion of facial skin and are less tolerant to facial dyschromia than White. The problems of ephelides (freckles), nevi of Ota, and melasma are common and difficult to treat. This article reviews laser treatment of pigmented lesions in Asians.

Facial Plastic Surgery Clinics of North America

RELATED INTEREST

Medical Engineering & Physics, May 2008 (Vol. 30, No. 4)
Mechanical Approach to Aging and Wrinkling of Human Facial Skin Based on the Multistage Buckling Theory
Kuwazuru O, Saothong J, and Yoshikawa N, *Authors*

THE CLINICS ARE NOW AVAILABLE ONLINE!

Access your subscription at:
www.theclinics.com

Comprehending and Improving the Aging Face

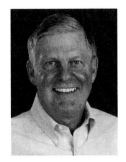

David A.F. Ellis, MD, FRCSC
Guest Editor

As facial plastic surgeons, we are highly skilled in correcting the aging face. Surgery to remove excessive fat bulges, hanging muscle in the neck, and excessive skin can show significant improvement. We can also, through injection techniques, augment lots of areas to help make patients appear younger, like depressed and collapsed cheeks. Moreover, aging skin and skin problems also need to be addressed and reviewed in great detail. This issue will tackle the aging skin and skin problems.

I would like to thank the authors sharing their expertise from both Canada and the United States for their contribution in making this issue as comprehensive as possible. This issue is fit for residents, staff, and practicing physicians in dermatology, facial plastic surgery, and general plastic surgery. The content of this issue is an excellent source of answers to questions that tend to show up in examinations. It is also useful for the early practicing surgeon and for ones that want to gain knowledge about the skin and its problems and to know about how lasers interface with the skin. Knowledge about skin is very important.

The surface of the skin is what we see when we look at people. The skin's quality can be measured in texture, brown patches, broken capillaries, and wrinkles. Hyperpigmented brown patches are definitely one of the signs of aging as are broken capillaries, rough texture, and wrinkles. Each of these problems is discussed in great detail so that the reader will understand the physiology, presentation, and possible degrees of improvement with treatment. Lax skin or elastosis is another aging skin problem that can be treated with nonsurgical technology. There is also an intraoperative laser technology that tightens the residual following a facelift. Astoundingly, it can be performed at the same time as a facelift. This is like "shrink wrapping" the skin. Other skin problems such as acne scarring and hirsutism are discussed.

In one section of this issue, the use of lasers in non-Caucasian skin ("Using Lasers for Specific Skin Types") is discussed. Many patients with Asian, Latino, and Black skin can have laser surgery to address their specific problems. Each of these three articles is very informative and gives the reader information on how to utilize lasers for ethnic skin problems.

The reader will have greater knowledge of the aging face, greater comprehension of how to improve common skin conditions, and additional skills to add to their surgical armamentarium—in hopes of providing his or her patients with the best possible outcome.

David A.F. Ellis, MD, FRCSC
Department of Otolaryngology
Head and Neck Surgery
University of Toronto
R. Fraser Elliott Building
190 Elizabeth Street, Room 3S-438
Toronto, ON M5G 2N2, Canada

Art of Facial Surgery
167 Sheppard Avenue West
Toronto, ON M2N 1M9, Canada

E-mail address:
ellis2106@gmail.com

facialplastic.theclinics.com

Facial Plast Surg Clin N Am 19 (2011) xiii
doi:10.1016/j.fsc.2011.06.001
1064-7406/11/$ – see front matter © 2011 Elsevier Inc. All rights reserved.

Aging Skin: Histology, Physiology, and Pathology

Jeannie Khavkin, MD[a],*, David A.F. Ellis, MD, FRCSC[a,b]

KEYWORDS

- Skin histology • Skin physiology • Skin aging
- Skin architecture • Photoaging

Skin is a complex organ covering the entire surface of the body. It provides a protective physical barrier between the body and the environment, preventing losses of water and electrolytes, reducing penetration by chemicals, and protecting against pathogenic microorganisms. The skin is important in regulation of body temperature and provides immunologic surveillance. It contains sensory and autonomic nerves and sensory receptors, which detect incoming stimuli of touch, vibration, pressure, temperature, pain, and itching.

Skin is an important component of outward beauty and is the focus of various cutaneous surgical and nonsurgical procedures. Skin changes associated with chronologic aging or photoaging, such as wrinkling, laxity, and changes in pigmentation, prompt patients to seek cosmetic procedures to improve the appearance of their skin. This article reviews skin histology and physiology as well as changes associated with cutaneous aging.

NORMAL SKIN ARCHITECTURE

Skin is organized into 3 layers: the epidermis, the dermis, and the hypodermis (**Fig. 1**). The fine structure of the skin shows considerable regional variations in epidermal and dermal thickness, distribution of epidermal appendages, and melanocyte content. Skin is glabrous or non–hair-bearing on the palms and soles, whereas hair-bearing skin covers the rest of the body.

Embryologically, the epidermis and its appendages develop from the surface ectoderm, and the dermis and hypodermis arise from mesoderm. During the fourth week of embryonic development, a single layer of ectoderm surrounds the embryo. This simple epithelium overlies a loosely organized layer of undifferentiated mesoderm known as mesenchyme. At about 6 weeks, the ectoderm and the underlying mesoderm begin to proliferate and differentiate. Hair follicles, nails, and glands begin to develop in the third month. By the end of the third month, regular bundles of collagen appear in the dermis. The embryonic connective tissue below the dermis develops into the subcutaneous layer of loose connective tissue characterized by fat islands.[1]

The Epidermis

The normal epidermis is a stratified squamous epithelium undergoing continuous renewal. The major cell in the epidermis is the ectodermally derived keratinocyte, making up approximately 95% of the epidermal cells. As the keratinocyte progressively moves from its attachment to the basement membrane to the skin surface, it forms several morphologically distinct epidermal layers: stratum basale or stratum germinativum, stratum spinosum, stratum granulosum, and stratum corneum (**Fig. 2**). On the palms and soles, an additional layer, stratum lucidum, can be identified between the stratum corneum and stratum granulosum. Other cell types found in the epidermis include melanocytes, Langerhans cells, and Merkel cells.

The authors have nothing to disclose.

[a] Division of Facial Plastic Surgery, Department of Otolaryngology-Head and Neck Surgery, University of Toronto, R. Fraser Elliott Building, 190 Elizabeth Street, Room 3S-438, Toronto, ON M5G 2N2, Canada
[b] Art of Facial Surgery, 167 Sheppard Avenue West, Toronto, ON M2N 1M9, Canada
* Corresponding author. 653 North Town Center Drive, Suite 308, Las Vegas, NV 89144.
E-mail address: jkhavkin@gmail.com

Facial Plast Surg Clin N Am 19 (2011) 229–234
doi:10.1016/j.fsc.2011.04.003

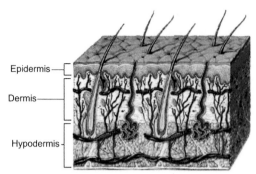

Fig. 1. The 3 layers of the skin: epidermis, dermis, and hypodermis. (*Courtesy of* A.D.A.M. Education, Atlanta, GA. Copyright © 2011 A.D.A.M., Inc.)

The basal layer is composed of a single layer of cuboidal cells, which rest on the basement membrane. Melanocytes can be seen between the basal cells of the epidermis. The basal cells divide, giving rise to the next layer: the prickle cell layer or stratum spinosum. This layer is usually 3 to 4 cells thick and is composed of polygonal cells with preformed keratin.[2] The desmosomal attachments between the cells appear as small spines, giving rise to the name stratum spinosum. The stratum spinosum is succeeded by stratum granulosum, which is usually 1 to 4 cells thick and derives its name from cytoplasmic keratohyalin granules. The outermost layer of the epidermis is stratum corneum composed of flattened keratinocytes that have lost their nuclei and cytoplasmic organelles.[1] These keratinocytes are shed in the process of epidermal turnover.

Melanocytes are derived from neural crest cells and migrate into the epidermis where they produce melanin. They are distributed among the basal keratinocytes with the ratio of 1 melanocyte to 4 to 10 basal cells. This ratio varies with anatomic location, with maximal density of

melanocytes on genital skin. Melanin is produced from tyrosine by the enzymatic activity of tyrosine kinase and is stored in melanosomes. Melanosomes are transported along the dendritic processes of melanocytes to adjacent keratinocytes, where they form an umbrella-like cap over the nucleus, protecting it from the injurious effects of UV light.[3] The ethnic variations in pigmentation are attributable to the different activity of melanocytes, not the difference in number of melanocytes. With age, melanocyte density decreases by 6% to 8% per decade, with higher density of melanocytes in sun-exposed skin than in non-exposed skin at all ages. This explains the generalized increase in pigmentation and simultaneous decrease in melanocyte density that often accompany aging.[4]

Langerhans cells are antigen-presenting cells derived from bone marrow. They make up 3% to 6% of all cells in the epidermis[3] and are found mainly within the spinous layer. The dendritic processes of Langerhans cells uptake antigens deposited on the skin, process them, and present them to T lymphocytes for activation of the immune response. The number of Langerhans cells increases during allergic reactions, such as contact hypersensitivity. With aging and chronic sun exposure, the number of Langerhans cells decreases, which may play a permissive role in the development of cutaneous carcinoma in individuals who are elderly with sun-damaged skin.[5]

Merkel cells are found in the basal layer of the epidermis and in the epithelial sheath of hair follicles. Merkel cells migrate from neural crest to the skin and have similar chemical and structural properties to an amine precursor uptake decarboxylation (APUD) cell.[6] Merkel cells are associated with sensory nerve endings in the skin and may function as mechanoreceptors.[4]

Epidermal appendages

Epidermal appendages are specialized epithelial structures located mainly in the dermis and hypodermis, but connected to the epidermis. They include pilosebaceous follicles, sweat glands, and apocrine glands. They play an important role in the epithelialization phase of wound healing.

Pilosebaceous unit The pilosebaceous unit consists of hair, hair follicle, sebaceous gland, and arrector pili muscle (**Fig. 3**). It is distributed throughout the integument, absent only in palms and soles and portions of the genitalia.

The hair follicle is composed of several segments: infundibulum, isthmus, lower follicle, and hair bulb. The topmost portion is the infundibulum, extending down from the skin to the opening

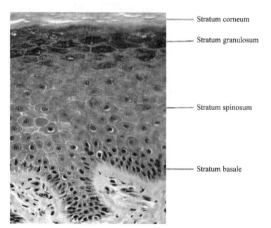

Fig. 2. Layers of the epidermis (hematoxylin-eosin, magnification ×40).

Stratum corneum

Stratum granulosum

Stratum spinosum

Stratum basale

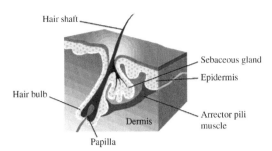

Hair shaft

Sebaceous gland

Epidermis

Hair bulb

Arrector pili muscle

Dermis

Papilla

Fig. 3. Pilosebaceous unit.

of the sebaceous duct into the hair follicle. The isthmus extends from the infundibulum to the bulge, the site of insertion of the arrector pili muscle into the follicle. The bulge contains stem cells of the hair follicle. Contraction of the arrector pili muscle causes the hair to be pulled from an oblique to a more vertical orientation in response to stimuli from the sympathetic nervous system. Clinically, contraction of the arrector pili muscle results in slight elevations of the skin or goose bumps. The lower follicle extends down to the top of the hair bulb and the hair bulb is the terminal portion of the hair follicle, which envelops the follicular papilla.

The papilla is a dermal structure containing a richly vascularized and innervated connective tissue and fibroblasts, important for hair growth.[3] The hair bulb contains the matrix cells that give rise to the hair and melanocytes responsible for hair pigmentation. Permanent hair removal requires damage to follicular stem cells in the bulge region of the hair follicle.

Hair growth exhibits a cyclical pattern. Anagen is the growth phase in which cells of the hair matrix are dividing rapidly. Catagen is the involutional phase in which cell division ceases, hair matrix regresses, papilla retracts to the level of the insertion of the arrector pili muscle, and capillary nourishment diminishes. During the resting phase, known as telogen, the follicle detaches from the papilla and contracts, eventually falling out. At any given time in one anatomical location, follicles are present in different phases of the cycle. Hairs in the anagen phase are susceptible to destruction by laser; therefore, repeated hair removal treatments are necessary to address new follicles coming into the anagen phase.

With aging, the rate of hair growth declines and hair diminishes in thickness. Gray hair appears as the result of decreased melanin production within the hair matrix.

Sebaceous glands empty into the hair follicle. In some areas, sebaceous glands are not associated with a hair follicle and open directly onto the skin's surface. These areas include the eyelids, areolae of the nipples, and vermilion border of the lips.

Sebaceous glands are present in most areas of the body with the exception of palms and soles, with highest density of sebaceous glands found on the face. They consist of an outer layer of basal cells and several layers of lipid-laden sebocytes. Sebocytes disintegrate toward the center of the gland, thus forming sebum, which empties into the hair follicle via a short duct. Sebum provides emollients for the hair and skin. The secretions of the sebaceous glands are under the influence of androgen hormones. The gland activity increases shortly after birth and subsides in the first few postnatal months. At puberty, there is a new rise in sebaceous gland activity associated with increased androgen output. Increased sebum production is a major factor in the pathophysiology of acne vulgaris.[7] Sebum secretion declines with age by about 23% per decade in men and 32% per decade in women.[8] The size of the sebaceous glands increases with age, despite decrease in sebum production.[9] This can result in large pores, as seen with age.

Sweat glands The eccrine glands are the main sweat glands in humans and play a vital role in the process of thermoregulation. They are found almost everywhere on the skin except the vermillion border of the lips and nail beds and have maximum density over palms, soles, axillae, and forehead.[3] With aging, the number and function of eccrine sweat glands decrease.

Each eccrine gland is composed of 3 parts: the secretory coiled gland, the dermal duct, and the intraepidermal spiral duct known as acrosyringium. The secretory gland is situated in the deep dermis or at the dermal-hypodermal junction. It is composed of secretory clear and dark cells surrounded by contractile myoepithelial cells. Clear cells produce sweat in response to cholinergic stimulation. Their secretions are discharged into the lumen of the gland through intercellular canaliculi. The excretory duct ascends through the dermis in a vertical fashion and spirals through the epidermis, opening directly onto the skin's surface.

Apocrine glands form as outgrowths of the pilosebaceous units. Unlike eccrine glands, they are present primarily in the axillae and in the anogenital region. Apocrine glands are also found in other areas of the body, such as the external auditory canal, eyelid, and breast. The apocrine gland consists of a coiled gland located in the subcutaneous fat, and a straight duct that ascends through the dermis and empties into the infundibulum of the hair follicle. The coiled gland consists of one layer of secretory cells around a large lumen, surrounded by myoepithelial cells.

Apocrine glands produce secretions by decapitation, a process where the apical portion of the secretory cell's cytoplasm pinches off and enters the lumen of the gland. Apocrine sweat is odorless initially and develops an odor when it comes in contact with bacterial flora on the surface of the skin.

The dermal-epidermal junction

The dermal-epidermal junction is a basement membrane synthesized by basal keratinocytes and dermal fibroblasts. It functions as a mechanical support for adhesion of dermis to the epidermis and as a barrier to chemicals and cells. The structure of the dermal-epidermal junction is complex, consisting of 4 distinct layers seen on electron microscopy.[3] The top layer contains the cell membrane of basal keratinocytes and their hemidesmosomes. Cytoskeletal filaments course through the basal cells and insert into the hemidesmosomes. The next layer is lamina lucida, which is traversed by anchoring filaments, and rests on top of lamina densa. The sub-basal lamina layer is a filamentous zone mainly made up of anchoring fibrils, which serve to anchor the epidermis and dermal-epidermal junction to the dermis.

The Dermis

The dermis is divided into 2 distinct regions: the upper papillary dermis and the lower reticular dermis. The papillary dermis is located just below the dermal-epidermal junction and forms conic upward projections known as dermal papillae. These projections interdigitate with epidermal rete ridges, increasing the area of dermal-epidermal interface and allowing for better adhesion between dermis and epidermis. The papillary dermis is composed of loosely arranged bundles of collagen, elastic fibers, fibrocytes, blood vessels, and nerve endings. The reticular dermis contains compact collagen fibers, thicker elastic fibers, deep part of epidermal appendages, and vascular and nerve networks.

Collagen is the major constituent of the dermis and is made of collagen fibers synthesized by fibroblasts. More than 90% of dermal fibers are made of interstitial collagen, mainly types I and III, providing tensile strength and mechanical resistance to the skin.

Elastic fibers are responsible for returning skin to its normal configuration after deformation and extend from lamina densa of the epidermal-dermal junction into the reticular dermis. The elastic fibers are thin in the papillary dermis but become thicker and more horizontally oriented in the reticular dermis. Reticulin fibers are also present in the dermis and consist of thin collagen fibers and fibronectin.

Dermal fibers and cells are embedded in the matrix of macromolecules known as ground substance. It consists of glycoproteins and proteoglycans and is abundant in the papillary dermis.

Cellular components of the dermis include fibroblasts, dermal dendrocytes, and mast cells. Fibroblasts are the main cells in the dermis synthesizing dermal fibers and the ground substance. They are abundant in the papillary dermis, but fewer in number in the reticular dermis. Fibrocytes are quiescent fibroblasts devoid of metabolic activity. Fibroclasts are fibroblasts with phagocytic activity toward collagen. Myofibroblasts are derived from fibroblasts and are involved in wound healing. Mast cells are derived from bone marrow and are distributed around blood vessels and adnexal structures of the papillary dermis. Dermal dendrocytes represent a heterogeneous population of mesenchymal dendritic cells and may act as phagocytes and antigen-presenting cells.

Vasculature

The skin has a rich vasculature consisting of 2 horizontally arranged networks: a superficial and a deep subdermal plexus. These networks originate from the perforator arteries of the underlying muscles and communicate via small vessels traversing the dermis vertically (**Fig. 4**). The subdermal plexus lies near the dermal-hypodermal junction and supplies hair follicles and sweat glands. The superficial plexus is derived from terminal arterioles and lies at the interface between the papillary and reticular dermis. The superficial plexus gives rise to a vascular loop that ascends to every dermal papilla as a precapillary arteriole, forms a turn of arterial and venous capillaries, and descends into the papillary dermis as a postcapillary venule. The venules form the superficial venular plexus, which connects with veins in subcutaneous fat. In some

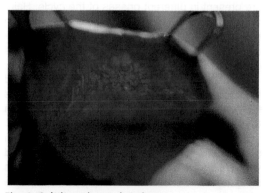

Fig. 4. Subdermal vascular plexus.

areas, arterioles and venules communicate directly via arteriovenous shunts bypassing the capillary circulation. These shunts are controlled by glomus cells innervated by adrenergic fibers.

Cutaneous vessels are composed of 3 layers similar to other vessels in the body. Endothelial cells are enveloped by the basement membrane containing enmeshed pericytes. They are surrounded by smooth muscle cells and connective tissue adventitia. Arterioles and venules of the deep dermis and hypodermis are larger than corresponding vessels of the superficial plexus, with more pericytes present.[3]

Lymphatics begin as blind-ended capillaries in the interstitial spaces of the dermal papillae and form a superficial and a deep plexus. Lymphatic vessels are lined by endothelial cells and lack basal lamina and pericytes. Superficial lymphatic vessels are valveless; deeper lymphatics have multiple valves and thicker walls. Lymphatics play an important role in regulation of interstitial fluid pressure, in removal of excess extracellular fluid, and in immune reactions.

Nerves

The skin is richly innervated by sensory and autonomic nerve fibers. The sensory nerves are afferent nerves that carry the sensation of pain, pressure, temperature, vibration, and itch. Specialized receptors are present in the skin to detect various stimuli. The encapsulated receptors include the Meissner and Vater-Pacini corpuscles. Meissner corpuscles are found in dermal papillae and function as mechanoreceptors mediating the sensation of touch. They consist of a cylindrical column of flattened laminar cells interspersed with terminal nerve fibers and surrounded by an adventitial capsule.[10] Vater-Pacini corpuscles are found at the dermal-hypodermal junction and function as receptors of pressure and vibration. They have a characteristic onionlike appearance, consisting of concentric lamellae wrapped around a single nerve fiber. The nonencapsulated receptors include free terminal nerve endings and Merkel cells.

The efferent nerves are autonomic and originate in the sympathetic nervous system. They innervate smooth muscles of blood vessels, glomus bodies, the arrector pili muscles, and eccrine and apocrine glands. They regulate vasomotor response, sweat production, and piloerection.

Hypodermis

The hypodermis is the deepest layer of the skin and lies below the dermis and above the underlying muscle. It insulates the body and protects it from mechanical injuries, as well as serves as a reserve energy supply. The main cells of the hypodermis are adipocytes arranged in lobules separated by connective tissue septae. The thickness of this layer shows anatomic and individual variation and reflects the nutritional status of the individual.

EFFECTS OF AGING

Cutaneous aging is characterized by intrinsic and extrinsic processes. Intrinsic or chronologic aging is genetically determined and is an inevitable process in the skin. Intrinsically aged skin is characterized by laxity and some exaggerated expression lines.

Histologically, the epidermis is thinner with flattening of the dermal-epidermal junction.[11] The loss of surface area of the dermal-epidermal interface contributes to increased skin fragility and reduced nutrient transfer between dermis and epidermis. Epidermal cell turnover decreases, which may account for slower wound healing and less effective desquamation. The dermis becomes atrophic with reduced numbers of fibroblasts and there is a decrease in subdermal adipose tissue. The number and diameter of collagen fiber bundles decreases with age and the ratio of type III collagen to type I collagen increases.[12]

Extrinsic aging is engendered by external factors, of which sun exposure is considered the most deleterious to the skin. Clinical signs of photoaging include dryness, rhytids, irregular pigmentation, loss of elasticity, telangiectasias, and areas of purpura. Histologically, photoaged skin is characterized by accumulation of elastin material just below the dermal-epidermal junction, known as elastosis. Epidermal atrophy and fragmentation of collagen and elastic fibers are also associated with photoaged skin.[13]

SUMMARY

The skin is a complex organ both structurally and functionally. Knowledge of skin histology and physiology fosters a better understanding of cutaneous changes associated with aging. In addition, it helps achieve an optimal cosmetic and functional outcome during surgical and nonsurgical procedures aimed to reverse the signs of cutaneous aging.

REFERENCES

1. McGrath JA, Eady RA, Pope FM. Anatomy and organization of human skin. In: Burns T, Breathnach S, Cox N, et al, editors. Rook's textbook

of dermatology. 7th edition. Malden (MA): Blackwell Publishing; 2004. p. 1–53.

2. Bennet RG. Anatomy and physiology of the skin. In: Papel ID, editor. Facial plastic reconstructive surgery. 2nd edition. New York: Thieme; 2002. p. 3–14.

3. Kanitakis J. Anatomy, histology and immunohisto-chemistry of normal human skin. Eur J Dermatol 2002;12(4):390–401.

4. Gilrecht BA, Blog FB, Szabo G. Effects of aging and chronic sun exposure on melanocytes in human skin. J Invest Dermatol 1979;73:141–3.

5. Thiers BH, Maize JC, Spicer SS, et al. The effect of aging and chronic sun exposure on human Langerhans cell populations. J Invest Dermatol 1984;82: 223–6.

6. Winkelman RK. The Merkel cell system and a comparison between it and the neurosecretory or APUD cell system. J Invest Dermatol 1977; 69:41–6.

7. Zouboulis CC. Acne and sebaceous gland function. Clin Dermatol 2004;22(5):360–6.

8. Jacobsen E, Billings JK, Frantz RA, et al. Age-related changes in sebaceous wax ester secretion rates in men and women. J Invest Dermatol 1985; 85:483–5.

9. Plewig G, Kligman AM. Proliferative activity of the sebaceous glands of the aged. J Invest Dermatol 1978;70:314–7.

10. Cauna N, Ross L. The fine structure of Meissner's touch corpuscles of human fingers. J Biophys Biochem Cytol 1960;8(2):467–82.

11. Montagna W, Carlisle K. Structural changes in aging human skin. J Invest Dermatol 1979;73:47–53.

12. Lovell CR, Smolenski KA, Duance VC, et al. Type I and III collagen content and fibre distribution in normal human skin during ageing. Br J Dermatol 1987;117:419–28.

13. Baumann L. Skin ageing and its treatment. J Pathol 2007;211(2):241–51.

Technical Characteristics of Fractional Light Devices

Kevin C. Smith, MD, FRCPC (Dermatology)[a],*,
G. Daniel Schachter, MD, FRCPC (Dermatology)[b,c]

KEYWORDS

- Fractional light devices • Fractional lasers
- Resurfacing devices • YSGG laser • Er-YAG laser
- CO_2 laser

This article deals with the technical characteristics of fractional light devices, fractional lasers, and light sources that cause their biologic effects by increasing the temperature of the target tissues to the point where the target is either killed (for example, where the target is a hair follicle or the lining of a blood vessel), or in other cases where the temperature of the target tissue is increased to the point where repair and remodeling systems are turned on but tissue is not killed.

Resurfacing devices act by causing ablation and/or coagulation. Coagulation produces a complex set of tissue effects, depending on the combination of temperature to which tissue is raised and duration of temperature rise. At one extreme, coagulation causes apoptosis and cell death; at the milder end of the spectrum, tissue exposed to lower energy (for example, because it is further away from the beam) may only be heated up to the extent that the tissue is injured but not destroyed, turning on repair and remodeling systems that contribute to the aesthetic benefits which the patient is seeking.

The light emitted by optical therapeutic devices can be either a single pure wavelength—generally produced by a laser—or a part of the visible and infrared spectrum (eg, produced by intense pulsed light [IPL] from a filtered flash lamp or light-emitting diodes [LED]). The energy is generally administered in pulses ranging in duration from milliseconds to seconds, and each pulse can range in shape from a square wave to a series of subpulses, depending on system design considerations and cost/performance trade-offs. The spot size can range from perhaps 100 microns in some fractionated ablative devices to several square centimeters in the case of many intense pulsed light devices.

The choice of technologies used in optical therapeutic devices depends to a great extent on what is most cost effective. There is no magic in "lasers," and over the years non-laser light sources have become increasingly effective—and cost-effective. In general, laser light is more expensive to produce and control, but has the advantage of allowing a much higher degree of precision when specifying the parameters shown in **Box 1**.

Precise control of the above parameters is valuable only up to a point; beyond that, extra precision adds cost without adding value.

The laser wavelengths and IPL/LED spectra used in these devices are chosen with careful

[a] Niagara Falls Dermatology and Skin Care Centre Limited, 6453 Morrison Street, Suite 201, Niagara Falls, ON L2E 7H1, Canada
[b] Department of Dermatology, Women's College Hospital, 208 Bloor Street, Suite 403, Toronto, ON M5S 3B4, Canada
[c] Department of Dermatology, University of Toronto Medical School, Toronto, ON, Canada
* Corresponding author.
E-mail address: ksmithderm@gmail.com

Facial Plast Surg Clin N Am 19 (2011) 235–240
doi:10.1016/j.fsc.2011.05.003

Box 1

Differences between fractional light treatment devices

1. Wavelength
2. Spot size
3. Spot pattern (**Fig. 1**)

   a. Grid versus random pattern

4. Density of spots: percent coverage of the treated area (**Fig. 2**)
5. Sequential adjacent versus nonsequential nonadjacent placement of spots, to minimize thermal load (bulk heating) on nontreated skin between spots (**Fig. 3**)
6. Pulse duration
7. Fluence
8. Degree of beam collimation
9. Beam homogeneity

   a. For example, top hat versus Gaussian energy distribution

10. Pulse characteristics

    a. Ranging from a simple square wave to a train of subpulses, the duration of which may be modulated to optimize the balance between ablation and coagulation; this is most commonly done with Er-YAG systems.

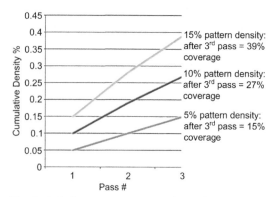

Fig. 2. It is important to note that when multiple passes are made using a fractional device, some pulses in the second and subsequent passes will hit areas that were already hit on a previous pass. The result is that the cumulative density will not be the simple sum of the densities of the passes, but will be a smaller number, equal to the number of unique areas treated per square centimeter.

Each of the items listed in **Box 1** is influenced by considerations of what is technically possible and what it financially feasible. Technical and financial tradeoffs define the design envelope within which engineers, physicians, and businesses must work to create a commercial piece of medical equipment having a satisfactory degree of safety, efficacy, reproducibility of results, and technical reliability.

Because these devices work by increasing the temperature of the target tissue, and because there can be some heating of nontarget tissue, it is necessary to design the equipment and to conduct treatments in a way that will minimize the risk of damage to nontarget tissues. As a practical matter, this often requires some degree of cooling to protect the surface of the skin. As a general rule, it is important to keep the surface of the skin below about 50°C, because even

attention to the degree to which they transfer energy to the intended chromophore, and taking into account the depth of the target and the depth to which the proposed wavelength or spectrum is capable of penetrating. The depth of penetration of a wavelength or spectrum is influenced by the degree to which it is absorbed (and scattered) by water and other tissue components (**Fig. 4**), and is also influenced by spot size (**Fig. 5**). The final effect of a given wavelength on target and nontarget tissue is strongly influenced by the factors listed in **Box 1**.

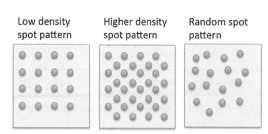

| Low density spot pattern | Higher density spot pattern | Random spot pattern |

Fig. 1. Fractional devices deliver energy either by laying down a grid pattern of pulses or a random pattern. Dot pitch refers to the number of pulses per square centimeter.

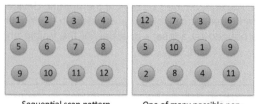

Sequential scan pattern   One of many possible non-sequential, non-adjacent scan patterns

Fig. 3. Sequential adjacent pulses at certain combinations of high power and/or high density may cause bulk heating. Nonsequential, nonadjacent pulse patterns may allow better heat dissipation and reduce the risk of bulk heating.

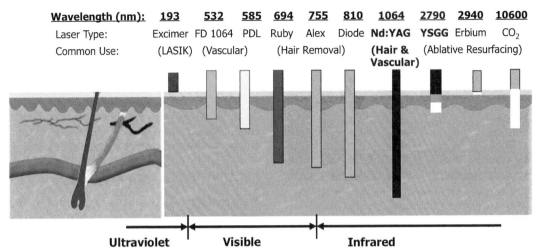

Wavelength (nm):	193	532	585	694	755	810	1064	2790	2940	10600
Laser Type:	Excimer	FD 1064	PDL	Ruby	Alex	Diode	**Nd:YAG**	**YSGG**	Erbium	CO$_2$
Common Use:	(LASIK)	(Vascular)		(Hair Removal)			**(Hair & Vascular)**	(Ablative Resurfacing)		

Ultraviolet   **Visible**   **Infrared**

Fig. 4. Scattering of light in the dermis decreases (so depth of penetration increases for a given spot size) as wavelength rises, up to about 1200 nm. Beyond 1200 nm, water becomes an important chromophore in the skin, and absorbs a great deal of energy, reducing depth of penetration of light beyond 1200 nm.

a few seconds at or above this temperature can cause death of skin components, including epidermal and dermal cells. It is important to remember that while it is often vital to cool the surface of the skin, it is counterproductive to cool the skin for too long before the energy pulse, because this would reduce the temperature of target tissues [for example, hair follicles or blood vessels] to the point that it will not rise to a sufficient temperature (generally above 80°C) for a fraction of a second when they absorb light energy and convert it to the heat that is necessary to kill the target.

Bulk heating refers to heating the entire surface of the skin, rather than a fraction of the surface. Bulk heating, for example during nonfractional CO$_2$ or Er-YAG laser resurfacing, can produce a dramatic improvement in the appearance of the treated area but is associated with increased down time and increased risks of complications like scarring, prolonged erythema, and pigment loss. Fractional ablative laser treatment avoids bulk heating, for example by using combinations of the elements shown in **Box 2** to keep the thermal load on normal skin between the spots below a level that would cause harmful heating. In general, the operator is only able to control the fluence and pattern density, and must be aware of the range of fluences and pattern densities that will produce optimal results with minimal risks on the individual being treated. The use of fluences and pattern densities that have a high risk of

> Effect of dermal scatter on beam propagation: larger spot sizes tend to lose a smaller proportion of their energy to scattering, and so can create thermal injury at greater depths.

Fig. 5. Small spot sizes are more strongly influenced by scattering of light in the dermis than are larger spot sizes, with the result that smaller spot sizes tend to have a lower depth of penetration for a given wavelength and fluence.

Box 2
Factors that influence the risk of bulk heating of the skin

1. Fluence
2. Spot size
3. Spot patterns (grid vs random) (see **Fig. 1**)
4. Pattern densities (see **Fig. 1**)
5. Sequences of spot delivery—for example, random spot delivery allows a slightly greater time for heat dissipation before an adjacent piece of skin is irradiated compared with sequential spot delivery (see **Fig. 3**).

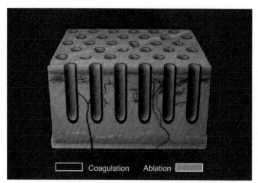

Fig. 6. Simple 3-dimensional diagram illustrating skin after treatment with fractional ablative laser.

causing bulk heating must generally be avoided. These parameters will vary with the characteristics of each individual device, and will also vary depending on the characteristics of the skin being treated (eg, skin on the lower two-thirds of the neck and the chest must be treated with lower fluences and pattern densities than would be appropriate on the face).

Increasing laser pulse energy increases depth of penetration and diameter of treated area

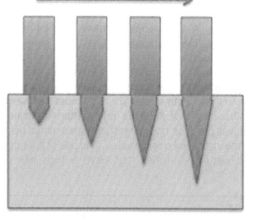

Fig. 7. In general, both the diameter and the depth of the fractional wound will increase in a fairly linear manner with increases in fluence. The energy level is chosen to produce a depth of penetration sufficient to treat the patient's problem ("put the energy where the target is"). For example, low energy/limited depth is appropriate for superficial lines and/or thin skin, for example on the eyelids. High energy/deep penetration is necessary for deep scars on the cheeks. It is important to realize that multiple passes at inadequate fluence will not give the depth of injury necessary to effectively treat a deep target.

Apart from lasers used for the treatment of tattoos (not the subject of this article), the chromophores targeted by lasers and light sources used for aesthetic treatment are melanin, hemoglobin, and water. While it is possible to target each of these chromophores with a range of wavelengths (in the case of lasers) or spectra (in the case of IPL and LED devices), the wavelength or spectrum chosen for a device will depend on the engineering and economic trade-offs already discussed.

ABLATIVE VERSUS NONABLATIVE

Fractional light devices that vaporize some of their target tissue are classified as ablative (**Fig. 6**). Devices that heat up but do not cause vaporization of tissue are considered nonablative. In some jurisdictions, the use of ablative devices is subject to more stringent regulation, and insurers may require higher premiums if such devices are used. A third group, comprised of the subablative devices, may be emerging. Subablative devices do not vaporize tissue, but cause a sufficient degree of subdermal coagulation that there is usually some desquamation or peeling for several days after treatment. Spot sizes used in fractional lasers and IPL devices can range in size from around 100 μmol to 1 mm or more. In general, larger spots are associated with greater discomfort, and may also be associated with the

> **Box 3**
> **Differences between fractional ablative lasers**
>
> 1. Depth and width of the zone of tissue ablation (see **Fig. 7**) influenced by
>   - Spot size
>   - Fluence
>   - Wavelength
>   - Pulse characteristics
> 2. Amount of normal tissue between zones affected by laser pulses (see **Fig. 1**)
> 3. Proportion between ablation and coagulation (see **Fig. 6**)
> 4. Grid versus random pattern (see **Fig. 1**)
> 5. Density (also referred to as dot pitch or percent coverage); it is important to realize the density of coverage does not increase in a linear manner with multiple passes, because during each pass after the first, some of the laser pulses will land on skin that has already received a pulse during a previous pass (see **Fig. 2**)
> 6. Sequential versus nonsequential delivery of laser spots to the skin (nonsequential delivery may have a lower risk of bulk heating the entire treated area) (see **Fig. 3**).

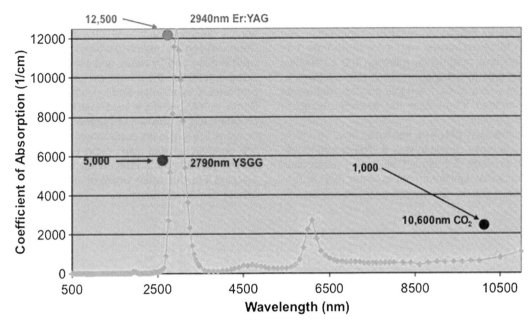

Fig. 8. Absorption of energy by water as a function of wavelength. 10,600 nm [CO_2 laser] has a low coefficient of absorption of approximately 1000, which produces a relatively high amount of coagulation in proportion to ablation. 2790 nm (YSGG laser) has an intermediate coefficient of absorption of approximately 5000, which produces a relatively balanced amount of ablation in proportion to coagulation. 2940 nm (Er-YAG laser) has a high coefficient of absorption of approximately 12,500, which produces a relatively high amount of ablation in proportion to coagulation. In some Er-YAG systems, the initial short ablative pulse of the Er-YAG is followed by 1 or more longer, lower powered coagulative pulses (**Fig. 5**), giving a final balance between ablation and coagulation approximating that produced by the YSGG laser (**Fig. 1**).

occasional development of pits after treatment. The use of random rather than grid patterns may make pits less obvious if they develop (see **Fig. 1**). The total area affected by the laser pulse (ablated zone, if any, plus the coagulated zone) is referred to as the microscopic treatment zone

(MTZ). In general, the width and depth of the MTZs increases in a fairly linear manner with increases in energy (**Fig. 7**).

Fractional ablative devices generally produce a higher degree of improvement with a smaller number of treatments than fractional nonablative devices. The trade-off is that aggressive fractional ablative treatments usually require more anesthesia with topical agents, cold air, and pretreatment of the patients with analgesics like

Thermal Zones by Wavelength
Assumes Sufficient Energy for Ablation

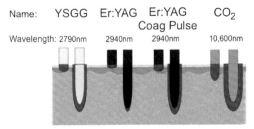

Fig. 9. The relative size of the zones of coagulation in this schematic diagram are shown in red. Note that in some variants of fractional ablative Er-YAG laser systems, 1 or more lower powered coagulative pulses, which are nonablative, follow the initial ablative pulse, and the effect of this series of pulses approximates the ablation/coagulation balance of the YSGG laser (**Fig. 10**).

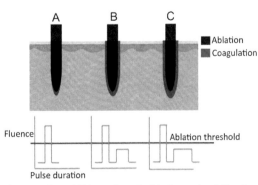

Fig. 10. The addition of a subablative pulse following the ablative pulse gives some Er-YAG systems an improved ratio of coagulation to ablation.

acetaminophen, ibuprofen, and occasionally narcotics. Fractional ablative treatments also tend to be associated with more down time than nonablative treatments, although the cumulative down time to get a given result may be lower in cases where fewer fractional ablative treatments are needed to produce the desired degree of improvement.

Differences between fractional ablative lasers include those shown in **Box 3**. The chromophore that accounts for almost all energy absorption in fractional light treatment is water (**Fig. 8**), because water is distributed quite homogenously throughout the top 1 to 2 mm of the skin, and is equally present in skin of all ages and ethnicities. Depending on the degree to which the wavelength used is absorbed by water, and depending on the pulse duration(s), the device will produce varying proportions of ablation and coagulation (**Fig. 9**). Some Er-YAG ablative fractional lasers can be programmed to follow the ablative pulse with 1 or more low-powered coagulative pulses, which are subablative and can improve the balance between ablation and coagulation in the Er-YAG systems (**Fig. 10**), which would otherwise produce almost exclusively ablation.

Standardized Photography for Skin Surface

Jeannie Khavkin, MD[a],*, David A.F. Ellis, MD, FRCSC[a,b]

KEYWORDS

- Dermatologic photography • Photographic documentation
- Photographic standards • Digital photography
- Facial resurfacing

High-quality photography is an essential part of any facial plastic surgery practice. Photographic documentation has a wide variety of clinical, research, and teaching applications and is also important for medicolegal purposes. Preoperative photographs assist in surgical planning and allow for effective communication of patients' perceptions and wishes. Comparison of preoperative and postoperative photographs allows surgeons and patients to accurately evaluate the outcome of the procedure. Review of photographic outcomes provides a surgeon with an opportunity for self-assessment and modification of surgical technique. In addition, photographs play an important role in advertising and marketing.

The prominent role of photography in facial cosmetic and reconstructive surgery places significant importance on using precisely defined standards during photodocumentation to achieve consistent and reproducible results. Standardized photography is especially important in facial resurfacing procedures where the changes are often subtle and variation in technique may demonstrate a clinical difference where none exists. In dermatologic photography, fine details, such as changes in skin texture, pigmentation, rhytids, and pore size, are evaluated to determine the efficacy of facial resurfacing procedures. The purpose of this review is to discuss how to obtain standardized, high-quality images of skin surface. Photographic variables, such as lighting, camera, exposure, focal length, white balance, and patient positioning, and their resultant effects on skin photography are discussed.

PHOTOGRAPHY EQUIPMENT
Camera

Digital single-lens-reflex (DSLR) cameras have replaced conventional 35-mm film cameras for most medical photography. The digital system is convenient to use because it allows for immediate viewing and evaluation of the images, many images can be taken without additional costs, and storage of images is quick and compact (**Fig. 1**).

Camera features should include a high-quality liquid crystal display screen for image review and an accessory shoe to connect with an external flash device. A gridded viewing screen is beneficial for consistent subject positioning. In terms of resolution, cameras with 5 megapixels or higher are sufficient for the purposes of medical photography.[1]

Lens

Lens selection is important for taking high-quality photographs and minimizing the amount of distortion. Lenses are classified by focal length. This measurement, defined in millimeters, is the distance between the optical center of the lens and the digital sensor when the lens is focused on

The authors have nothing to disclose.
[a] Department of Otolaryngology-Head and Neck Surgery, University of Toronto, R. Fraser Elliott Building, 190 Elizabeth Street, Room 3S-438, Toronto, ON M5G 2N2, Canada
[b] Art of Facial Surgery, 167 Sheppard Avenue West, Toronto, ON M2N 1M9, Canada
* Corresponding author. 653 North Town Center Drive, Suite 308, Las Vegas, NV 89144.
E-mail address: jkhavkin@gmail.com

facialplastic.theclinics.com

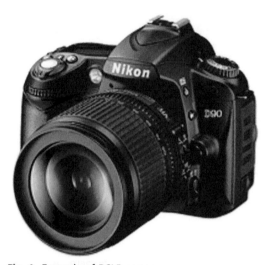

Fig. 1. Example of DSLR camera.

infinity. This distance relates to the distance that the camera must be from the subject for the subject to be in focus.

Most DSLR cameras come equipped with a zoom lens, which allows the photographer to change the focal length without changing lenses. If working with a zoom lens, it is imperative to use the *same* focal length for preoperative and postoperative documentation to avoid inconsistencies. Fixed focal length lenses are also available and some authors recommend using a fixed focal length lens to ensure image consistency.[2] Macro lenses are designed for near-focusing and allow capture of facial details. For medical portraiture, a macro lens with a focal length of 90 to 105 mm is recommended to capture relevant details of facial anatomy.[1,2] The range is extended to 120 mm for close-up dermatologic photography.[3] Lenses with shorter focal lengths, such as 50 to 55 mm, create a noticeable midface distortion (**Fig. 2**).

Exposure

Exposure control plays a fundamental role in creating a high-quality image. To obtain consistent exposure, automatic exposure settings should be avoided. The camera mode should be set to manual and 3 camera variables that determine exposure must be set by the photographer: f-stop setting, shutter speed, and ISO.

The amount of light that strikes the image sensor depends on aperture setting, also referred to as f-stop, and shutter speed. The aperture, much

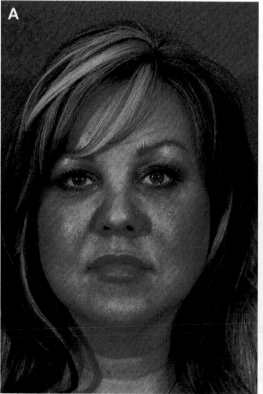
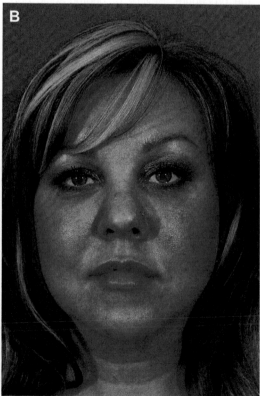

Fig. 2. (*A*) Photograph taken using 105-mm lens. (*B*) Photograph taken using 55-mm lens creates noticeable distortion, such as increase in nasal size.

like the pupil of the eye, controls the amount of light that passes through the lens. Shutter speed, much like a blink, determines the length of time the light is allowed to hit the sensor. Proper aperture and shutter speed selection is critical for achieving accurate reproduction of the subject matter.

F-stop number represents the ratio of the focal length of the lens to the diameter of the lens diaphragm opening. The larger the f-stop number, the smaller the diameter of the lens opening, the less light is allowed to strike the camera sensor. Each f-stop setting lets in half as much light as the next lower setting. The aperture of the camera also affects the depth of field, or the distance over which objects in the picture appear sharply focused. The larger the f-stop, the greater the depth of field. Typically, f/16 is desirable to ensure that all facial features are in focus. Patients with darker pigmentation may require f-stop to be lowered by half to 1 setting to brighten the image.[4] To select an appropriate f-stop for a given studio setup, a series of test shots should be taken at varied f-stops. These images can then be examined to select the appropriate setting.

Shutter speed affects the amount of light that enters the camera and controls the amount of movement seen in the photograph. For most photography in the office studio, shutter speed should be set to 1/60 seconds, a standard flash sync speed.[2]

ISO setting controls sensitivity of the camera sensor to light. The higher the ISO, the more sensitive the sensor is to light. In medical portraiture, an ISO of 200 is ideal to produce high-quality images.

BACKGROUND

The purpose of the background is to eliminate distractions and to place full focus on patients. For medical photography, a medium to light blue background is ideal. Blue background is visually pleasing in black and white or in color photography, provides sufficient patient-background separation, complements all skin tones, does not overwhelm patients, and allows for a greater depth of field. Having the same blue background in all preprocedure and postprocedure photographs guarantees that changes in skin color are not reflective of the change in the lighting. A white background produces harsh shadows, whereas black background diminishes 3-dimensional quality of the image.[4] The background should be without folds or creases and made of nonreflective material, such as matt paint, wallpaper, or cloth.

LIGHTING

Lighting is a major variable that affects ultimate quality of the image. There are several lighting techniques that can be employed in medical photography.

Using a single flash unit, such as a camera-mounted flash, produces harsh and uneven lighting (**Fig. 3**).

Using a ring flash tends to create an even, flat lighting, but may wash out color and skin tones.[3] In rhinoplasty photography, a stronger light source is desirable to highlight details of the nasal anatomy. In contrast, for facial rejuvenation and resurfacing procedures and to capture facial redness and pigmentation, soft, even, diffuse light, devoid of shadows and sharp lines, is used. These lighting conditions are achieved by using multiple flash units and soft boxes or umbrellas, which act as diffusers to eliminate shadows and provide even lighting.[5]

Most investigators recommend using 2 light sources placed at 45° angles to patients.[6–8] Additionally, a single backlight mounted centrally above, 1 to 3 ft from the background, or 2 backlights directed at 45° angles toward the background should be used to eliminate shadows in the background.[5,6] Patients should be positioned at least 2 to 3 ft from the background.[5] Light diffusers, such as soft boxes or umbrellas, should be placed in front of the main lights to provide even, soft lighting to the face (**Fig. 4**).

An understanding of color temperature and white balance is important in achieving appropriate color balance of the images. Different light sources have different color temperatures, containing different amounts of red, green, and blue light (**Fig. 5**).

White balance tells the camera which combination of red, green, and blue light should be perceived at pure white under given lighting conditions. Because lighting in the medical office studio is often mixed, white balance should be set to automatic to produce truest color results. If all the light in the medical studio comes from strobes, camera white balance may be set to flash.[2]

Electronic strobes are ideal light sources for medical photography studio.[2] Other light sources include ambient light, such as overhead fluorescent lighting, and tungsten flood lights. These light sources may produce inaccuracies in skin tones. For example, images taken in fluorescent lighting may have a slight greenish tint to them, whereas tungsten lighting produces a yellow/orange hue. Strobe lights produce light at 5500 K, which is sufficient to overpower any uncontrollable ambient light; however, every attempt should still be made to minimize ambient light, both natural and artificial.

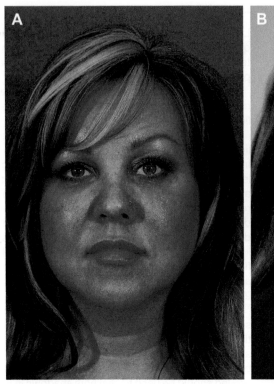
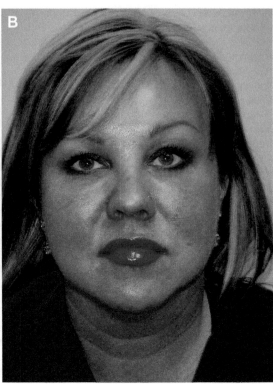

Fig. 3. (*A*) Soft light with 2 flashes at 45°. (*B*) Strong, harsh single flash directed at patient creating uneven brightness and color.

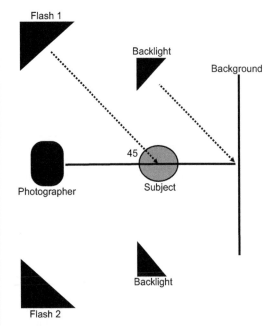

Fig. 4. Suggested setup for a medical photography studio. The light sources are set up at 45° to the subject. Backlights are used to eliminate shadows in the background.

PATIENT POSITIONING

Patient positioning is an important factor in achieving consistency and capturing pertinent anatomic details. All photographic distractors, such as hats, eyeglasses, jewelry, and scarves, should be removed. Patients should be advised to wear clothing in dark shades because light clothing may change the color tone by reflecting more light. Patients' hair should be pulled away from the face to expose the forehead and both ears. Makeup is acceptable as long as it is not distracting or excessive. Importantly, because fine

Type of Light	Color Temperature (K)	
Candle Flame	1,500	Red Hue
Incandescent	3,000	↑
Sunrise, Sunset	3,500	
Midday Sun, Flash	5,500	
Bright Sun, Clear Sky	6,000	
Cloudy Sky, Shade	7,000	↓
Blue Sky	9,000	Blue Hue

Fig. 5. Color temperature of different sources of light.

rhytids and skin irregularities may be camouflaged by makeup, it is recommended that all makeup be removed before photography for resurfacing procedures.[9]

Facial expression can affect fine details of skin appearance. Smiling can accentuate periorbital wrinkles and nasolabial folds. Neutral facial expression is necessary to accurately access topography of the skin.[3] Importantly, patients should be photographed with the same facial expression, whether smiling or neutral, before and after the procedure.

The position of the head and neck and the direction of the gaze must be standardized to prevent distortion. Sommer and Mendelsohn[10] demonstrated that small variation in patient positioning can affect photographic interpretation. Specifically, neck extension or head protrusion can improve jaw line and reduce the appearance of submental soft tissue. Direction of gaze is also important to obtain accurate photographs. Having patients look up will improve the appearance of periorbital wrinkles.[3]

Identical patient positioning should be used during each photography session. The Frankfort plane has been used as a method of standardizing the horizontal plane in lateral, oblique, and frontal views.[10] This imaginary line drawn from the top of the tragus to the infraorbital rim should be parallel to the floor. Because infraorbital rim is a bony landmark, it is not always easily found as a surface landmark and may need to be palpated

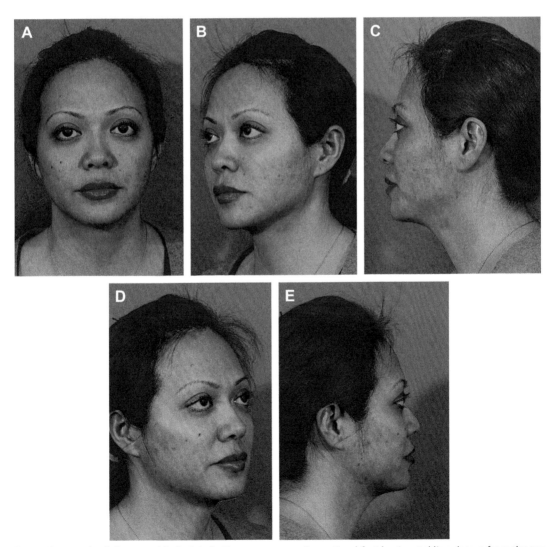

Fig. 6. Five standard views used in facial plastic surgery procedures. Frankfort horizontal line drawn from the top of the tragus to the infraorbital rim is used to guide proper head positioning. (*A*) Frontal view. (*B*) Right obilique view. (*C*) Right lateral view. (*D*) Left oblique view. (*E*) Left lateral view.

and marked for proper positioning. Using a grid-line display in the viewfinder may also aid in obtaining the proper Frankfort plane.

For the frontal view, patients commonly tilt their head to either left or right. The midsagittal plane in the viewfinder should also be used to align the head position in frontal views. On lateral view, patients tend to lift their neck out of the Frankfort plane or rotate their head toward or away from the camera. Rotation toward the camera is detected when the other eye is visible. Slight rotation away from the camera is harder to detect.

Maneuvers to ensure the proper lateral view involve asking patients to open their mouth and verifying the correct position by direct line of sight across the 2 oral commissures.[11] Superimposing the eyelashes may also be used.[12]

Standardization of the oblique view can either be achieved by aligning medial canthus with the oral commissure or aligning the tip of the nose with the lateral cheek (**Fig. 6**).

Standardization of photographic technique is critical for facial resurfacing procedures. Details of skin texture, rhytids, pore size, and pigmentation need to be captured and accurately assessed. Five views of patients are recommended with close-ups of the areas that are specifically addressed. The timing of photography is also important. If a series of treatments is planned, follow-up photographs need to be taken immediately before the next treatment to minimize edema and erythema.[3]

Photographs should be taken at the same distance to ensure uniform magnification. The axis of the camera lens should be maintained at patients' eye level and in the same plane.[2] Patients should be seated comfortably in a swivel chair. Markings on the floor may be placed to indicate the position of the patients' stool and foot placement. It may be helpful to place markers at specific sites around the room for patients to fixate their gaze and head position for frontal, lateral, and oblique views.

SUMMARY

Photography is an integral part of facial plastic surgery practice. Standardized photodocumentation allows for evaluation of surgical outcomes and for effective communication between physicians and patients. In dermatologic procedures, fine details, such as pore size, skin texture, and rhytids, are evaluated by photographic analysis. Capturing these subtle changes requires consistent, standardized photographic technique.

REFERENCES

1. Swamy RS, Most SP. Pre- and postoperative portrait photography: standardizedphotos for various procedures. Facial Plast Surg Clin North Am 2010; 18:245–52.
2. Neff LL, Humphrey CD, Kriet JD. Setting up a medical portrait studio. Facial Plast Surg Clin North Am 2010;18:231–6.
3. Shah AR, Dayan SH, Hamilton GS. Pitfalls of photography for facial resurfacing and rejuvenation procedures. Facial Plast Surg 2005;21(2):154–61.
4. Kontis TC. Photography in facial plastic surgery. In: Papel ID, editor. Facial plastic and reconstructive surgery. 2nd edition. New York: Thieme; 2002. p. 116–24.
5. Galdino GM, DaSilva D, Gunter JP. Digital photography for rhinoplasty. Plast Reconstr Surg 2002; 109:1421–34.
6. DiBernardo BE, Adams RL, Krause J, et al. Photographic standards in plastic surgery. Plast Reconstr Surg 1998;102(2):559–68.
7. Archibald DJ, Carlson ML, Friedman O. Pitfalls of nonstandardized photography. Facial Plast Surg Clin North Am 2010;18:253–66.
8. Persichetti P, Simone P, Langella M, et al. Digital photography in plastic surgery: how to achieve reasonable standardization outside a photographic studio. Aesthetic Plast Surg 2007;31:194–200.
9. Henderson JL, Larrabee WF, Krieger BD. Photographic standards for facial plastic surgery. Arch Facial Plast Surg 2005;7:331–3.
10. Sommer DD, Mendelsohn M. Pitfalls of nonstandardized photography in facial plastic surgery patients. Plast Reconstr Surg 2004;114:10–4.
11. Davidson TM. Photography in facial plastic and reconstructive surgery. J Biol Photogr Assoc 1979; 47(2):59–67.
12. Thomas JR, Tardy ME Jr, Przekop H. Uniform photographic documentation in facial plastic surgery. Otolaryngol Clin North Am 1980;13(2):367–81.

Fractional CO$_2$ Laser Resurfacing

Paul J. Carniol, MD[a],*, Sanaz Harirchian, MD[a], Erin Kelly[b]

KEYWORDS

- CO$_2$ laser • Fractionated laser • Skin resurfacing
- Fractionated laser resurfacing

The advent of lasers in the 1960s led to a paradigm shift in skin rejuvenation. The carbon dioxide (CO$_2$) laser was designed at Bell Laboratories (Murray Hill, NJ, USA) by Patel in 1964.[1] Medical applications of CO$_2$ lasers started in the latter 1970s. These lasers were found to provide significant advantages when dealing with pediatric airway problems.[2] In 1993, using high-energy CO$_2$ lasers, the first skin resurfacing was performed. By 1998 they had become popularized for skin rejuvenation; however, by that time it also had become apparent that there were risks of significant complications.[3]

The CO$_2$ laser emits an invisible infrared beam at a 10,600-nm wavelength, which is strongly absorbed by the chromophore, water (absorption coefficient, 800 cm^{-1}). Light energy from the CO$_2$ laser is absorbed by intracellular and extracellular water, resulting in coagulative necrosis and skin vaporization. A single pulse of the CO$_2$ laser with fluences of 4 J/cm^2 to 19 J/cm^2 ablates 20 μm to 40 μm depth of skin.[4] The depth of penetration can be changed by altering the laser fluence and/or pulse duration. Altering these also affects the surrounding zone of thermal injury.

The high-energy pulsed resurfacing CO$_2$ laser utilizes the laser biophysics concept of thermal relaxation time (TRT). This is the time required for the target tissue to lose 50% of its heat to surrounding tissue. The TRT for 20 μm to 30 μm of skin is approximately 1 ms. Selective heating of the target chromophore, water, is achieved when utilizing a laser pulse duration time shorter than the TRT. With pulse duration of less than 1 ms and an energy fluence of 4 J/cm^2 to 19 J/cm^2, the pulsed CO$_2$ laser selectively vaporizes 20 μm to 40 μm of tissue.[4]

The high-energy pulsed resurfacing CO$_2$ laser is the gold standard for modern ablative laser therapy. There also was a second basic type of CO$_2$ laser, which used a computer-controlled optomechanical flash scanner for resurfacing. This device, the FeatherTouch/SilkTouch (Sharplan Lasers, Allendale, NJ, USA) is of historical interest only because Sharplan was acquired by Lumenis (Palo Alto, CA, USA) and these lasers are no longer manufactured; it used a rapid scan with a focal spot of a continuous wave CO$_2$ laser over the skin, with a dwell time of less than 1 ms.

Resurfacing CO$_2$ lasers have been effective in the treatment of facial rhytides and scarring. Most reports found significant, 50% to 90%, improvement.[5,6] Studies also reported improvement in scars. Although ablative high-energy pulsed CO$_2$ laser therapy has been shown effective, there is a risk of associated complications. These include infection, persistent or prolonged erythema, delayed hypopigmentation, hypertrophic scars, ectropion, and scleral show.[3] Over time, considering the possibility of postresurfacing prolonged erythema and the risks of complications, other lasers were developed. These included nonablative lasers, fractional nonablative lasers, and, most recently, fractional ablative lasers.

FRACTIONAL PHOTOTHERMOLYSIS

The first laser to use fractional photothermolysis was nonablative. All fractional lasers create spaced columns of treated tissue rather than treating an entire area. Between these treated columns the tissues are not lasered; however, these unlasered adjacent tissues are subject to bulk heating effects.

[a] Department of Otolaryngology Head and Neck Surgery, New Jersey Medical School-UMDNJ, 185 South Orange Avenue, Newark, NJ 07103-2757, USA
[b] Wake Forest University, 1834 Wake Forest Road, Winston-Salem, NC 27106, USA
* Corresponding author.
E-mail address: pjclaser@aol.com

Facial Plast Surg Clin N Am 19 (2011) 247–251
doi:10.1016/j.fsc.2011.05.004
1064-7406/11/$ – see front matter © 2011 Published by Elsevier Inc.

The first fractional device was a 1550-nm laser, the Fraxel SR (Solta Medical, Hayward, CA, USA).[7]

Subsequently, ablative fractional lasers were created. In contrast to the nonablative fractional lasers, these devices vaporize columns of epidermis and part of the dermis as well as producing adjacent tissue heating. As with the nonablative fractional lasers, there is viable epidermis and dermis in the adjacent untreated areas. The percentage of the area that is vaporized varies, depending on the parameters that are set by the laser surgeon.

Initial healing after ablative fractional resurfacing occurs by more than one mechanism. Keratinocyte migration from the adjacent tissue into ablated areas occurs within the first 24 to 48 hours. This rapid epithelialization is associated with the decreased risk of infection, erythema, and scarring as well as a faster recovery time.[8] Furthermore, there are the beneficial effects of the adjacent fibroblasts and stem cells.[7,9] This results in wound remodeling with neocollagenesis and elastic fibrin formation with subsequent skin tightening and improved appearance.[10]

Currently, there are several fractionated CO_2 lasers available. These include Fraxel re:pair, Juvia, Affirm CO_2, Active FX, Deep FX, Pixel CO_2 OMNIFIT, MiXto SX, and Matrix.[9,11] Different fractional CO_2 lasers can vary in treatment spot diameter, pulse energy, and treatment depth. There is controversy as to whether a particular fractionated laser is more effective than the others. In one study, with limited follow-up,[12] there was no significant difference in outcome between the lasers that were evaluated.

For any one fractionated CO_2 laser, an increase in fluence increases penetration depth. Increasing pulse duration increases adjacent nonlasered tissue heating effects. Increasing microspot density increases the percentage of treated area. The issue

of optimal depth of penetration for this procedure is controversial. In general, the first author (PJC) prefers a smaller microspot size, shorter pulse duration, and higher fluence. One study found that the time for reepithelialization was the same in patients treated with superficial fractional and in those treated with deep fractional CO_2 laser resurfacing.[13]

INDICATIONS FOR FRACTIONAL CO_2 LASER

Currently, fractional CO_2 lasers are used for treatment of photoaging (rhytides, dyschromia, lentigines, and skin laxity) (**Fig. 1**) and scarring (acne, traumatic, and surgical). Significant improvement has been reported for treatment of periorbital/perioral fine rhytides. These facial skin aging changes are less amenable to improvements with rhytidectomy.[13] Fractional CO_2 laser resurfacing is effective for treatment of facial fine-moderate rhytides and static wrinkles. Dynamic rhytides have less predictable results and can be combined with neurotoxins for treatment of the dynamic component to optimize the results. There are varying reports on the use of fractional CO_2 lasers for the cervical region. In one limited study,[14] there were no significant problems with fractional laser resurfacing of the neck. In contrast, another retrospective study reported on significant scarring.[13]

CONTRAINDICATIONS

Current contraindications to fractional CO_2 laser therapy include, but are not limited to, active bacterial, viral, or fungal infections in the area, which are treated. Although oral isotretinoin use within the past 6 months is a contraindication, some laser surgeons suggest waiting longer, up to 12 months before laser therapy. There are no current data to

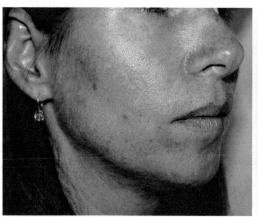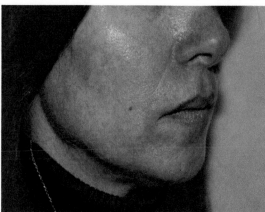

Fig. 1. This woman was treated for facial aging changes with a fractionated laser. The photo on the left is pretreatment. The photo on the right is 1 year after fractional CO_2 laser resurfacing. (*Courtesy of* Paul J. Carniol, MD, Summit, NJ.)

support the exact time frame. The first author favors waiting 12 months. Other relative contraindications include collagen vascular disease, previous scarring after cutaneous laser resurfacing, immunosuppresion, history of keloid or hypertrophic scar formation, prior radiation therapy, other autoimmune cutaneous diseases (ie, vitiligo and psoriasis), and gold therapy. Some surgeons perform fractional resurfacing when performing a surgical procedure in the same area whereas others suggest waiting for the completion of initial healing. This controversy usually relates to whether a laser resurfacing procedure should be combined with rhytidectomy.

PREPARATION FOR PROCEDURE

For each aspect of any patient's treatment, each surgeon must decide what is best. As with many procedures, there is no one cookbook-type approach. The first author usually starts prophylactic antiviral therapy 1 day prior to fractional CO$_2$ laser resurfacing. This is continued for 2 to 5 days after the procedure. The use of oral antibiotics varies. Some surgeons use them routinely whereas others do not. There are no definitive studies in the literature about the efficacy of prophylactic antibiotics for fractionated resurfacing. The first author does not always use prophylactic antibiotics. He has patients cleanse their skin with a dilute water and white vinegar solution to inhibit the growth of some types of bacteria and fungus in association with recovery. The utility of periprocedural antifungals is not uniformly agreed on for fractional resurfacing. One article endorses prophylactic fluconazole due to promotion of reepithelialization.[15]

ANESTHESIA

The first author has found that topical medication and use of a chiller device provide adequate anesthesia for fractional CO$_2$ laser resurfacing. The topical anesthesia contains 6% lidocaine and 6% tetracaine. This is not occluded. He does not use local anesthesia.

POST PROCEDURE CARE

As described previously, the first author typically places patients on a brief course of antivirals starting 24 hours prior to the laser treatment. This is continued until initial healing is completed. All patients are asked to wash the lasered area with a mildly acidic vinegar solution 2 to 3 times a day. The first author has his patients make this solution by adding 1 teaspoon of white vinegar to 2 cups of water. Rather than use prophylactic antibiotics for all patients, he reserves antibiotics for selected

patients. Topical antibiotics are not used due to the greater risk of contact dermatitis post resurfacing. Instead Aquaphor™ (Beiersdorf, Wilton, CT, USA) is applied 2 to 3 times a day to the treated area. Patients are advised to avoid the sun for several weeks after the procedure to diminish the risk of hyperpigmentation. Typically, initial recovery requires 4 to 7 days. As soon as the initial recovery is completed, the patients stop the topical Aquaphor, any antivirals, and antibiotics.

RESULTS OF FRACTIONAL CO$_2$ LASER

Preliminary data on fractionated CO$_2$ lasers show favorable clinical outcomes, although the data are limited. Clinical improvement in rhytides and scars is similar to that in reports with traditional ablative CO$_2$ laser treatments. An article published in 2007 on 55 patients treated with fractional CO$_2$ laser, Active FX, reported significant improvement in photoaging 3 months postlaser, with minimal side effects and short downtime.[16] In another study, 10 patients with Fitzpatrick skin types I to III with photodamaged skin were treated with a single pass of fractionated CO$_2$ laser at energy levels of 80 mJ to 100 mJ. Not only was photoaging significantly clinically improved but also biopsies indicated neocollagenesis and fibrosis.[17] In another study, 15 patients, ages 31 to 81, with facial rhytidosis, hyperpigmentation, and skin laxity, and 1 patient with acne scarring were treated 3 to 5 times at 3-week intervals. Patients received 2 passes with fractional CO$_2$ laser during each treatment session. Treatment areas included the face,[7] periocular region,[5] perioral region,[2] and malar region.[1] Patients were followed for 3 months post-treatment, and biopsy specimens were obtained before treatment and at 3, 7, and 14 days post-treatment. Patients received an average of 3.5 total treatments. Three months post-treatment, good to excellent improvement in photodamage was observed in 92% of patients, good to excellent reduction in rhytides in 85%, and good to excellent improvement in pore sizes and skin laxity in 79%. Histologic analysis after a single treatment indicated neocollagenesis.[18] Fractionated CO$_2$ has also shown excellent results on atrophic acne scars, although not as profound an effect as with rhytides. Thirteen patients received 2 to 3 treatments of fractionated CO$_2$ laser at 1-month to 2-month intervals, with pulse energies of 20 mJ to 100 mJ and densities of 100 to 400 mtz/cm^2. There was a mean improvement in the depth of scars of 66.8%, ranging from 43% to 79.9%.[19]

Besides equivalent clinical outcomes, fractionated CO$_2$ laser has the added advantage of expanded treatment areas, such as the periorbital region. Although traditional ablative CO$_2$ laser has been avoided in the periorbital region due to risks of ectropion, various studies have reported the safety of fractionated CO_2 laser. Kotlus and colleagues[10] evaluated 15 patients treated with dual-depth fractional CO_2 laser, pulse energy of 5 mJ to 7.5 mJ used on upper eyelid and 7.5 mJ to 10 mJ on lower eyelid with density of 10% to 15%; on noneyelid skin, pulse energy of 15 mJ with density of 15% to 20% was used. The treatment boundary was from 1 mm of brow cilia to 1 mm of upper eyelash line and within 2 mm of lower eyelash line, with 2 treatment passes performed. In 6-month follow-up, there was a mean improvement in rhytidosis 53.1% and skin redundancy 42%. No ectropion complications were reported. Two of 15 patients had hyperpigmentation, which resolved with topical 4% hydroquinone and sunscreen.

Due to the quicker recovery and the lower complication rate, fractionated CO_2 laser has increased in popularity. The long-term efficacy of fractionated CO_2 laser is still being evaluated. Ortiz and colleagues[20] evaluated patients treated with fractional CO_2 laser, with clinical follow-up at 2 years post-treatment. Ten patients (6 acne scar and 4 photodamaged), ages 24 to 63 years, with Fitzpatrick scale skin types I to V and treated with fractionated CO_2 laser, were followed for 2 years post-treatment. Acne scar patients maintained 83% of their improvement at 2 years compared with 3 months post-treatment, whereas photodamaged patients maintained 67% of their improvement. The investigators not only conclude that fractional CO_2 laser is effective in management of photodamage and acne but also support the long-term efficacy of fractionated CO_2 laser resurfacing.

Although the current literature demonstrates the clinical efficacy of fractionated CO_2 laser resurfacing, there is no uniform consensus on laser settings, number of treatments, number of passes, or clinical endpoints. Data on the different fractionated lasers are mixed.[21] These different settings and treatment protocols may be associated with different risks of complications and side effects, although this has not been evaluated.

The rates of post-treatment viral infection are significantly lower in 0.3% to 2% of cases compared with 2% to 7% rates with traditional ablative CO_2 treatment. Rates of bacterial superinfection are also decreased from 0.5% to 4.5% to 0.1% after fractionation.[22,23] Acneiform lesions are also significantly lower, ranging from 2% to 10%. Postinflammatory hyperpigmentation (PIH) is a well-described phenomenon after traditional CO_2 ablative therapy. Rates of PIH from fractionated CO_2 laser vary in the literature, with some investigators reporting no PIH complications[24] others 1% to 32% of patients, depending on treatment parameters and Fitzpatrick scale skin types.[10,23] Some cases of PIH were successfully managed with 4% hydroquinone and sunscreen.[25]

Hypertrophic scarring has been reported with fractionated lasers.[13,26] Focal areas of persistent erythema may be the first clinical signs of hypertrophic scarring. Risks factors for hypertrophic scarring may include infection, overlapping laser passes resulting in stacking, multiple treatment sessions, history of hypertrophic scarring or keloid formation, and a prior history of radiation.

SUMMARY

Fractionated CO_2 lasers are a new treatment modality for skin resurfacing. These lasers have been shown efficacious in treating facial photoaging changes and scars. These lasers have an improved safety and recovery profile compared with traditional CO_2 laser resurfacing. Precise treatment parameters vary between patients, the pathology treated, and the details of the particular laser.

REFERENCES

1. Stellar S, Polanyi TG. Lasers in neurosurgery: a historical overview. J Clin Laser Med Surg 1992;10:399.
2. Shapshay S, Simpson G. Lasers in bronchology. Otolaryngol Clin North Am 1983;16(4).
3. Bridenstine JB, Carniol PJ. Managing post resurfacing complications. In: Carniol PJ, editor. Laser skin rejuvenation. Philadelphia: Lippincott-Raven; 1998.
4. Goldman MP, Fitzpatrick RE. CO2 laser surgery. In: Goldman MP, Fitzparick RE, editors. Cutaneous laser surgery the art and science of selected photothermolysis. St Louis (MO): Mosby-Year Book; 1994.
5. Fitzpatrick RE, Goldman MP, Satur NM, et al. Pulsed carbon dioxide laser resurfacing of photoaged facial skin. Arch dermatol 1996;132:395–402.
6. Alster TS, Garg S. Treatment of facial rhytides with a high-energy pulsed carbon dioxide laser. Plast Reconstr Surg 1996;98:791–4.
7. Manstein D, Herron GS, Sink RK, et al. Fractional photothermolysis: a new concept for cutaneous remodeling using microscopic patterns of thermal injury. Lasers Surg Med 2004;34:426.
8. Hantash BM, Bedi VP, Chan KF, et al. Ex vivo histological characterization of a novel ablative fractional resurfacing device. Lasers Surg Med 2007;39:87–95.
9. Cohen SR, Henssler C, Johnston J. Fractional photothermolysis for skin rejuvenation. Plast Reconstr Surg 2009;124:281–90.
10. Kotlus BS. Dual-depth fractional carbon dioxide laser resurfacing for periocular rhytidosis. Dermatol Surg 2010;36:623–8.
11. Allemann IB, Kaufman J. Fractional photothermolysis—an update. Lasers Med Sci 2010;25:137–44.

12. Dover J. Comparison of four fractional devices. Presentation, American society of laser medicine and surgery, annual meeting. Phoenix (AZ); 2010.

13. Avram MM, Tope WD, Yu T, et al. Hypertrophic scarring of the neck following ablative fractional carbon dioxide laser resurfacing. Lasers Surg Med 2009; 41:185–8.

14. Tierney EP, Hanke CW. Ablative fractionated CO2 laser resurfacing for the neck: prospective study and review of the literature. J Drugs Dermatol 2009;8(8):723–31.

15. Conn H, Nanda VS. prophylactic fluconazole promotes reepithelialization in full-face carbon dioxide laser skin resurfacing. Lasers Surg Med 2000;26:201–7.

16. Clementoni MT, Gilardino P, Muti GF, et al. Nonsequential fractional ultrapulsed CO2 resurfacing of photoaged facial skin: preliminary clinical report. J Cosmet Laser Ther 2007;9:218–25.

17. Berlin AL, Hussain M, Phelps R, et al. A prospective study of fractional scanned nonsequential carbon dioxide laser resurfacing: a clinical and histopathologic evaluation. Dermatol Surg 2009;35:222–8.

18. Katz B. Efficacy of a new fractional Co2 laser in the treatment of photodamage and acne scarring. Dermatol Ther 2010;23:403–6.

19. Chapas AM, Brightman L, Sukla S, et al. Successful treatment of acneiform scarring with Co2 ablative fractional resurfacing. Lasers Surg Med 2008;40: 381–6.

20. Ortiz AE, Tremaine AM, Zachary CB. Long-term efficacy of a fractional resurfacing device. Lasers Surg Med 2010;42:168–70.

21. Karsai S, Raulin C. Comparison of clinical outcome parameters, the patient benefit index and patient satisfaction after ablative fractional laser treatment of peri-orbital rhytides. Lasers Surg Med 2010;42: 215–23.

22. Metelitsa AI, Alster TS. Fractional laser skin resurfacing treatment complications: a review. Dermatol Surg 2010;36:299–306.

23. Grabber EM, Tanzi EL, Alster TS. Side effects and complications of fractional laser photothermolysis: experience with 961 treatments. Dermatol Surg 2008;34:301–5.

24. Tan KL, Kurniawati C, Gold MH. Low risk of post-inflammatory hyperpigmentation in skin types 4 and 5 after treatment with fractional co2 laser device. J Drugs Dermatol 2008;7:747–77.

25. Spriprachya-anunt S, Marchell NL, Fitzpatrick RE, et al. Facial resurfacing in patients with Fitzpatrick skin type IV. Lasers Surg Med 2002;30:86–92.

26. Ross RB, Spencer J. Scarring and persistent erythema after fractionated ablative co2 laser resurfacing. J Drugs Dermatol 2008;7:1072–3.

YSGG 2790-nm Superficial Ablative and Fractional Ablative Laser Treatment

Kevin C. Smith, MD, FRCPC (Dermatology)[a],*,
G. Daniel Schachter, MD, FRCPC (Dermatology)[b,c]

KEYWORDS

- YSGG laser • Superficial resurfacing
- Fractional ablative laser

The 2790-nm wavelength yttrium-scandium-gallium-garnet (YSGG) laser was introduced for aesthetic purposes under the trade name, Pearl, by Cutera in 2007. Like 10,600-nm CO_2 and 2940-nm erbium:yttrium-aluminum-garnet (Er:YAG) ablative resurfacing lasers, the YSGG 2790 nm uses as its chromophore water in the top 1 mm of the skin (**Fig. 1**).

YSGG 2790 nm was chosen by Cutera because it was considered to produce a better blend of coagulation and ablation than the CO_2 laser, which deposits a large amount of coagulation-causing thermal energy in the skin for a given amount of ablation, or the Er:YAG laser, which deposits little thermal energy in the skin for a given amount of ablation (**Fig. 2**). Some Er:YAG lasers can be made to produce a train of subpulses, which, at appropriate parameters, can produce a greater degree of coagulation in proportion to ablation (**Fig. 3**), so approximate the ratio of ablation to coagulation created by the YSGG. All 3 types of fractional lasers are capable of penetrating more than 1 mm into the skin.

During fractional resurfacing, thermal energy is useful to the extent that it turns on repair and remodeling systems in the skin and coagulates

blood vessels to limit pinpoint bleeding. Too much thermal energy can cause a burn, with attendant risks of scarring, pigment loss, and prolonged healing. Not enough thermal energy can result in reduced skin tightening and remodeling and troublesome pinpoint bleeding during the procedure.

In clinical use, the Pearl superficial resurfacing laser has proved effective and well tolerated for the correction of superficial brown epidermal dyschromia and superficial fine lines and scars, and the Pearl Fractional laser produces excellent improvement in both dyschromia and improvement of deeper lines and moderately deep acne scarring. The 2 laser treatments can be combined in a single treatment session, either on different parts of the face or on the entire face, depending on a patient's needs and priorities (**Fig. 4**).

The risks of treatment using the YSGG lasers are similar to other ablative and fractional ablative resurfacing lasers. The risk of bulk heating, which can cause scarring and pigment loss, seems to be lower with YSGG than in CO_2 fractional ablative lasers and perhaps lower than Er:YAG fractional ablative systems when they are operated with a high level of coagulation. Scarring and pigment

[a] Niagara Falls Dermatology and Skin Care Centre Limited, 6453 Morrison Street, Suite 201, Niagara Falls, ON L2E 7H1, Canada
[b] Department of Dermatology, Women's College Hospital, 208 Bloor Street, Suite 403, Toronto, ON M5S 3B4, Canada
[c] Department of Dermatology, University of Toronto Medical School, Toronto, ON, Canada
* Corresponding author.
E-mail address: ksmithderm@gmail.com

Facial Plast Surg Clin N Am 19 (2011) 253–260
doi:10.1016/j.fsc.2011.05.005

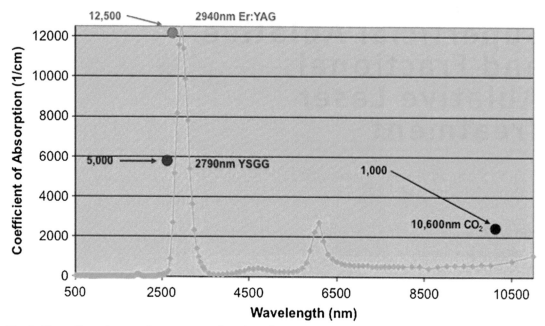

Fig. 1. Absorption of energy by water as a function of wavelength. Energy from the 10,600-nm CO_2 laser has a low coefficient of absorption by water of approximately 1000, which produces a high amount of coagulation in proportion to ablation. 2790-nm (YSGG) laser energy has an intermediate coefficient of absorption of approximately 5000, which produces a balanced amount of ablation in proportion to coagulation. 2940-nm (Er:YAG) laser energy has a high coefficient of absorption at approximately 12,500, causing a high amount of ablation in proportion to coagulation. In some Er:YAG systems, the initial short ablative pulse of the Er:YAG is followed by 1 or more longer, lower-powered coagulative pulses (see **Fig. 2**), giving a final balance between ablation and coagulation approximating that produced by the YSGG laser (see **Fig. 3**).

loss have been reported after fractional CO_2 laser[1] but as of late 2010 not with Pearl fractional YSGG, probably because the Pearl Fractional ablative system delivers a lower thermal load to the skin. All fractional ablative lasers can occasionally cause superficial pitting of the skin (**Fig. 5**), and

this can persist for many months after treatment and occasionally is permanent. The cause of this pitting has not been determined, and an effective treatment protocol for it has not been defined. The risk of pitting may increase with spot size.

ACTUAL USE OF YSGG LASERS
The Consultation

When considering the range of treatments a patient might benefit from, YSGG superficial resurfacing laser comes into play with patients who have brown epidermal dyschromia and/or fine lines or superficial acne scarring **Fig. 6**. Such patients might benefit from a series of 3 to 6 intense pulsed light treatments but might benefit more (and with only 1 or 2 treatments) from YSGG resurfacing.

Patients need to understand that it took several years for their skin to get to the point where corrective treatment was needed, and patients need to allow approximately 4 to 5 days for sunburn-like social downtime, after which makeup can usually be worn, plus another week or two of somewhat pink skin (**Fig. 7**). Usually, the greatest degree of inflammation and erythema occurs at 48 to 72 hours after treatment. Patients should expect that they usually see improvement by

Thermal Zones by Wavelength
Assumes Sufficient Energy for Ablation

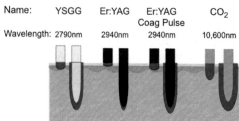

Name:	YSGG	Er:YAG	Er:YAG Coag Pulse	CO_2
Wavelength:	2790nm	2940nm	2940nm	10,600nm

Fig. 2. The relative sizes of the zones of coagulation in this schematic diagram are shown in red. Note that in some variants of fractional ablative Er:YAG laser systems, 1 or more lower-powered coagulative pulses, which are nonablative, follow the initial ablative pulse, and the effect of this series of pulses approximates the ablation/coagulation balance of the YSGG laser.

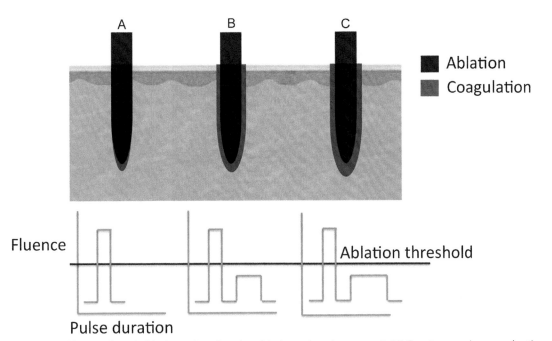

Fig. 3. The addition of a subablative pulse after the ablative pulse gives some Er:YAG systems an improved ratio of coagulation to ablation.

approximately 3 weeks, and maximum improvement is reached by 3 to 6 months after treatment.

In a more severe case (see **Fig. 7**), patients might have more severe brown dyschromia together with many fine and moderate lines or perhaps moderate superficial acne scarring (see **Fig. 7**).

In such cases, YSGG fractional laser treatment might be most appropriate. If there is a great deal of brown dyschromia, patients might want to consider YSGG ablative laser treatment or intense pulsed light treatment on the same day or on a different day in addition to fractional treatment.

Patients who are preparing for YSGG fractional ablative treatment should expect that there will be some pinpoint bleeding during and immediately after the treatment and that there may in occasional cases be considerable pinpoint bleeding, which may persist to some extent for up to 24 hours. This may be more severe and persistent in people who have ruddy complexions and many superficial telangiectasia. It may be wise to correct the erythema and telangiectasia in such individuals by using intense pulsed light followed by Nd:YAG laser before proceeding to fractional ablative laser resurfacing.

Patients should plan for 4 to 7 days of sunburn-like social downtime following YSGG fractional ablative resurfacing, after which makeup can usually be worn during 1 to 3 weeks of somewhat pinker-than-usual skin. Usually, the greatest degree of inflammation and erythema occurs at 48 to 72 hours after treatment. Patients should expect that they would be able to see the grid pattern of tiny laser dots in at least some places on their faces for approximately a week and occasionally longer. Rarely, there may be some evidence of this pattern weeks or even months after treatment (see **Fig. 5**).

It can be helpful to show patients a series of photos of patients 1 hour, 1 day, 2 days, 1 week, and several weeks after treatment, so they know what to expect.

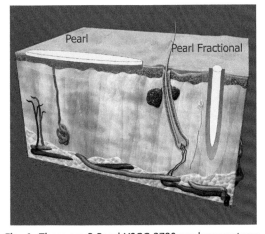

Fig. 4. There are 2 Pearl YSGG 2790-nm laser systems, one optimized for superficial resurfacing and the other for fractional ablative resurfacing. Either or both systems can be used in a single treatment session, depending on a patient's needs and priorities.

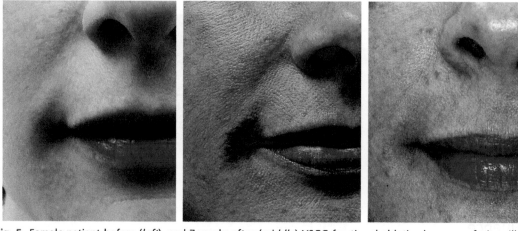

Fig. 5. Female patient before (*left*), and 7 weeks after (*middle*) YSGG fractional ablative laser resurfacing, illustrating pitting of the skin. Patient was treated a second time with YSGG fractional ablative laser resurfacing at low fluence [60 mJoules] and high density (5), three passes, and had marked resolution of pitting (*right*) at five months after the second procedure.

The benefits of treatment with either type of YSGG laser can last for many years, but patients may want or need retreatment sooner if they continue to have UV exposure (see **Fig. 7**) and/or are smokers. Patients who stop smoking a couple of weeks before treatment and refrain from smoking for a month after treatment may respond better and also have a lower risk of delayed healing or infection.

It is vital to take high-quality digital photos and to print these photos out and keep them in the chart for quick reference during a treatment session and at follow-up visits. A full discussion of office photography is beyond the scope of this article. I find it useful to have anterior and oblique photos, taken both with flash (for best color rendition) and without flash but with symmetric overhead lighting (for example, with a patient standing between 2 overhead fluorescent lights) for best skin texture and skin fold images.

On the Day of Treatment

When patients arrive for treatment, their understanding the procedure and postprocedure care should be confirmed. Patients should expect to be in the office for up to 3 hours: approximately 1 hour of anesthetic cream application, approximately

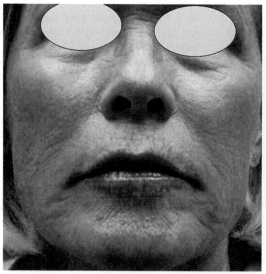
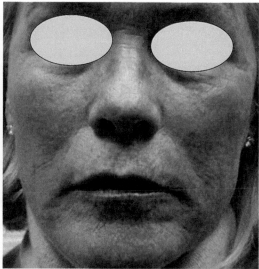

Fig. 6. Woman with brown dyschromia and superficial fine lines and acne scarring before and after Pearl resurfacing.

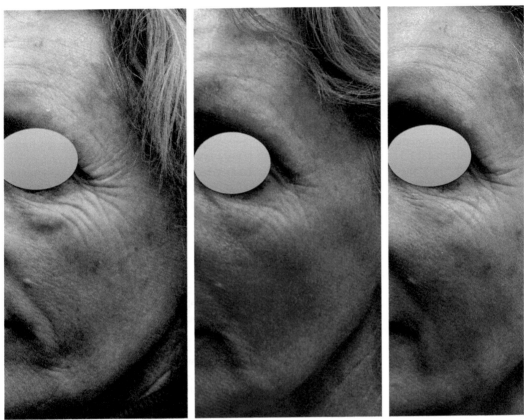

Fig. 7. Fifty-year-old woman with a long history of sun exposure. Shown before treatment with Pearl Fractional ablative resurfacing laser (*left*), 10 days after treatment (*middle*), and 2 years after treatment (*right*).

1 hour for treatment with either the Pearl or Pearl Fractional laser, and approximately 1 hour after treatment. Patients are welcome to have someone drive them to the appointment, but most of my patients drive themselves to and from the treatment session.

I have found it helpful to give patients two 500 mg Tylenol Rapid Release™ gel caps together with two 400 mg Advil™ liquid gel caps as soon as they arrive. There may be an additive analgesic effect from the combination of acetaminophen and ibuprofen,[2] and these medications do not cause sedation. The gel caps release the medication rapidly so a good blood and brain level is obtained by the time the procedure starts.

As long as there are no contraindications, such as asthma, I also give my patients one or two 40 mg tablets of propranolol. This is a highly lipid-soluble β-blocker that crosses the blood-brain barrier efficiently and reduces anxiety without causing sedation by blocking β-receptors in the central nervous system, notably on the amygdala.[3] The addition of ʟ-theanine 200 mg to propranolol has further improved patient relaxation during the procedure[4] without causing sedation. The side-

effect profiles of these medications are benign when the medications are taken as a single dose by otherwise healthy people.

Patients are then offered a chance to go to the bathroom, and the location of the bathroom is pointed out so they can find their way if they wish to go later.

Patients then scrub the face thoroughly with soap, for example, BioClenz 4, which contains 4% chlorhexidine, and water, removing all oils and makeup. It is explained that this is important for the anesthetic cream to penetrate as deeply as possible into the skin.

After the face is dried:

- A head band is applied to keep hair off the forehead
- Patients lay back and are made comfortable on an examination table
- Patients are draped with a towel
- Patients are given a large Kleenex Super-Strength tissue™ to hold, in case they want to wipe their eyes
- It is explained to patients that they should be careful to avoid getting the anesthetic

cream in their eyes, because it is irritating (pH approximately 8.4), and they should avoid licking their lips because the cream makes their tongue and mouth numb.

Thick, adherent anesthetic cream containing 23% lidocaine, 7% tetracaine, and 0.2% clobetasol propionate is then applied from the hairline all the way down to 2 cm below the jawline, using a tongue depressor, rather like icing a cake. Cream should be kept at least 1.5 cm away from the lower eyelid margins and should not be applied to the upper eyelids. Local anesthetic can be injected if desired to perform laser treatment on the eyelids.

The pharmacy adds 0.2% clobetasol propionate when compounding anesthetic cream because it is a potent vasoconstrictor.[5] This vasoconstriction improves the depth and duration of topical anesthesia and also reduces the severity and duration of pinpoint bleeding during fractional ablative resurfacing. A single 1-hour application of 0.2% clobetasol propionate does not seem to interfere with healing after YSGG laser treatment nor does it seem to produce an increased risk of infection. Other vasoconstrictors, such as phenylephrine, should be avoided because they can cause prolonged mydriasis if any gets into the eyes.

A good rule of thumb is that the anesthetic cream should be applied so thickly that the skin cannot be seen. This ensures that there is a good partition coefficient between the cream layer and the skin, driving the medication from the cream into the skin.

A timer is set for 66 minutes, and a second timer is set for 20 minutes. Patients are checked every 20 minutes, and the anesthetic cream is redistributed and if necessary more anesthetic cream is applied to maintain a thick layer. There is music and a selection of reading materials in the room where the patients wait while the anesthetic cream takes effect.

At approximately 66 minutes after application of the anesthetic cream, patients are offered another chance to go to the bathroom; then they walk to the room where the laser procedure is performed and are made comfortable on the procedure table. Towels are laid under the head and draped over the chest. The power table is adjusted to a height that is optimal for operator comfort and to reduce operator fatigue. It is good to tell patients before each adjustment of the power table so they are not surprised by sudden movements of the table.

The laser, smoke evacuator, and Cryo 5 cold air blower are all turned on and briefly explained to patients, then bright overhead lights, which are helpful for safe and effective laser treatment, are turned on. The exhaust fan is turned on because there is a substantial heat load from the various pieces of equipment, 2 or 3 people, and bright lights. The background music level is adjusted to be heard above the sound of the equipment running in the room.

I wear 3× bar loupes while treating patients, making it easier to monitor the laser-tissue interactions and reducing operator fatigue.

If necessary, local anesthetic is injected to prevent discomfort when the eyelids are treated. If the eyelids are to be treated, steel shields must be inserted to protect the cornea in case the laser beam penetrates the eyelid. It is vital to avoid getting any anesthetic cream on the corneal shields, because the high pH of the cream (approximately 8.4) may cause severe corneal burns. Medium-sized Cox II H corneal shields (oculoplastik.com) are a popular choice. The insertion and removal of these is simple, but a full discussion of the issues surrounding the use of corneal shields is beyond the scope of this article. Helpful videos can be viewed at oculoplastik.com/videos.

It is useful to print out large copies of patients' pretreatment photos and hang them up in the laser treatment room to refer to during treatment. It can also be helpful to mark the photos before treatment, indicating the fluence, density, and number of passes planned in each area of the face. It can also be useful to mark patients' face and jawline while the patient is upright, after the face is washed, and several minutes before anesthetic cream is applied. This reminds the laser operator of landmarks and areas requiring changes in parameters. The best marker is a red medium-point Sharpie™, which persists better than purple surgical markers but which can be removed easily using alcohol swabs or isopropyl alcohol after the procedure. Any residual pink blends in with the post-treatment skin color and is not a problem for patients.

Before starting to treat patients, it is wise to demonstrate the sound of the laser by firing it at a tongue depressor, so patients know what it sounds like, holding the tongue depressor approximately 20 cm from the patient's ear when this is done.

When removing anesthetic cream, it is vital to remove all of the cream so there is no residue on the skin. Cream residue on the skin absorbs and wastes laser energy and spatters back on to the laser window, causing both wastage of laser energy and interference with the beam profile. It is important to check the laser window every few minutes and clean it if necessary. If a good job is done removing the cream from the skin, a case may be completed without having to clean the laser window.

I scrape off the bulk of the anesthetic cream using a tongue depressor; then, I wipe the skin down with a dry towel to remove more of the cream and follow this with a moist towel wipe and finally a dry towel. A large stack of 20 × 20 cm face cloths is kept for this purpose.

Because pinpoint bleeding can occur and because blood runs downwards, it is best to start fractional ablative laser treatment in the most inferior part of the section being treated, working upwards, so if there is any bleeding it does not get in the way of the laser beam. If there is bleeding, the application of a vasoconstrictor, such as xylometazoline nasal spray, after the section is completed may reduce the bleeding to some degree. Apart from that, simply wait while the clotting cascade eventually brings the bleeding to a halt. Occasionally patients do not have much pinpoint bleeding during or immediately after the procedure but report that there was some pinpoint bleeding a few hours later, after they got home. Perhaps this happens when the vasoconstricting effect of the clobetasol propionate wears off.

Both Pearl and Pearl Fractional lasers have integrated smoke evacuators, leaving my assistant free to hand me moist towels, wipe away blood, hold pressure on areas of pinpoint bleeding, and attend to patient comfort. It is best to perform resurfacing procedures with a patient lying on a power table, so that the patient can be kept at the ideal height for the operator, reducing operator fatigue and the resulting risk of operator error.

In all areas, two or sometimes three passes at approximately 30° to each other are made. To avoid bulk heating the skin, which could increase the risk of scarring, slow healing, or depigmentation, it is wise to allow at least 10 seconds between passes on any point on the skin, so the skin can cool down between passes.

The anesthetic effect begins to decline within minutes after the cream is removed and can decline to a significant extent within 10 or 20 minutes. For this reason, the face is treated one section at a time and anesthetic cream is removed from each section just before it is treated.

In general, it is best to treat the eyelids and periocular area first. This minimizes the risk that anesthetic cream will get in the patient's eyes and cause discomfort. After the eyelids are treated, the ocular shields are removed, and steel goggles are put on the patient for the rest of the treatment. Durette IV external shields, also from oculoplastik.com, are ideal for this purpose because both the nose and temple pieces are made of steel and easily swivel up or down out of the way when treating the nose or temples. The eyelid and periocular skin is thin, and so

should be treated with 2-3 passes at density 2 and 120 J/cm^2 or less. The right and left forehead are then treated, usually at 120 J/cm^2, density 2, two passes.

Next, it is good to treat the posterior cheeks, from the midpupillary line back to the preauricular area. This is less sensitive than the central face and forehead, so is less anxiety provoking for patients and allows the anesthetic cream to stay on the more sensitive areas for a longer time. The cheeks are generally treated at density 2, 160 J/cm^2 to 200 J/cm^2.

After the right and left posterior cheeks have been treated, I treat the right and left medial cheeks and nose and finally the perioral area. If a patient has deep perioral rhitids, I sometimes inject a perioral anesthetic block using 1% lidocaine with epinephrine to allow comfortable administration of 2 to 3 passes at 160 J/cm^2 to 200 J/cm^2, density 2 to 3. I find it helpful the stretch the skin while it is being lasered, in particular in the perioral area.

Patient discomfort is assessed from time to time during the procedure using the verbal pain scale: "On a scale of 0 to 10, with 0 being no pain and 10 being the worst possible pain, what number would you say the treatment is now?" If the score is 5 or higher, I take this as a sign that the patient is having excessive discomfort and start to direct cold air from the Cryo 5 cold air machine on to the skin which is about to be treated. Because this machine takes several minutes to start producing cold air, it should be turned on before the start of the procedure, so it is immediately available if needed. I set the Cryo 5 cold air blower on maximum airflow and set the time to 60 minutes, so that it does not time out during the procedure and need to be restarted. Avoid blowing cold air up a patient's nose because patients find this uncomfortable or frightening.

When treating along the jawline, it is best to feather the treated area, for example by reducing the fluence from 160 J/cm^2 on the cheek to 120 J/cm^2 on the jawline and 80 J/cm^2 under the jawline. This creates a gradual transition between the appearance of the treated and untreated areas. Another approach when making the transition at the jawline is to hold the handpiece 5° to 10° away from perpendicular to the skin, so the laser beam is slightly oblique and so has a somewhat reduced fluence as I pass over and below the jawline.

When treatment is completed, the laser and Cryo 5 cold air blower are turned off and patient goggles gently removed. It is nice to have a glass of ice-cold water waiting for patients. If there is any pinpoint bleeding, it is gently wiped away.

Patients are then given a large hand mirror and invited to check their face. Patients are usually relieved to see that they look normal. It is important at this point to explain again that the face will become somewhat red and swollen over the next 24 to 48 hours and then improve until the 4-day to 7-day mark, at which point the use of makeup may be resumed. It is wise for patients to sleep the night after treatment with the head elevated on 2 or 3 pillows, so there is less swelling, in particular of the eyelids, during the night.

A thin layer of Vaseline™ is applied to the treated areas, and patients are given the rest of a 90-g tube to take home. Patients are advised to stand for 5 to 10 minutes in a warm shower twice a day and let the water run over their face, gently massaging their face with bare fingers—no soap, no washcloths. After patting their face dry, patients should apply another thin layer of Vaseline to lock in the moisture and prevent dryness. Vaseline can usually be stopped by approximately days 4 to 5, and patients can start using their favorite moisturizer. Vaseline has the advantage of containing no preservatives or other chemicals, which could cause contact or irritant dermatitis.

It is good to phone patients the evening after a procedure, or the next day, to check on their progress. Patients are invited to call any time if there are problems or questions and informed that my cell phone number is on the answering machine at my office, so they can reach me at any time.

Patients are usually seen for follow-up at 2 to 4 days, 2 to 3 weeks, and 2 to 3 months.

REFERENCES

1. Fife DJ, Fitzpatrick RE, Zachary CB. Complications of fractional CO2 laser resurfacing: four cases. Lasers Surg Med 2009;41(3):179–8.
2. Mehlisch DR, Aspley S, Daniels SE, et al. A single-tablet fixed-dose combination of racemic ibuprofen/paracetamol in the management of moderate to severe postoperative dental pain in adult and adolescent patients: a multicenter, two-stage, randomized, double-blind, parallel-group, placebo-controlled, factorial study. Clin Ther 2010;32:1033–49.
3. van Stegeren AH, Everaerd W, Cahill L, et al. Memory for emotional events: differential effects of centrally versus peripherally acting beta-blocking agents. Psychopharmacology (Berl) 1998;138:305–10.
4. Lu K, Gray MA, Oliver C, et al. The acute effects of L-theanine in comparison with alprazolam on anticipatory anxiety in humans. Hum Psychopharmacol 2004;19(7):457–65.
5. Sommer A, Veraart J, Neumann M, et al. Evaluation of the vasoconstrictive effects of topical steroids by laser-Doppler-perfusion-imaging. Acta Derm Venereol 1998;78:15–8.

Versatility of Erbium YAG Laser: From Fractional Skin Rejuvenation to Full-Field Skin Resurfacing

J. David Holcomb, MD

KEYWORDS

- Erbium YAG laser • Laser resurfacing
- Ablative fractional resurfacing

Despite alternative methods for skin rejuvenation, including nonablative fractional laser therapy, photorejuvenation, photodynamic therapy, medium and deep chemical peels, ablative fractional laser therapy, and other treatments, full-field (complete surface coverage) ablative laser therapy remains popular for patients seeking maximum improvement with a single treatment. Ablative laser skin resurfacing (LSR) wavelengths include 2790 nm (erbium:yttrium-scandium-gallium-garnet or Er-YSGG), 2940 nm (erbium:yttrium-aluminum-garnet or Er-YAG), and 10,600 nm (carbon dioxide or CO_2). Of these, the Er-YAG laser wavelength is an excellent choice for improvement of a variety of skin conditions and features of aging, including dyschromia, actinic photodamage, solar elastosis, acne and traumatic scarring, fine lines and mild to moderate rhytidosis, coarse skin texture, and skin laxity.[1–7]

Similar therapeutic benefits, including skin tightening, are well established with the carbon dioxide and Er-YSGG wavelengths[8–12]; however, overall benefit, including rhytid effacement, skin tightening, and long-term improvement has long been considered by many physicians to be superior with the CO_2 wavelength.[13–15] Even so, traditional multipass ablative full-field CO_2 LSR has declined in popularity owing to a number of factors, including higher risk of postresurfacing sequelae and

complications, extended posttreatment recovery time, and increasing popularity and effectiveness of the alternative skin-resurfacing modalities enumerated previously.[10,16,17] And when directly comparing full-field resurfacing lasers, it is the author's opinion that the Er-YAG laser is an indispensible tool with an acceptably low risk-to-benefit ratio that, with appropriate functionality, enables physicians to effectively treat aging skin and other conditions in patients with a greater diversity of skin types.

The first Er-YAG laser was introduced commercially in 1997. In practice, the first Er-YAG skin-resurfacing lasers proved to be effective for soft tissue ablation but not for soft tissue coagulation. The initial excitement about the 2940-nm alternative wavelength diminished with the realization that the first-generation devices required multiple passes to ablate into the upper dermis and that on reaching this depth, significant bleeding caused difficulty with completion of treatments and also reduced the ablation efficiency of the device at that point during treatment.[15,18] Second-generation Er-YAG lasers (circa 1999) avoided unchecked bleeding by adding a long-pulse or variable-pulse feature designed to provide significant soft tissue coagulation ability.[15]

The flexibility to deliver Er-YAG laser energy for "pure" ablation or "pure" coagulation as well as

Financial Disclosures and/or Conflicts of Interest: Lutronic, Inc—Medical Advisory Board, Equipment Discount, Honoraria, Stock Options.
Holcomb Facial Plastic Surgery and Institute for Integrated Aesthetics, 1 South School Avenue, Suite 800, Sarasota, FL 34237, USA
E-mail address: drholcomb@srqfps.com

a user-determined blend of ablation and coagulation to precise tissue depths led to recognition of these devices (those with long-pulse or variable-pulse modes) as extremely versatile. Full-field ablative Er-YAG LSR options that remain relevant more than a decade later (even with the interim development of many other useful treatment modalities) include superficial (partial epidermal), moderate depth (ablation into upper dermis), and deep skin peels (mid-papillary dermis or deeper) and combinations with other treatment modalities (eg, superficial peel and photorejuvenation).

The benefits of nonablative fractional laser treatment (including wavelengths of 1410, 1450, 1540, 1550, and more recently 1927 nm) profoundly influenced the approach to laser skin rejuvenation and also led to use of this novel type of energy delivery with the ablative laser wavelengths.[19,20] Reduction of initial posttreatment recovery time (compared with traditional full-field LSR; dramatic for nonablative fractional resurfacing [NFR] and modest for ablative fractional resurfacing [AFR]), extension of these treatment modalities to additional skin types and conditions, widespread patient acceptance, and significant demand has legitimized this alternative approach.[21,22]

Nonetheless, an area of current interest is the middle ground between pure AFR and pure full-field LSR, where the potential for very significant improvement, while preserving at least some of the benefits of AFR and of LSR, exists by combining these very different approaches to delivery of laser energy to the skin. The advantages of dual-wavelength (CO_2 and Er-YAG) LSR have been explored in detail in the past.[23–26] By partial extension, a novel approach currently in use by the author and others involves concurrent dual-wavelength, dual-modality laser skin rejuvenation wherein CO_2 AFR deep dermal ablation immediately precedes or immediately follows full-field Er-YAG LSR.

ER-YAG LASER TISSUE INTERACTION

The Er-YAG laser wavelength has the highest absorption coefficient for water among the ablative laser wavelengths (Fig. 1) with approximately 12 times and 5 times greater absorption in water versus CO_2 and Er-YSGG, respectively. During LSR, water serves as the primary tissue target wherein light energy is transduced into heat energy that is then quickly absorbed by the surrounding tissues, including collagen. The

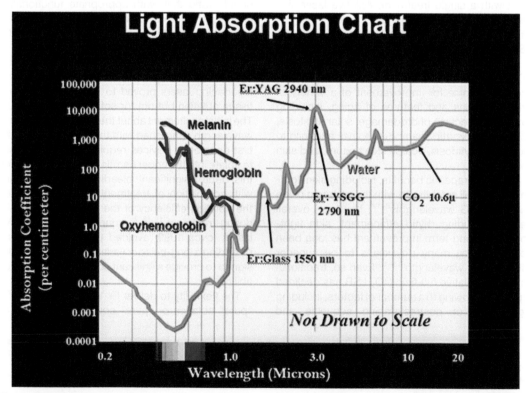

Fig. 1. Optical absorption of water versus wavelength. Log scale of water absorption versus wavelength. Absorption at 2940 nm (Er-YAG) corresponds with a water absorption peak. Absorption at 2940 nm is approximately 5 times greater than that for 2790 nm (Er-YSGG) and 12 times greater than that for 10,600 nm (CO_2).

characteristic tissue interactions that define each of the ablative resurfacing lasers are related to their relative absorption by water but also several other factors. The continuum of responses to heating of biologic tissues includes hyperthermia, coagulation, carbonization, and vaporization and each of these may be observed during LSR. In general terms, higher water absorption is correlated with greater tissue ablation (vaporization), whereas lower water absorption is correlated with greater tissue coagulation.

Distinct zones of tissue injury occur following cutaneous application of laser energy with ablative properties (**Fig. 2**), including vaporization zone (superficial for full-field and central for microfractional techniques), irreversible injury zone (coagulation; intermediate for full-field and for microfractional techniques), and reversible injury zone (hyperthermia; deep for full-field and peripheral for microfractional techniques). Carbonization may also occur (most likely with CO_2 laser wavelength) if tissue heating continues beyond the coagulation stage and the tissue is not vaporized.[27]

LSR tissue response is affected by wavelength (with tissue-specific absorption coefficient and optical penetration depth), tissue, and energy delivery factors. The optical penetration depth reflects that level in the tissue where laser irradiation has decreased by approximately 60% from its peak value incident at the tissue surface (or about 20 μm for the CO_2 and 1 μm for the ablative erbium lasers).[28] Energy delivery factors include power (W or watts), spot size, pulse duration, radiant exposure (RE), and power density. RE (energy density or fluence) reflects energy delivered to a unit of tissue expressed in joules per centimeter squared (J/cm^2). Power density is determined by the ratio of fluence over exposure time. Increased fluence

during short-pulse and long-pulse Er-YAG LSR increases depth of ablation and coagulation but correlation of device settings and histologic effect diminishes in long-pulse mode after the initial pass.[29] Excessive fluence during Er-YAG LSR may be a major contributing factor for unfavorable outcomes with repeated passes using long-pulse mode.

Other tissue factors include thermal relaxation time and wavelength and tissue-specific ablation threshold. Thermal relaxation time refers to the time needed for 50% reduction of the achieved peak tissue temperature. Although skin thermal relaxation time of 1 millisecond is widely quoted in the literature, Ross and colleagues[28] suggest that it may be significantly longer for the CO_2 laser (and by extension long-pulse Er-YAG laser). Ablation threshold, radiant energy required to vaporize tissue, is dependent on wavelength and tissue type. For human skin, the ablation threshold is much lower for the Er-YAG than for the CO_2 laser (1.6 vs 5.0 J/cm^2).[28] In general, pulse durations shorter than thermal relaxation time and energy densities equal to or greater than ablation threshold limit thermal spread and related collateral tissue damage, whereas longer pulse durations and subablative laser fluences accomplish the opposite.

From a practical standpoint, the laser surgeon is able to modulate tissue response to desired effect by exerting control over energy density (reflecting selected parameters for power, pulse duration, and spot size) and energy delivery method. With short-pulse durations, the early Er-YAG skin resurfacing lasers were optimized (beyond the native properties inherent to this wavelength) for efficient tissue ablation but poor tissue coagulation. Increasing the fluence with these systems resulted

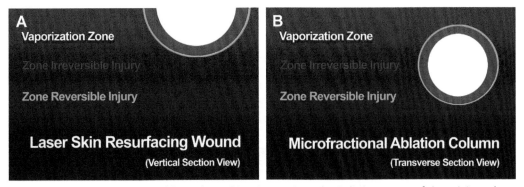

Fig. 2. Zones of tissue injury after ablative laser skin rejuvenation. The 3 distinct zones of tissue injury observed with both full-field and ablative fractional laser skin resurfacing include vaporization zone, irreversible injury zone, and zone of reversible injury. The zones are planar or tangential (*A*) with full-field resurfacing and perpendicular or axial (*B*) with ablative fractional resurfacing. The width of the irreversible injury zone is relatively narrow with short-pulse energy delivery but can be widened with long-pulse energy delivery.

in increased depth of tissue ablation but also re-sulted in significant bleeding upon reaching the microvasculature of the upper papillary dermis. The subsequent generation of Er-YAG skin-resur-facing lasers added a long or variable pulse feature with a low fluence to increase the coagulation effect and reduce intraprocedure bleeding. This "long" pulse effect was achieved by developing the ability to entrain or stack multiple subablative pulses close together that in aggregate resulted in a dramatic shift in tissue behavior with excellent coagulation. The ability to create nearly pure abla-tive or coagulative effects, as well as a user-defined (problem-specific) blend of these tissue effects with second-generation Er-YAG skin resur-facing lasers, brought this wavelength squarely to the forefront of skin rejuvenation technologies.

Er-YAG radiant laser energy may be delivered via a traditional scanning handpiece (eg, full-field skin resurfacing), fixed spot (eg, lesion ablation), or via fractional handpiece (also scanned). Frac-tional laser energy delivery was applied to the Er-YAG wavelength following introduction of AFR with the CO_2 wavelength and involves creation of multiple microscopic ablation columns at fixed distances apart and leaving normal, uninjured tissue in the intervening spaces. The same tissue effects (ablation, coagulation, ablation + coagula-tion) may be achieved; however, the orientation of effects is perpendicular to the target (vs planar with scanned full-field LSR) such that ablation is central, coagulation is paracentral, and reversible tissue injury is peripheral (see **Fig. 2**).

During Er-YAG AFR with the Sciton ProFraction-al XC handpiece (Sciton, Inc, Palo Alto, CA, USA),

energy is delivered with a spot size of 430 μm with total surface area coverage of up to 11% with a single pass and with available treatment depth (up to 1500 μm) well beyond the typical depth achieved with traditional full-field ablative LSR. Increasing the pulse energy and/or stacking short pulses increases treatment depth in short-pulse mode, whereas use of long-pulse mode increases the width of the irreversible injury zone and enhances tissue remodeling. **Figs. 3** and **4** high-light representative histology with variable treat-ment depth (see **Fig. 3**, short-pulse Er-YAG AFR) and variable levels of irreversible thermal injury (see **Fig. 4**, short-pulse and long-pulse Er-YAG AFR with fixed treatment depth).

INDICATIONS—FULL-FIELD LSR, SPOT TREATMENT, AND AFR

Contemporary indications for Er-YAG full-field ablative LSR include actinic photodamage, dys-chromia, fine lines, mild to moderate rhytidosis, mild skin laxity, acne or traumatic scarring, and coarse skin texture. Er-YAG full-field ablative LSR indications extend primarily to Fitzpatrick skin types I and II; however, Fitzpatrick skin types III and IV may be successfully treated with the understanding that more conservative treatment parameters are generally indicated and that the potential for postinflammatory hyperpigmentation (PIH) following treatment is higher.

Spot treatment (eg, 2-mm spot) with the Er-YAG laser in pure ablate mode may be used for a variety of skin lesions with excellent outcomes among all skin types. Lesions amenable to removal using

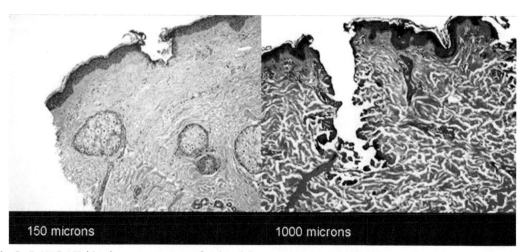

150 microns   1000 microns

Fig. 3. Er-YAG AFR histology at more superficial and deeper treatment depths. Short-pulse Er-YAG ablative frac-tional resurfacing laser treatment depth adjusted via alteration of pulse energy and sequential pulsing (pulse stacking) to enable routine skin rejuvenation (eg, depth 150 to 250 μm) and more aggressive treatments (eg, 700 to 1000 μm) for acne scarring. The left image represents treatment depth of 150 μm; the right image represents treatment depth of 1000 μm. (*Courtesy of* Jason Pozner, MD.)

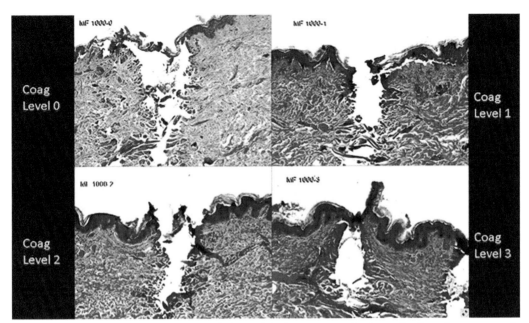

Fig. 4. Er-YAG dual-mode (short and long pulse) AFR histology. Long-pulse (coagulate) mode progresses from coagulate setting of 0 (*upper left*) up to 3 (*lower right*) with uniform treatment depth of 1000 µm.

this approach include seborrheic keratoses, benign (including pigmented) moles, skin tags, small superficial intradermal cysts, and even solitary dilated pores or deep (eg, ice-pick) acne scars. Other conditions (eg, syringoma, xanthelasma) may require additional intervention, but ablation of the skin over these lesions using Er-YAG spot energy delivery is a very useful adjunct.

The general goal for Er-YAG spot treatment is to ablate just past the lesion(s) while sparing as much normal remaining tissue as possible to minimize the potential for scar formation.[30] In contrast, treatment of a solitary dilated pore or deep acne scar involves essentially creating a circular ablation column through the entire thickness of the skin down to the subcutaneous fat. The superficial aspect of the transcutaneous ablation column may be closed with a 6-0 fast-absorbing gut horizontal mattress cutaneous suture or the wound may be left to heal by secondary intention. Secondary intention healing of the transcutaneous ablation column occurs rapidly with cicatricial wound contraction. The potential for dermal scarring may be further minimized by superficial closure, but healing and results have been very good with both methods.

Indications for Er-YAG AFR partially overlap those for ablative LSR. Single-session improvements with the Sciton ProFractional XC handpiece at maximum coverage (11%) are limited (even at maximum coverage with double pass, 22%), however, compared with full-field techniques with 100% coverage. AFR should not be used as

a definitive therapeutic method for treatment of actinic keratoses. Similarly, patient expectations for resolution of dyschromias should be realistic for the partial skin surface coverage typical of a single AFR treatment. Improved single-session results may be obtained with preexisting diffuse dyschromia by combining AFR with a superficial laser skin peel (partial epidermal or transepidermal). Improved single-modality results with Er-YAG AFR alone may be obtained in a single session with multiple passes or via a series of treatments over multiple sessions.[20,31] Er-YAG AFR may be performed for skin types I through VI. PIH following fractional laser skin rejuvenation may occur with ablative and nonablative wavelengths and has been correlated with skin type (more likely with darker skin) and increased density but not depth of microfractional ablation/coagulation columns/zones.[32]

ER-YAG LASER SKIN REJUVENATION TECHNIQUES

Spot treatment with the Sciton Er-YAG laser 2-mm spot is typically performed in pure ablate (short-pulse) mode. The laser surgeon selects treatment depth (generally 10 µm per pulse) and treatment speed (generally 10 to 40 Hz or pulses per second). Spot treatment of superficial seborrheic keratoses may not require anesthesia. For deeper lesions, infiltrated local anesthesia is necessary for pain control and to minimize bleeding. Bleeding varies with final treatment depth. Very light bleeding may be ignored or treated with topical aluminum chloride solution (25%). More significant bleeding may require light application of bipolar cautery. The wound(s) are then covered with an occlusive ointment or with paper tape. Re-epithelialization generally occurs within 4 to 7 days after treatment. For transcutaneous ablation of large pores or deep scars, the wound can be left to heal by secondary intention or closed with a single horizontal mattress cutaneous suture.

At a minimum, Er-YAG AFR with the Sciton Pro-Fractional XC handpiece requires topical anesthesia. A single pulse delivers 4 spots each with diameter of 430 μm and the scanner is very quick. Delivering 4 spots simultaneously increases total surface area coverage per pulse (4 times compared with a single 430-μm spot and 12.8 times compared with a single 120-μm spot) and increases treatment speed but also affects patient comfort. Additional measures (eg, regional nerve blockade, oral and/or intramuscular analgesia/sedation) to minimize discomfort are also generally necessary and also affected by treatment depth and density. Treatment may be subregional (eg, traumatic scarring), regional (eg, bilateral cheeks for acne scarring), or full face (eg, photodamage and coarse skin texture). Treatment depth of 1000 μm or more may be useful for deep acne or traumatic scarring, whereas treatment depth of 250 μm is acceptable for generalized skin rejuvenation.

Greater treatment density (eg, 22%—double pass) may lead to noticeable improvement with fewer sessions versus less-aggressive treatment densities. Adding peripheral tissue heating with the coagulation feature (graded over levels 1, 2, and 3) may decrease bleeding and enhance skin tightening and tissue remodeling. The skin is covered with saline-moistened gauze immediately following treatment until initial bleeding subsides. The skin is then kept moist with an occlusive ointment (eg, Skin-Medica Restorative Ointment, SkinMedica Inc, Carlsbad, CA, USA) for 5 to 7 days after treatment or until re-epithelialization is complete.

Full-field Er-YAG LSR with the Sciton Tunable Resurfacing Laser (TRL, formerly Contour) may be performed under general anesthesia, intravenous sedation, or oral/intramuscular analgesia/sedation. Except for general anesthesia cases, topical anesthesia (eg, 20% lidocaine, 5% prilocaine gel) is typically used for initial preparation for the procedure. The topical anesthetic is placed over the treatment area(s) and then occluded with plastic wrap for 1 hour. Regional nerve (frontal, external nasal, infraorbital, mental, labial, great auricular) and peripheral ring blockade (eg, 0.5% lidocaine, 0.25% marcaine, 1:200,000 epinephrine)

are very helpful along with direct subcutaneous infiltration of the eyelids and portions of the cheeks and perioral areas that are not adequately anesthetized with the preceding measures.

Treatment depth and number of passes during full-field Er-YAG LSR are adjusted according to pretreatment skin rejuvenation goals and regional condition and pathology of the skin. Facial skin is thicker over the forehead, medial cheeks, nose, and perioral areas and thinner over the posterior cheeks and eyelids.[33] The first or initial pass is typically performed in pure ablate mode with the goal of full ablation of the epidermis and exposure of dermal collagen in the upper papillary dermis. By varying the fluence (eg, 20 J/cm^2 for 80-μm depth for the eyelids; eg, 30 J/cm^2 for the forehead, cheeks, nose, and perioral areas for 120-μm depth), the laser surgeon can remove part or all of the epidermis with the first pass in pure ablate (short-pulse) mode. First-pass technique is demonstrated in Video 1.

By adding (blending) coagulation mode (eg, eyelids at 80-μm ablation plus 50-μm coagulation for total treated tissue depth of 130 μm; forehead, cheeks, and perioral areas at 100 to 200 μm ablation plus 50-μm to 100-μm coagulation for total treated tissue depth of 150 to 300 μm) for the second pass, both additional depth of ablation and controlled heating of collagen in the upper to mid-papillary dermis are achieved. Additional passes (third and occasionally fourth) may occasionally be performed for more severe conditions in lighter skin types and in areas where the skin has greater thickness (eg, perioral). The skin is covered with saline-moistened gauze immediately following treatment until initial bleeding subsides. The skin is then kept moist with an occlusive ointment (eg, SkinMedica Restorative Ointment) or with a hydrocolloid dressing (eg, Vigilon, C. R. Bard, Inc, Murray Hill, NJ, USA) for 5 to 7 days after treatment or until re-epithelialization is complete.

Full-field resurfacing may be performed for various indications (eg, atrophic acne scarring) on darker skin types, but the risk for prolonged erythema and ultimately PIH is significant.[34] For mild dyschromia and photodamage, superficial intraepidermal Er-YAG "micro" laser skin peels are well tolerated with topical anesthesia, require minimal downtime, and deliver impressive results with regard to improvements in surface skin texture and tone.[35–37]

ER-YAG LASER SKIN REJUVENATION OUTCOMES

Outcomes for Er-YAG laser ablation of skin lesions are generally very good. Occasionally, thicker lesions may not be completely ablated and re-treatment may be warranted. Assessment of results is fairly straightforward with attempted removal of individual lesions. Assessment of Er-YAG AFR or LSR results, however, may present a challenge if the improvement is subtle. Carefully obtained before and after photographs with make-up removed, similar lighting, and similar focal points is essential for adequate comparison and assessment of results.

Another option, VISIA Complexion Analysis (Canfield Scientific, Canfield Imaging Systems, Fairfield, NJ, USA), enables quantification of changes in facial skin compared with baseline findings. VISIA Complexion Analysis includes assessment of fine lines and rhytids, pore size, brown dyspigmentation, and deeper UV photodamage, as well as cutaneous vasculature (redness). Routine use of the VISIA Complexion Analysis improves patients' understanding of skin health, favorably shapes reasonable expectations for improvement with various procedures, and also guides patients' skin rejuvenation treatment programs at both the procedure and skin care levels.

Fig. 5 shows improvement in a large left cheek traumatic scar after multiple Er-YAG AFR sessions. Improvement of traumatic and acne scars can be dramatic with serial AFR. Scars that involve a large area in a confluent fashion (normal tissue absent except at periphery) may be subject to delayed healing and worsening of the scar if the central (interior) portion of the scar is treated. A useful alternative is to treat the periphery such that portions of the adjacent normal tissue and scar tissue are treated with the goal of gradually recruiting normal tissue (replacing abnormal tissue) from the periphery over multiple sessions in a centripetal fashion. Fig. 6 shows substantial improvement in overall skin tone and texture, including marked rhytid reduction following full-face Er-YAG LSR.

ER-YAG LASER SKIN REJUVENATION COMPLICATIONS

Complications related to Er-YAG cutaneous laser irradiation are best subcategorized with regard to onset and causation. Laser surgeons' success in dealing with these issues hinges on pretreatment patient education, primary prevention (to the extent possible) and early identification, and appropriate management. Initial patient education should document patient responsibilities for wound care, normal timelines for healing, and reasonable expectations for improvement (so that prolonged erythema, incomplete rhytid effacement, or partial dyschromia resolution are not perceived as adverse events), as well as the potential for complications (adverse outcomes that are not anticipated; eg, delayed healing, wound infection, scar formation). **Table 1** outlines complication types by causation and onset with the most common complications observed within each time period.

Ocular injury related to periorbital Er-YAG laser irradiation is most likely to involve injury to the cornea. Primary prevention involves use of water-based ocular lubricant and polished stainless steel corneal shields. Experienced physicians may opt for water-based ocular lubricant and multiple folded layers of saline-dampened gauze along with physically holding the eyelid closed during periorbital LSR. In the event of a significant corneal injury, urgent ophthalmology consultation is necessary.

Oxygen ignition is a potentially lethal complication that should be avoided through routinely incorporated safety measures. With general anesthesia, a laser-safe endotracheal or laryngeal mask airway must be used and it is also advisable to enlist the cooperation of the anesthesia team to reduce the concentration of oxygen during delivery of laser energy. With intravenous sedation, oxygen tubing should be removed during delivery of laser energy. Additional safety measures may include wrapping the endotracheal tube or laryngeal mask airway tube with a saline-soaked sterile towel. In the event of oxygen ignition, external effects may be limited to first-degree or second-degree burns if the fire is quenched nearly immediately. The outcome can be far worse if the fire also involves the airway.

It is apparent that many of the acute, subacute, and late complications of laser skin rejuvenation are directly related to decisions made during treatment. Overly aggressive treatment (overtreatment) may lead to excessive tissue devitalization and increased risk for infection, delayed healing, and scar formation. Overly conservative treatment (undertreatment) may lead to lack of tangible results and failure to meet patient expectations with regard to anticipated improvements in skin tone, texture, and rhytid effacement. Uneven treatment may lead to mixed results with variegation in tone and texture and possibly lines of demarcation between adjacent treatment areas. In considering overall treatment goals, it is helpful to consider each patient treatment as a continuum with regard to total energy applied to the skin. The therapeutic window wherein desired results are obtained is relatively narrow but the subtherapeutic and supratherapeutic windows are very wide.

Corneal exposure may occur following periorbital Er-YAG LSR but is very unlikely following periorbital Er-YAG AFR. Corneal exposure is more likely with one or more predisposing conditions

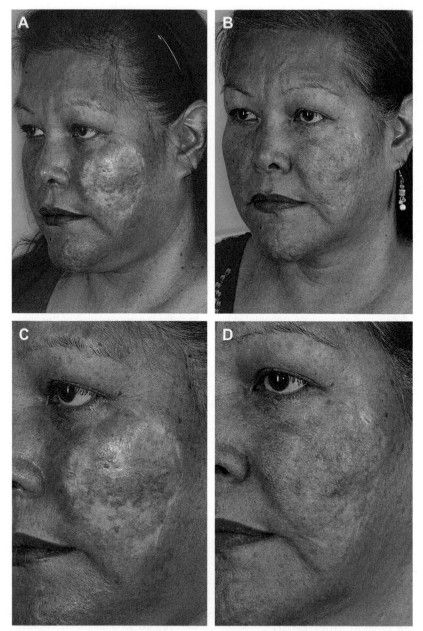

Fig. 5. Er-YAG AFR for traumatic scarring over left mid-cheek. Er-YAG ablative fractional laser skin resurfacing for traumatic scarring (50-year-old female, Fitzpatrick skin type IV) over left central cheek. *A, C* before and *B, D* after 14 short-pulse Er-YAG AFR treatments (11% coverage and 400-μm treatment depth). Close-up views (*C* and *D*) demonstrate dramatic improvement in skin quality with elimination and reduction of scarring and related improvements in skin tone and texture.

and aggressive periorbital treatment parameters. Predisposing conditions include prior upper and/ or lower blepharoplasty, marginal eyelid closure, lower eyelid laxity or malposition, and anterior position of the globe (relative to the inferior orbital rim). In some cases, anticipatory management of existing lower eyelid laxity (eg, lateral cantho-plasty) may prevent lower eyelid malposition even while safely enabling more effective laser treatment parameters (greater energy density). Mild lagophthalmos or mild lower eyelid retraction may be temporary; however, if either of these conditions persists or worsens, oculoplastic evaluation may be warranted. The cornea should be supported with appropriate ocular lubricants until symptoms resolve.

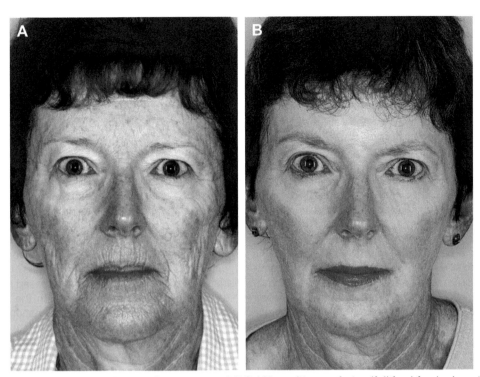

Fig. 6. Er-YAG full-face laser skin resurfacing. Er-YAG full-field laser skin resurfacing (full face) for dyschromia, rhytidosis, perioral lines, and skin laxity (68-year-old female, Fitzpatrick skin type II) (*A*). Ablation and coagulation settings (A/C) were adjusted for each treatment region: forehead (first pass: 120 A/0 C; second pass: 100 A/25 C; third pass: 50 A/50 C); periorbital (first pass: 80 A/0 C; second pass: 60 A/50 C; third pass: 60 A/50 C); cheeks (first pass: 120 A/0 C; second pass: 100 A/50 C); perioral (first pass: 120 A/0 C; second pass: 100 A/50 C; third pass: 140 A/50 C); (fourth pass: 50 A/100 C). Desired treatment goals met with marked improvement of all indications. Moderate erythema lasting more than 4 months was observed. Mild hypopigmentation is evident (*B*).

Normal initial healing, ie, time for re-epithelialization, following Er-YAG AFR and LSR is generally 3 to 5 and 4 to 7 days, respectively. Delayed re-epithelialization may result from overtreatment, desiccation, infection, secondary wounding, or decreased activity of pilosebaceous units (eg, isotretinoin use in the past 12 months; prior external beam radiation therapy) but may rarely also be idiopathic or the result of contact dermatitis (eg, reaction to petroleum or other topical substances that may not have been provided or recommended by the treating physician). Primary prevention is

Table 1
Laser skin resurfacing causation and onset

Causation	Onset Intraoperative	Onset Acute <14 Days	Onset Subacute 14–60 Days	Onset Late >60 Days
Device malfunction	Ocular injury	Corneal exposure	Corneal exposure	Corneal exposure
Environmental	Oxygen ignition	Delayed healing	Delayed healing	Delayed healing
Iatrogenic	Overtreatment	Dermatitis	Dermatitis	Dermatitis
Idiopathic	Undertreatment	infection	Dyschromia	Dyschromia
Patient induced	Uneven treatment	—	Failure to meet expectations	Failure to meet expectations
Physiologic	—	Milia	Milia Prolonged erythema Scarring	Milia Prolonged erythema Scarring

Abbreviation: —, no data.

facilitated by a careful medical history, reasonable treatment parameters, appropriate prophylactic antibiotic and antiviral coverage, adequate wound care, and avoidance of any secondary trauma (eg, scratching during sleep).

In the event that delayed healing does occur, it is typically a focal delay in one or more discrete areas and much more attention to the patient's condition becomes necessary to work toward an optimal outcome. Depending on level of patient cooperation and the appearance of the wound(s), daily wound evaluation may be appropriate. Findings may include wound desiccation, superficial or deeper skin devitalization, biofilm, early granulation tissue, and no evidence of continuing re-epithelialization. Treatment may require debridement and alteration of topical wound care with a variety of options including silver nitrate (for focal treatment of granulation tissue), one-quarter strength sodium hypochlorite wet to dry dressing changes, silver sulfadiazine or Biafine Topical Emulsion. Most problematic wounds ultimately close with an appropriate regimen. In more severe circumstances, minor surgical wound closure may be considered. The final texture and tone of the skin in the affected area may not be optimal (eg, atrophic, hypertrophic, dyspigmented) and secondary laser treatment(s) may become necessary.

Dermatitis is more often a subacute problem, but may result from reaction to ingredients (including petrolatum) in the occlusive balm used to facilitate re-epithelialization. Restorative Ointment (SkinMedica, Inc) is a non–petrolatum-containing occlusive balm that incorporates plant-based oils as a suitable alternative during initial healing. Dermatitis during the subacute phase may result from contact hypersensitivity. Definitive treatment most often involves removal of the offending substance(s) and replacement with a nonirritant alternative. More severe reactions may require topical and/or oral steroid (eg, short burst and taper) treatment. Other conditions that may be seen include folliculitis, heat rash (miliaria rubra), and inflammatory acne flair.

Infection may be of bacterial, fungal, or viral origin and may manifest in a variety of ways, including colonization of desquamative debris, adherent biofilm, edema, and erythema extending beyond the laser treatment area (typical of cellulitis), purulent exudate, fluid-filled vesicles, and so forth. If the patient has been on prophylactic antibiotic and antiviral coverage, a change in therapy is likely warranted. In particular, an acutely worsening condition may require intravenous antibiotic and/or antiviral therapy.

Milia, small white cystic lesions that form with blockage of pores and prevention of normal egress of skin sebum and debris, may form during any of the stages of healing. Milia may occur as a result of extended use of occlusive balm recommended for initial healing. As the skin continues to heal, pore blockages may occur from changes within the skin that are very superficial or relatively deeper such that the lesions may respond to treatment with an exfoliant or may require manual debridement. The phenomenon is usually temporary and may be improved with alteration of the skin care regimen.

Dyschromia is much more likely following Er-YAG LSR versus Er-YAG AFR and may involve either an abnormal increase or decrease in skin pigment. More aggressive full-field laser skin resurfacing treatments with long pulsed systems and greater thermal damage has been correlated with induction with pigmentary disorders in Fitzpatrick skin types III and above.[38] Increased melanin deposition has been correlated with the healing response following laser skin rejuvenation where inflammatory mediators may upregulate tyrosinase activity.[39] So-called postinflammatory hyperpigmentation (PIH) has been correlated with increased density of microthermal zones with nonablative fractional resurfacing in darker skin types.[32] Although PIH may occur with Er-YAG LSR, this phenomenon is less likely with Er-YAG AFR, at least in pure ablation (short-pulse) mode. Although more likely with darker skin types (eg, Fitzpatrick types III, IV, V), PIH may also occur with lighter skin types (eg, Fitzpatrick types I, II) following laser skin rejuvenation treatments.

PIH may be averted or reduced in severity via the following:

1. pretreatment with a tyrosinase inhibitor
2. careful selection of procedure including appropriate modifications to treatment settings for each patient's skin condition and Fitzpatrick skin type
3. early identification and appropriate intervention in the event PIH develops.

For patients with darker skin types who also desire more aggressive laser skin rejuvenation treatments, a regimen consisting of topical application of 4% hydroquinone twice daily for 1 month before treatment has been successful in reducing the incidence and severity of PIH. For patients with darker skin types, Er-YAG AFR treatment with conservative microablation zone density and optional combination with a superficial Er-YAG laser skin peel is a reasonable method to achieve incremental improvements in skin texture and moderate improvements in skin tone while reducing the likelihood of PIH.

In the event that PIH becomes evident, often between 4 and 8 weeks after treatment, the natural history tends to be one of slow resolution over several months, presuming no additional factors are independently stimulating melanin production (eg, sun exposure, contact dermatitis). Alone or in combination, initial treatment of PIH typically involves appropriate photoprotection, topical tyrosinase inhibition, and/or topical steroid therapy but various chemical skin-peeling regimens are also commonly used.[39]

Hypopigmentation may be observed following Er-YAG LSR but is unlikely and has not been reported following Er-YAG AFR. Following deep, diffuse (nonfractionated) skin injury, hypopigmentation after Er-YAG LSR may present in a delayed fashion and may be permanent. Skin depigmentation has been attributed to melanocyte injury and suppressed melanogenesis but the precise mechanism is unknown.[40] The area(s) of hypopigmentation may appear relatively worse if juxtaposed to skin with significant accumulated melanin pigment (eg, frequent sun exposure). No universally efficacious therapy has been identified to ameliorate postresurfacing hypopigmentation but some success has been obtained recently in a small study where NFR treatments preceded topical therapy with bimatoprost ophthalmic solution 0.03% (twice a day) and tretinoin 0.025% (every night).[41]

Failure to meet expectations with a particular treatment can be frustrating for patient and physician alike. Digital pretreatment and posttreatment patient photographs (including several photographs at each posttreatment visit) are not only a necessary part of the medical record but also invaluable as a tool for patient teaching. Comparison of the pretreatment and posttreatment photographs often reveals improvements in skin tone and texture that a particular patient may not have yet appreciated. The VISIA Complexion Analysis (VCA) system is a more sophisticated method for patient education that also enables comparison and quantification of changes in the skin over multiple visits. As such, VCA can also help to guide patient treatment decisions both at topical skin care and procedure levels.

Posttreatment erythema generally declines gradually over several weeks to several months following Er-YAG LSR and much more quickly following Er-YAG AFR. Ablation and coagulation depth are directly correlated with severity and duration of postresurfacing erythema. Redness is typically more pronounced in severity and duration in patients with lighter skin types. Severity and duration of postresurfacing erythema may be reduced with photobiomodulation treatments and/or topical steroid or antioxidant (eg, ascorbic acid) therapy. Extremely protracted postresurfacing erythema may precede development of PIH, as well as permanent hypopigmentation. Although not a treatment goal, postresurfacing erythema of relatively short duration may be desirable for many patients. This secondary goal may be achieved along with modest to very significant improvements in skin tone and surface texture with relatively more superficial Er-YAG LSR and/or Er-YAG AFR treatments.

Scarring is not common with Er-YAG LSR and has not been reported with Er-YAG AFR. Scarring may be atrophic or hypertrophic in nature. Atrophic scarring is very unlikely with Er-YAG cutaneous laser use but may follow infection with tissue devitalization, resulting in impaired reformation of the normal skin layers or with excessive ablation depth. Focal hypertrophic scarring after Er-YAG LSR may occur with excessive energy density delivered at the dermal level in more permissive tissues (eg, eyelids).

ADJUNCTIVE ER-YAG LASER SKIN REJUVENATION

Er-YAG LSR is a valuable adjunct for cervicofacial rhytidectomy and facial contouring procedures (eg, soft tissue augmentation; laser-assisted facial contouring). Patients' perception of facial rejuvenation success, in terms of number of years that features of aging appear to be reversed, increases significantly when LSR is completed with facelift surgery compared with facelift surgery alone.[42] Numerous studies have demonstrated the safety of concurrent facial surgery and skin resurfacing, including treatment of elevated flaps.[43–45] Nonetheless, it is prudent to reduce treatment depth and energy density over elevated flaps (especially longer cutaneous flaps) and to consider staging of rhytidectomy and skin-resurfacing procedures in the event that flap viability becomes questionable.[45]

SUMMARY

For the laser surgeon, the Er-YAG laser is an invaluable tool that delivers unsurpassed ablation efficiency, and with appropriate functionality (quasi long-pulse feature) provides sufficient tissue coagulation to remodel deep rhytids. As such, the 2940-nm wavelength is well suited for routine laser skin rejuvenation in full-field, fractional, and point-beam modes with additional benefits, including applicability to diverse skin types, short healing times, and a low likelihood of energy-related complications.

SUPPLEMENTARY DATA

Supplementary data related to this article can be found online at doi:10.1016/j.fsc.2011.04.005.

REFERENCES

1. Kutlubay Z, Gokedemir G. Treatment of atrophic facial acne scars with the Er:YAG laser: a Turkish experience. J Cosmet Laser Ther 2010;12(2):65–72.
2. Tay YK, Kwok C. Minimally ablative erbium:YAG laser resurfacing of facial atrophic acne scars in Asian skin: a pilot study. Dermatol Surg 2008;34(5):681–5.
3. Tanzi EL, Alster TS. Treatment of atrophic facial acne scars with dual-mode Er:YAG laser. Dermatol Surg 2002;28(7):551–5.
4. Teikemeier G, Goldberg DJ. Skin resurfacing with the erbium:YAG laser. Dermatol Surg 1997;23(8):685–7.
5. Bass LS. Erbium:YAG laser skin resurfacing: preliminary clinical evaluation. Ann Plast Surg 1988;40(4):328–34.
6. Perez MI, Bank DE, Silvers D. Skin resurfacing of the face with the Erbium:YAG laser. Dermatol Surg 1998;24(6):653–8.
7. Weiss RA, Harrington AC, Pfau RC, et al. Periorbital skin resurfacing using high energy erbium:YAG laser: results in 50 patients. Lasers Surg Med 1999;24(2):81–6.
8. Tanzi EL, Alster TS. Side effects and complications of variable-pulsed erbium:yttrium-aluminum-garnet laser skin resurfacing: extended experience with 50 patients. Plast Reconstr Surg 2003;111(4):1524–9.
9. Adrian RM. Pulsed carbon dioxide and long pulse 10-ms erbium-YAG laser resurfacing: a comparative clinical and histologic study. J Cutan Laser Ther 1999;1(4):197–202.
10. Rostan EF, Fitzpatrick RE, Goldman MP. Laser resurfacing with a long pulse erbium:YAG laser compared to the 950 ms pulsed CO_2 laser. Lasers Surg Med 2001;29(2):136–41.
11. Khatri KA, Ross V, Grevelink JM, et al. Comparison of erbium:YAG and carbon dioxide lasers in resurfacing of facial rhytides. Arch Dermatol 1999;135(11):1416–7.
12. Ross EV, Miller C, Meehan K, et al. One-pass CO2 versus multiple-pass Er:YAG laser resurfacing in the treatment of rhytides: a comparison side-by-side study of pulsed CO2 and Er:YAG lasers. Dermatol Surg 2001;27(8):709–15.
13. Fitzpatrick RE. Maximizing benefits and minimizing risk with CO2 laser resurfacing. Dermatol Clin 2002;20(1):77–86.
14. Newman JB, Lord JL, Ash K, et al. Variable pulse erbium:YAG laser skin resurfacing of perioral rhytides and side-by-side comparison with carbon dioxide laser. Lasers Surg Med 2000;26(2):208–14.
15. Zachary CB. Modulating the Er:YAG laser. Lasers Surg Med 2000;26(2):223–6.
16. Tanzi EL, Alster TS. Single-pass carbon dioxide versus multiple-pass Er:YAG laser skin resurfacing: a comparison of postoperative wound healing and side-effect rates. Dermatol Surg 2003;29(1):80–4.
17. Riggs K, Keller M, Humphreys TR. Ablative laser resurfacing: high-energy pulsed carbon dioxide and erbium:yttrium-aluminum-garnet. Clin Dermatol 2007;25(5):462–73.
18. Weinstein C. Computerized scanning erbium:YAG laser for skin resurfacing. Dermatol Surg 1998;24(1):83–9.
19. Hantash BM, Bedi VP, Chan KF, et al. In vivo histological evaluation of a novel ablative fractional resurfacing device. Lasers Surg Med 2007;39(2):96–107.
20. Lapidoth M, Yagima Odo ME, Odo LM. Novel use of erbium:YAG (2940 nm) laser for fractional ablative photothermolysis in the treatment of photodamaged facial skin: a pilot study. Dermatol Surg 2008;34(8):1048–53.
21. Tierney EP, Kouba DJ, Hanke CW. Review of fractional photothermolysis: treatment indications and efficacy. Dermatol Surg 2009;35(10):1445–61.
22. Reddy BY, Hantash BM. Emerging technologies in aesthetic medicine. Dermatol Clin 2009;27(4):521–7.
23. Millman AL, Mannor GE. Combined erbium:YAG and carbon dioxide laser skin resurfacing. Arch Facial Plast Surg 1999;1(2):112–6.
24. Goldman MP, Manuskiatti W. Combined laser resurfacing with the 950-microsec pulsed CO2 + Er:YAG lasers. Dermatol Surg 1999;25(3):160–3.
25. Collawn SS. Combination therapy: utilization of CO2 and Erbium:YAG lasers for skin resurfacing. Ann Plast Surg 1999;42(1):21–6.
26. Goldman MP, Marchell N, Fitzpatrick RE. Laser skin resurfacing of the face with a combined CO2/Er:YAG laser. Dermatol Surg 2000;26(2):102–4.
27. Ross EV, Domankevitz Y, Skrobal M, et al. Effects of CO2 laser pulse duration in ablation and residual thermal damage: implications for skin resurfacing. Lasers Surg Med 1996;19:123–9.
28. Ross EV, McKinlay JR, Anderson RR. Why does carbon dioxide resurfacing work? A review. Arch Dermatol 1999;135(4):444–54.
29. Pozner JM, Goldberg DJ. Histologic effect of a variable pulsed Er:YAG laser. Dermatol Surg 2000;26(8):733–6.
30. Kaufmann R. Role of Erbium:YAG laser in the treatment of aged skin. Clin Exp Dermatol 2001;26(7):631–6.
31. Dierickx CC, Khatri KA, Tannous ZS, et al. Micro-fractional ablative skin resurfacing with two novel erbium laser systems. Lasers Surg Med 2008;40(2):113–23.
32. Kono T, Chan HH, Groff WF, et al. Prospective direct comparison study of fractional resurfacing using different fluencies and densities for skin rejuvenation in Asians. Lasers Surg Med 2007;39(4):311–4.

33. Ha RY, Nojima K, Adams WP Jr, et al. Analysis of facial skin thickness: defining the relative thickness index. Plast Reconstr Surg 2005;115(6):1769–73.

34. Ko NY, Ahn HH, Kim SN, et al. Analysis of erythema after Er:YAG laser skin resurfacing. Dermatol Surg 2007;33(11):1322–7.

35. Khatri KA, Machado A, Magro C, et al. Laser peel: facial rejuvenation with a superficial erbium:YAG laser treatment. J Cutan Laser Ther 2000;2(3):119–23.

36. Christian MM. Microresurfacing using the variable-pulse erbium:YAG laser: a comparison of the 0.5- and 4-ms pulse durations. Dermatol Surg 2003; 29(6):605–11.

37. Pozner JN, Goldberg DJ. Superficial erbium:YAG laser resurfacing of photodamaged skin. J Cosmet Laser Ther 2006;8(2):89–91.

38. Kim YJ, Lee HS, Son SW, et al. Analysis of hyper-pigmentation and hypopigmentation after Er:YAG laser skin resurfacing. Lasers Surg Med 2005; 36(1):47–51.

39. Taylor S, Grimes P, Lim J, et al. Postinflammatory hyperpigmentation. J Cutan Med Surg 2009;13(4): 183–91.

40. Helm TN, Shatkin S Jr. Alabaster skin after CO2 laser resurfacing: evidence for suppressed melanogenesis rather than just melanocyte destruction. Cutis 2006;77(1):15–7.

41. Fitzpatrick R. Repigmentation of hypopigmented scars. Presented at the American Society for Laser Medicine and Surgery 30th Annual Conference. Phoenix (AZ), April 16–18, 2010 [abstract: 92].

42. Roberts TL III, Pozner JN, Ritter E. The RSVP facelift: a highly vascular flap permitting safe, simultaneous, comprehensive facial rejuvenation in one operative setting. Aesthetic Plast Surg 2000;24(5):313–22.

43. Weinstein C, Pozner J, Scheflan M, et al. Combined Erbium:YAG laser resurfacing and face lifting. Plast Reconstr Surg 2000;107(2):593–4.

44. Alster TS, Doshi SN, Hopping SB. Combination surgical lifting with ablative laser skin resurfacing of facial skin: a retrospective analysis. Dermatol Surg 2004;30(9):1191–5.

45. Holcomb JD, Kent KJ, Rousso DE. Nitrogen plasma skin regeneration and aesthetic facial surgery: multi-center evaluation of concurrent treatment. Arch Facial Plast Surg 2009;11(3):184–93.

Treatment of Acne Scarring

Jaggi Rao, MD, FRCPC

KEYWORDS

- Acne vulgaris • Acne scarring • Laser treatment

ACNE PATHOPHYSIOLOGY

Acne vulgaris, popularly known as acne, is an inflammatory dermatosis of the pilosebaceous unit (ie, the hair follicle and its associated sebaceous gland) and is characterized by the presence of comedones (whiteheads and blackheads), inflammatory papules and pustules, cysts, and nodules. Acne is believed to be caused by the interplay of 4 separate pathophysiologic factors: (1) keratin dysadhesion along the follicular epithelium resulting in the formation of a keratin plug or microcomedone, (2) increased sebum production by the sebaceous gland, (3) bacterial overgrowth, and (4) inflammation (**Fig. 1**).[1] Trigger factors known to contribute to acne formation include exogenous factors, such as occlusive agents (skincare products, makeup, and so forth), and endogenous factors, such as androgen hormones and specific medications (eg, antiseizure drugs).[1]

Acne vulgaris is by far the most prevalent skin disorder, with more than 80% of adolescents and young adults affected.[1] Almost everyone experiences some form and degree of acne during a lifetime. Unfortunately, when acne resolves, it has a tendency to scar the skin, often creating significant physical and psychological sequelae. An understanding of the nature of acne scarring and the role of modern therapies to reduce its disfiguring appearance can have a positive impact on the quality of life of patients.

ACNE SCARRING PATHOPHYSIOLOGY

Acne scarring occurs when active acne irreversibly injures the microscopic structure of the skin to the point that its appearance is altered in terms of color, texture, or both. Altered skin texture and color can offer a sharp contrast with surrounding nonscarred skin, attracting attention from the human eye.

Acne scarring is more likely after certain forms of acne vulgaris, with specific skin types, and in particular anatomic locations. Typically, acne scarring is commonly seen after acne that has been characterized by deep inflammation, nodules, or cysts. In these forms of acne, inflammation resulting from follicular rupture and expulsion of sebum, bacteria, and keratin into the dermis of the skin ultimately causes skin surface abnormalities. In some cases, inflammatory injury to the dermis may cause deposition of new collagen that creates uneven surface elevations. In other cases, resolution of cysts and nodules may cause tethering of the skin surface, resulting in small crypts or depressions.[2] Inflammation may also cause injury to pigmented epithelia, causing melanin to be released into the dermis, which results in brown pigmentation. In some postacne individuals, blood vessels may become permanently dilated as part of a wound healing response at the sites of focal inflammation; for an observer, this is perceived as areas of persistent redness.

Patients with darker skin types (Fitzpatrick scale skin types IV, V, and VI) are more prone to acne scarring compared with those who have white skin. Dark-skinned individuals are more prone to postinflammatory hyperpigmentation due to more pigment that may be released into the dermis as the result of skin injury. This is visible as focal and persistent areas of brown pigmentation in areas of prior inflammation. Darker skin types are also more susceptible to the formation of

Disclosures: Dr Rao serves has served as a consultant and speaker for Cutera, Cynosure, Lumenis, and Sciton.
Division of Dermatology and Cutaneous Sciences, University of Alberta Dermatology Centre, University of Alberta, 2-125 Clinical Sciences Building, Edmonton, Alberta T6G 2G3, Canada
E-mail address: jrao@ualberta.ca

Facial Plast Surg Clin N Am 19 (2011) 275–291
doi:10.1016/j.fsc.2011.04.004
1064-7406/11/$ – see front matter © 2011 Elsevier Inc. All rights reserved,

facialplastic.theclinics.com

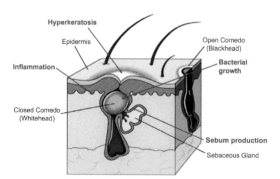

Fig. 1. Pathophysiologic factors in the development of acne vulgaris.

Box 1
Acne scarring classification

- Color
  - Normal color
  - Red
  - Brown
  - White (hypopigmented or depigmented)
- Texture
  - Normal texture
  - Elevated
    - Hypertrophic
    - Keloid
  - Depressed (or atrophic)
    - Icepick
    - Boxcar
    - Rolled

hypertrophic and keloid scars as a result of injury to the skin. It may be that these skin types are genetically more prone to collagen deposition post–skin injury, mediated by the release of profibrotic chemical messengers, such as transforming growth factor β.[2]

Anatomic site of active acne can also predict the likelihood and type of acne scarring that may result. Acne of the forehead and mid to upper cheeks typically results in small icepick scars that may be persistently red in white skin types and brown in darker skin types.[2] Acne of thicker areas of skin, such as the lower face (lower cheeks, chin, and jawline), usually results in larger and deeper scars. Acne of the angle of the jaw, sternal and upper chest, shoulders, and upper back has a tendency to result in hypertrophic and keloid scars. Acne of the lower back tends to yield larger, depressed scars.[2]

CLASSIFICATION AND NATURE OF ACNE SCARRING

Of the many systems advocated to classify acne scarring,[3] the author uses a unique compiled system based on both color and texture, which he considers the most practical as pertaining to subsequent management (**Box 1**). When new acne scarring modalities arise, they can be readily added to this classification scheme.

This classification system has two major categories: color and texture. Every acne scar can be broken down and categorized according to these two components, both of which must be considered and addressed independently to attain improvement of the visible quality of the scar. The elements of a scar's color and texture must be considered in relative contrast to the surrounding normal skin of the same individual at the same anatomic site. In this classification scheme, there should not be active inflammation. If inflammation exists, it can interfere with

understanding the nature of the scar and reduce treatment efficacy. Active inflammation should first be resolved to determine the correct classification of acne scarring. Active inflammation is usually characterized by a purple discoloration, focal elevation of the skin, and tenderness.

Scar Color

For a scar's color to be considered normal, it must be the same color as the surrounding background skin in the same anatomic site. If a scar is not of normal color, it contrasts with the surrounding background skin in the same anatomic site and can be red, brown, or white.

Scars may appear red due to either persistent inflammation (which is not true scarring and should be eliminated before scar treatment) or permanently dilated small blood vessels (capillaries) beneath the skin's surface (**Fig. 2**). Dilatation of blood vessels is part of the skin's normal healing response to dermal injury, designed to provide oxygen, chemical factors, and nutrients necessary for the skin to adequate recover from the injury. Red blood cells contain hemoglobin, which is red in color. Increased amounts of red blood cells within areas of dilated blood vessels give the skin surface above this area a varying degree of skin surface redness. Deeper and highly concentrated capillaries create a dull red skin surface appearance, whereas superficial and less concentrated blood vessels make the scar appear bright red. Redness within acne scars may be self-limited but can take months to years to resolve.

Brown scars are due to either melanin deposition at the site or hemosiderin pigmentation

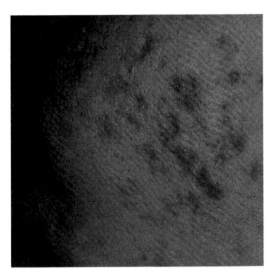

Fig. 2. Example of red acne scarring.

(Fig. 3). Melanin deposition is often due to the inflammatory injury that acne creates. Seen especially in darker individuals, melanin has the tendency to become incontinent from skin epithelium, depositing into the dermis and creating persistent pigmentation as perceived on the surface by an observer. Skin injury through acne can also stimulate greater melanin transfer to other cells within the skin's epithelium, contributing to the brown appearance of the scar. Melanin pigmentation may be self-limited but can take months to years to fully resolve.

Hemosiderin is an iron oxide compound that results from extravasated red blood cells at the site of skin injury. When blood vessels are persistently dilated, it becomes more possible for red blood cells and red blood cell fragments to exit the confines of the capillaries that contain them and deposit within the skin's dermis. If this occurs, the free hemoglobin that results ultimately degrades to release iron constituents that, when combined with tissue oxygen, stain the skin brown. This form of brown scarring is usually more persistent than melanin deposition because hemosiderin exists in small, inert particles that often evade the skin's clearance system, in many ways similar to the application of a cosmetic tattoo.

White scars are possible, not as part of the natural healing process of acne, but as the result of manipulation from the patient (eg, scratching, pinching the skin) (Fig. 4). It is important to distinguish between scars that are truly white and those that may appear white due to a background of pigmentation (eg, melasma, tanned skin, or sun damage). If there is doubt as to what is normal skin and what is not, a small biopsy may be performed and the specimen treated with a Fontana-Masson stain to identify melanocytes or a Melan-A stain to identify hyperpigmentation. Truly white color in scars is due to either a complete or partial absence of melanin pigment or a thick fibrosis of the skin's dermis. Melanin pigment may be decreased by inflammation that has completely or partially destroyed the melanocytes that generate melanin. Usually, this is due to a more immune-specific inflammation than is typically seen with acne but more commonly seen with concomitant skin conditions, such as vitiligo. Scarring from chicken pox (varicella) and other

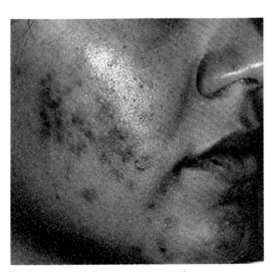

Fig. 3. Example of brown acne scarring.

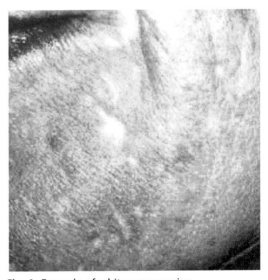

Fig. 4. Example of white acne scarring.

inflammatory or fibrotic conditions (eg, lichen sclerosus or morphea) can result in white scars due to destruction of the dermal epidermal junction and underlying fibrosis but is rare in acne vulgaris.

Scar Texture

For a scar's texture to be considered normal, it must be along the same plane as the surrounding background skin in the same anatomic site. If a difference can be felt in skin texture overlying the scar, it is not considered normal according to the classification scheme. Inflammation and active acne must be resolved to perform scar classification, because inflammation itself can cause textural anomalies and alter the true perception of scar texture.

If a scar is not of normal texture, it contrasts with the surrounding background skin in the same anatomic site and can be either elevated or depressed. Elevated scars can be further classified as either hypertrophic or keloid. Hypertrophic scars are those where the scar tissue has vertical growth only; that is, the lateral confines of the scar do not extend beyond the injury or defect that has initiated the scar. A hypertrophic scar has, by definition, has the same surface area as the inflammatory papule, nodule, or cyst that was its precursor. In contrast, keloid scars have vertical and lateral growth. They are typically more spherical in surface contour and extend beyond the confines of the injury. Keloids are seen more commonly on the shoulders, angle of the jaw, sternal chest, and any areas where there has been cartilaginous injury (such as the ears). Both hypertrophic and keloid scars are the result of excessive collagen deposition at the site of skin injury, the fibrosis of which has elevated the skin surface focally. Although elevated scars may soften or flatten with time, they are not expected to completely resolve without intervention (**Fig. 5**).

Depressed or atrophic scars occur when the skin contour has dropped beneath the plane of the surrounding skin at the site of skin injury. Depressed acne scars can be classified as (1) icepick, (2) boxcar, or (3) rolled in nature. In icepick scarring, the scar has an acute angle at this base and is usually small (less than 2 mm in width) and superficial (less than 1 mm in depth). Icepick scars typically occur in multiples as a result of focal collagen injury from prior inflammatory acne (**Fig. 6**). Boxcar acne scars have right angles and therefore appear crateriform in contrast to icepick scars. Boxcar scars may be several millimeters in diameter and can be as deep as 2 mm (**Fig. 7**). Rolled scars are characterized by shallow, rolled, nonangled borders and can be several millimeters

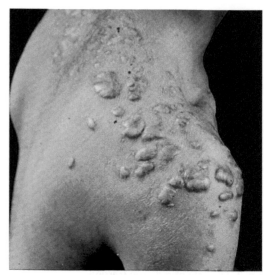

Fig. 5. Example of hypertrophic and keloid acne scarring.

deep. Rolled scars are usually larger in diameter than both icepick and boxcar scars and typically do not occur in clusters (**Fig. 8**). Rolled scars are the result of a deep cyst or nodule that has involuted or retracted. When cysts or nodules are chronically present in the dermis, adhesions tend to form that affix the lesion in place relative to the surface of the skin. A physical reduction in lesion size results in a tethering of the surface contour directly above the lesion, resulting in the typical rolled morphology. After adhesions have broken down, the skin surface typically takes on a rippled or undulated appearance. Generally,

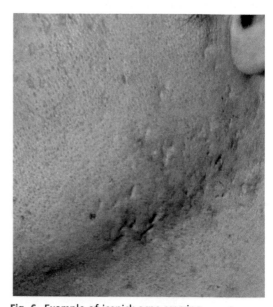

Fig. 6. Example of icepick acne scarring.

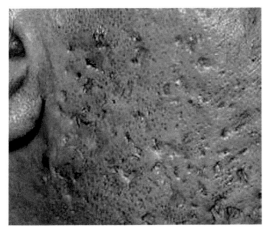

Fig. 7. Example of boxcar acne scarring.

the natural history of all forms of depressed scars is gradual and partial improvement of depth and surface area, but usually not complete normalization of skin contour.

LASER MANAGEMENT OF ACNE SCARRING

Choosing the optimal modality for treatment of an individual patient's acne scarring depends on a thorough understanding of many factors, including the type and degree of scarring and the anatomy involved as well as the patient's skin type. Treating clinicians should also consider a patient's tolerance for procedures and their outcome expectations. The author attributes treatment options according to the type of scarring that is present. The general philosophy is to normalize both the color and texture of individual acne scars to resemble the color and texture of surrounding normal tissue.

Table 1 illustrates various treatment options considered by the author for the various types of

acne scarring according to the classification system described previously. Of the various treatment options, this article discusses only the laser options for scar improvement, in particular the usefulness of lasers in normalizing scar color and texture. Thorough knowledge and experience of these laser modalities and their use may lead to creative therapeutic combinations, which may yield faster results with greater improvement. A discussion of multiple modality synergies, however, is beyond the scope of this article.

Table 2 outlines the steps required to perform a successful acne scarring consultation.

Normalization of Scar Color

Red color
Erythema or redness of scar tissue accentuates the depth of a scar and focuses an observer's attention, but removal of the redness can make a scar seem less deep and noticeable, even if the depth and size are unchanged. Erythema is the result of dilated capillaries beneath the skin surface. The intensity of the erythema is dependent on (1) the concentration of blood vessels within the scar, (2) the average caliber or lumen size of the blood vessels at the site, and (4) the distance of the blood vessels from the skin surface (ie, their depth). Bright erythema within scars is suggestive of vessels that are not concentrated, have a relatively small diameter lumen, and are in the superficial dermis (relatively close to the skin surface). Dull erythema is typically seen in scars where blood vessels are concentrated, large caliber, and deep. These clinical signs may be useful in selecting appropriate treatment modalities to normalize erythema.

Lasers and light sources that may be used to reduce the red coloration of acne scars include the pulsed dye laser (PDL), the potassium-titanyl-phosphate (KTP) laser, intense pulsed light (IPL), and the neodymium:yttrium-aluminum-garnet (Nd:YAG) laser. Usually, 3 to 4 or more treatments are required, at approximately 1-month intervals.

PDL PDL has been the gold standard for treating the erythema of acne scarring.[4] This laser has an output wavelength of 585 nm or 595 nm, depending on the property of the particular rhodamine dye used as the lasing medium for a given device. Both wavelengths specifically target oxyhemoglobin within red blood cells, by approximating a major hemoglobin absorption peak at 577 nm (**Fig. 9**). Because tissue penetration increases with longer wavelengths in the visible spectrum, the 595-nm PDL is more commercially popular because it offers the advantage of deeper tissue penetration

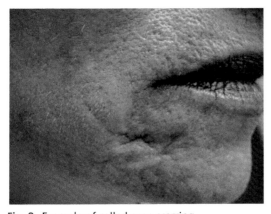

Fig. 8. Example of rolled acne scarring.

Table 1
Acne scarring treatment options

Color	Color Treatment Options	Texture	Texture Treatment Options
Normal	No treatment necessary	Normal texture	No treatment necessary
Red	• Topical treatment 　○ Vasoconstrictors 　○ Camouflage • Vascular-Targeting Laser Treatment 　○ PDL 　○ IPL 　○ Nd:YAG laser 　○ Microsecond-Pulsed Nd:YAG laser	Elevated (Hypertrophic and keloid)	• Topical Treatment 　○ Topical corticosteroids 　○ Topical imiquimod • Physical Treatment 　○ Intralesional corticosteroids 　○ Intralesional 5-FU 　○ Occlusive dressings 　○ Surgical excision • Fractionated Ablative Laser Treatment 　○ Fractionated Er:YAG laser 　○ Fractionated YSGG laser 　○ Fractionated CO_2 laser • Confluent Ablative Laser Treatment (with Surgical Excision) 　○ Er:YAG laser 　○ YSGG laser 　○ CO_2 laser
Brown	• Topical Treatment 　○ Lightening creams 　○ Topical retinoids 　○ Chemical peels 　○ Camouflage • Physical Treatment 　○ Microdermabrasion 　○ Micropuncturing • Pigment-Targeting Laser Treatment 　○ IPL 　○ Q-Switched lasers (ruby, alexandrite, Nd:YAG lasers) 　○ Microsecond-Pulsed Nd:YAG laser • Confluent Ablative Laser Treatment 　○ Er:YAG laser 　○ YSGG laser • Fractionated Ablative Laser Treatment 　○ Fractionated Er:YAG laser 　○ Fractionated YSGG laser		
White	• Topical Treatment 　○ Tacrolimus 　○ Pimecrolimus 　○ Camouflage • Phototherapy 　○ UV light therapy (PUVA, UVA1, NBUVB, BBUVB) • Physical Treatment 　○ Surgical excision • Pigment Stimulation Laser Treatment 　○ Excimer laser • Fractionated Ablative Laser Treatment 　○ Fractionated Er:YAG laser 　○ Fractionated CO_2 laser 　○ Fractionated YSGG laser	Depressed (Icepick and boxcar)	• Topical Treatment 　○ Chemical peels 　○ Camouflage • Physical Treatment 　○ Microdermabrasion 　○ Dermabrasion 　○ Soft tissue fillers 　○ Profibrotic agents 　○ Volumizing agents 　○ Punch excision • Confluent Ablative Laser Treatment 　○ Er:YAG laser 　○ YSGG laser 　○ CO_2 laser • Confluent Non-Ablative Laser Treatment 　○ PDL 　○ IPL 　○ Microsecond-Pulsed Nd:YAG laser

(continued on next page)

Table 1
Acne scarring treatment options (*continued*)

Color	Color Treatment Options	Texture	Texture Treatment Options
White (*continued*)		Depressed (Icepick and boxcar) *continued*	○ Q-switched Nd:YAG laser ○ 1320 nm laser ○ 1440 nm and 1450 nm lasers ○ 1540 nm and 1550 nm lasers • Fractionated Ablative Laser Treatment 　○ Fractionated Er:YAG laser 　○ Fractionated YSGG laser 　○ Fractionated CO_2 laser • Fractionated Non-Ablative Laser Treatment 　○ Fractionated 1440 nm and 1450 nm laser 　○ Fractionated 1540 nm and 1550 nm laser
		Depressed (Rolled)	• Physical Treatment 　○ Soft tissue fillers 　○ Profibrotic agents 　○ Volumizing agents 　○ Surgical excision 　○ Subcision • Confluent Non-Ablative Laser Treatment 　○ Pulsed dye laser 　○ Intense pulsed light 　○ Microsecond-Pulsed Nd:YAG laser 　○ Q-Switched Nd:YAG laser 　○ 1320 nm laser 　○ 1440 nm and 1450 nm lasers 　○ 1540 nm and 1550 nm lasers • Fractionated Ablative Laser Treatment 　○ Fractionated Er:YAG laser 　○ Fractionated YSGG laser 　○ Fractionated CO_2 laser • Fractionated Non-Ablative Laser Treatment 　○ Fractionated 1440 nm and 1450 nm lasers 　○ Fractionated 1540 nm and 1550 nm lasers

Abbreviations: BBUVB, broadband UVB; 5-FU, 5-fluorouracil; NBUVB, narrowband UVB; PUVA, psoralen plus UVA; UVA1, long-wave UVA.

without significantly compromising vascular selectivity.

The PDL is indicated for scars that have superficial blood vessel dilatation (**Fig. 10**). Generally, flat red scars respond better than elevated ones, but PDL treatments can also have the potential of softening indurated thick scars. Although nonpurpuric settings can reduce erythema, more treatments are usually required to achieve the same effect seen with purpuric parameters. PDL treatments may be safely performed on all skin types (with additional caution encouraged in darker-skinned individuals) and over hair-bearing areas without fear of follicular destruction. Dynamic cooling in the form of forced air or cryogen spray may be used to improve tolerability of laser treatment but may reduce efficacy by diminishing photocoagulation of blood vessels.

Table 2
The acne scarring consultation

Step	Activity
1.	Thorough and careful examination of the patient.
2.	Categorize the patient's acne scars according to the Color and Texture Classification shown in **Box 1**.
3.	Identify and prioritize the patient's primary concerns.
4.	Formulate management strategies based on • Options listed **Table 1**, based on Color and Texture Classification • Availability of these treatment modalities • Personal comfort, knowledge and experience of these modalities • Patient concerns It is preferable to have more than one strategy to discuss with the patient.
5.	Discuss • The goals of treatment • Merits and disadvantages of each treatment strategy and its individual components ○ Downtime ○ Financial and time cost ○ Possible side effects ○ Post-treatment care ○ Pain and other symptoms • Expectations (especially extent and timeline of projected skin improvement) • Scheduling and follow-up
6.	Together with the patient, agree on a treatment plan, and develop a therapeutic alliance with them to increase compliance and patience during the treatment course.

With PDL treatment of red acne scars, purpura is advocated as an endpoint. Purpura is the clinical sign of extravasated red blood cells and indicates immediate vascular photocoagulation. Usually in healthy individuals, purpura lasts a maximum of 7 to 10 days and resolves without sequelae. When using PDL, purpura can be achieved by using large spot sizes (7 to 10 mm), short pulse durations (less than 3 ms), and high fluences (greater than 6 J/cm^2) with minimal to no dynamic cooling.

When treating scars that are both elevated and red, PDL is suggested after addressing texture to maximize efficiency and efficacy. Theoretically, however, PDL treatment may also stimulate collagen production around targeted superficial vessels, improving skin contour as well. PDL is safe to use on ethnic skin with minimal postinflammatory hyperpigmentation, even at purpuric settings.

KTP laser The KTP laser, also known as a frequency-doubled Nd:YAG laser, has an output wavelength of 532 nm, which has a high target specificity for the first peak of the oxyhemoglobin absorption curve (see **Fig. 9**). As such, the KTP laser is ideal for erythema where the causative dilated capillaries are superficial.[5] Erythema that is caused by deeper vessels has limited improvement with the KTP laser, the penetrative depth of which is confined to the papillary dermis of the skin. Generally, KTP lasers cause only mild, if any, purpura. Similar to PDL, the KTP laser is safe to use on ethnic skin with minimal postinflammatory hyperpigmentation.

The KTP laser is especially successful for scar erythema with spot sizes of 4 mm to 5 mm, pulse durations of 20 ms to 30 ms, and fluences of 6 J/cm^2 to 9 J/cm^2.

IPL IPL devices are not true lasers. Instead, noncoherent light of multiple wavelengths (approximately 500–1200 nm) is released by a flashlamp within the device, which is then confined to narrower ranges of wavelengths by filters that simulate the monochromatic nature of true laser light. IPL devices have the great benefit of larger spot sizes that allow for larger surface areas to be treated deeper and more quickly. Also, wide range manipulation of pulse duration and fluences is possible with IPL devices. As such, IPL can treat several conditions, sometimes at the same time (eg, erythema and superficial pigmentation of the skin) but is often limited in treating any one condition optimally due to absorption competition from multiple tissue targets and its inherently poor specificity compared with true lasers. Purpura is rare with IPL treatment; however, care must be taken to prevent postinflammatory hyperpigmentation in darker skin types.

IPL treatments are useful in reducing superficial erythema in those who have flat acne scars.[6] Although parameters vary greatly depending on the individual patient, typical settings are 560-nm to 650-nm filters, 2.4 ms to 4.0 ms, single pulsed or double pulsed, and 15 J/cm^2 to 30 J/cm^2, depending on a patient's background skin pigmentation. Multiple treatments may be required to achieve patient satisfaction, typically at 1-month intervals.

Nd:YAG Nd:YAG lasers may be useful in treating deep erythema of scars due to dilated blood vessels within the deep dermis. Purpura is rare

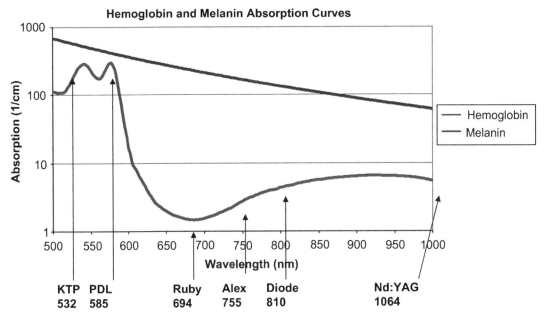

Fig. 9. Hemoglobin and melanin absorption curves with the superimposition of various lasers with their output wavelengths.

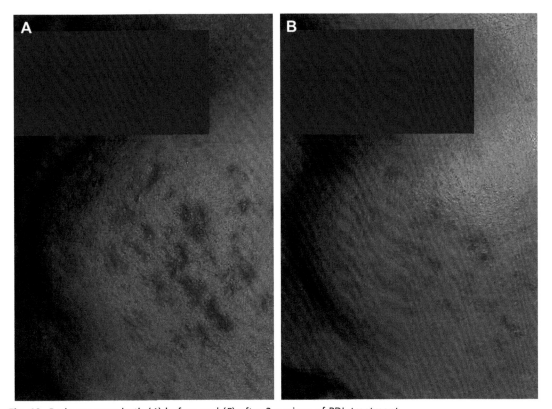

Fig. 10. Red acne scars both (*A*) before and (*B*) after 2 sessions of PDL treatment.

with Nd:YAG laser treatment and, in general, darker skin types may be treated safely. Usually for the erythema of acne scarring, however, Nd:YAG lasers penetrate the skin well-beyond the target depth of these superficial vessels in question.

To achieve success in reducing superficial erythema, new microsecond-pulsed Nd:YAG lasers have shown good results by bulk heating the papillary dermis through small spot size (5 mm), short pulse durations (0.3 ms), low fluence (14 J/cm^2), and quick (5–10 Hz) repeated laser bursts.[7] With these parameters, temperature increases in the superficial dermis not only cause reduction in erythema but also stimulate collagen production without inducing injury to surrounding tissue. This laser may be used for any skin type.

Brown color

Hyperpigmentation of acne scars is common, particularly in individuals of darker skin types. Often this gives the impression that active acne is still present to an observer. Although hyperpigmentation often improves with time, treatment with one or a combination of modalities can expedite clearance.

Laser options to treat the hyperpigmentation of scars include IPL, quality-switched (Q-switched) lasers, microsecond-pulsed Nd:YAG laser, both confluent and fractionated ablative erbium:YAG (Er:YAG) lasers, and yttrium-scandium-gallium-garnet (YSGG) lasers. The nonablative lasers and IPL target that part of the melanin absorption curve where there is minimal competition with hemoglobin absorption. The ablative lasers work by physically removing pigment from the skin either via exfoliation (eg, confluent ablative lasers) or transepidermal elimination (eg, fractionated ablative lasers). With any laser treatment of hyperpigmentation, concomitant use of lightening creams is advocated to increase pigment loss and prevent further pigment gain. Post–laser treatment sun avoidance and sunscreen use (even during cloudy weather) are advocated for several weeks to prevent repigmentation.

IPL IPL devices, with their ability to vary output wavelength, pulse duration, and fluence, can treat several skin conditions, including superficial pigmentation.[8] Special care must be taken to protect the epidermis from overheating, which could cause pigment incontinence and further darkening of the skin. Various forms of concomitant cooling of the skin during laser treatment may achieve this, and it is critical to use cooling to provide safe IPL treatment in patients with brown scars. Parallel cooling in modern IPL systems is usually provided through the use of

a sapphire window handpiece that provides surface cooling to approximately 5°C.

Although parameters vary depending on individual patients, typical settings are 640-nm or higher filters, 4.0 ms to 6.0 ms, single pulsed or double pulsed, and 10 J/cm^2 to 25 J/cm^2, depending on a patient's background skin pigmentation. Multiple treatments may be required to achieve patient satisfaction, typically at 1-month intervals. Because the therapeutic window of treating brown scars with IPL is narrow, IPL devices are not advocated as first-line therapy for this condition.

Q-switched lasers Q-switched lasers have the unique property of extremely short pulse durations in the order of nanoseconds. This feature allows Q-switched lasers to target very small pigment cells and particles, such as melanocytes (pigment cells containing melanin), hemosiderin (endogenous iron oxide) particles, and exogenous tattoo materials, which typically contain metal oxides and carbon. The Q-switched lasers that are useful for treating skin pigmentation, listed in order of decreasing pigment absorption, are the Q-switched ruby laser (694 nm), the Q-switched alexandrite laser (755 nm), and the Q-switched Nd:YAG laser (1064 nm).[9] As such, the Q-switched ruby laser is more effective for low-contrast pigmentation that is more commonly seen with acne scars. All of these lasers operate at wavelengths where there is good absorption by brown pigment and minimal competition with hemoglobin absorption.

When using Q-switched lasers, the only variable parameters are spot size (which generally ranges between 3 and 6 mm) and fluence (which can range between 1 and 6 J/cm^2). The endpoint of treatment is mild but not excessive superficial crusting. For treatment of brown scars, care must be taken to use the lowest energy settings possible to achieve pigment reduction. Test spots are advocated with review after 1 week to determine the effect of the test. Too much energy can easily be delivered to the scar, which may result in punctate bleeding, cell rupture, scarring, and increased pigmentation. Unfortunately, parallel cooling is ineffective with Q-switched lasers because tissue disruption occurs faster than any form of cooling can diminish it.

Nd:YAG laser Microsecond-pulsed Nd:YAG lasers may be useful in treating hyperpigmented flat or depressed scars that are often seen as the sequelae of acne vulgaris and varicella (**Fig. 11**). These lasers use a small spot size (5 mm), very short pulse durations (0.3 ms), low fluence (14 J/cm^2), and quick (5–10 Hz) repeated laser bursts. With these parameters, the 1064-nm wavelength

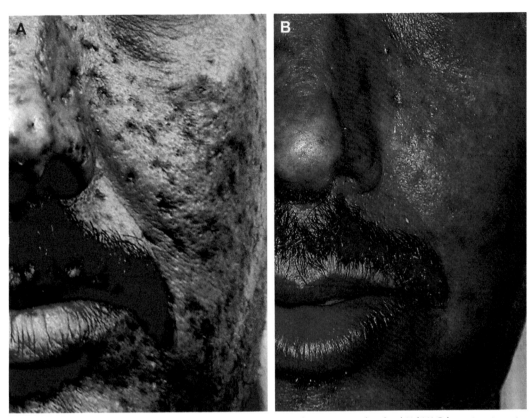

Fig. 11. Brown scars both (*A*) before and (*B*) after 3 sessions of microsecond-pulsed Nd:YAG laser treatment.

targets pigment to a small degree while also targeting small blood vessels to reduce erythema and stimulating collagen production without inducing injury to surrounding tissue. This laser may be used for any skin type.[7]

Confluent ablative Er:YAG and YSGG lasers Confluent laser treatment involves laser light striking the entire surface of the skin in a given area. In contrast, fractionated laser treatment involves treating a fraction of the skin's surface in a given area. Confluent ablative Er:YAG (2940-nm) and YSGG (2790-nm) lasers have the capacity to reduce superficial pigmentation when used in full-contact mode, because they have tremendous water absorption capacity, which translates into almost complete vaporization of surface tissue with minimal collateral heating (**Fig. 12**). Unlike the carbon dioxide laser, which in contrast has tremendous collateral heating capacity, the Er:YAG and YSGG lasers do not cause much damage to surrounding tissue during ablation, which in turn minimizes the risk for further pigmentation.[10] With these two lasers, approximately 30 μm of the skin's epidermis is ablated, inducing substantial exfoliation of the epidermis and, in many cases, improvement of superficial

hyperpigmentation. Test spots should be used whenever using any ablative laser on darker skin types.

Confluent and fractionated ablative Er:YAG and YSGG lasers Fractionated lasers, in contrast to full-surface laser resurfacing, treat only a fraction of the skin's surface, releasing laser light at high peak power to create channels in skin tissue.[11] These channels can be manipulated by laser parameters to vary channel depth, diameter, and spacing to treat several skin conditions. When using ablative fractionated lasers (Er:YAG, YSGG, and carbon dioxide lasers), channels are physically ablated, leaving true air channels representing vaporized tissue as well as an avenue for surrounding pigment to potentially leave via transepidermal elimination. Nonablative fractionated lasers do not leave true air channels, only coagulated, heated tissue through which pigment cannot escape. To treat deep pigmentation, wavelengths that have high absorption by water are preferable to reduce collateral heat damage and possible sequelae that may result. Also, ablative channels with minimally coagulated walls theoretically allow for greater transepidermal elimination of surrounding pigment. For these reasons, the Er:YAG

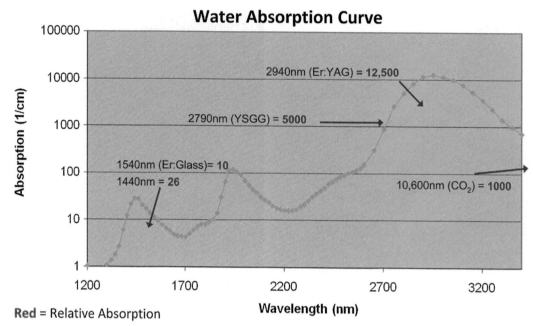

Fig. 12. Water absorption curve with the superimposition of various lasers with their output wavelengths and relative absorption coefficients.

and YSGG fractionated lasers are better for pigment reduction than fractionated carbon dioxide lasers.

White color

Excimer lasers To stimulate pigmentation with the goal of normalizing the color of white scars, ultra-violet (UV) light can be useful.[12] UV light stimulates melanogenesis in areas where melanocytes are intact. In areas where melanocytes are few to none, UV light can stimulate melanocytes to migrate to these deficient areas, increasing pigment at the site. Excimer, or excited dimer, lasers have a wavelength in the UV range (308 nm), providing concentrated melanin stimulation to white scars. If there is no improvement after 5 to 10 sessions of excimer laser therapy, treatment should be deemed unsuccessful and other modalities should be considered.

Fractionated ablative lasers Fractionated ablative lasers of all kinds (Er:YAG, YSGG, and carbon dioxide) have the capacity to improve the appearance of white scars, creating air channels that ultimately contract to possibly reduce the surface area of the white scars to make them appear smaller in diameter.[11] Although there is a limit as to how much contraction occurs after fractionated treatment, repeated sessions with any of these lasers can improve the surface area of white discoloration and, therefore, the scar's contrast with normal surrounding skin.

Normalization of Scar Texture

Elevated (hypertrophic and keloid) scars

In general, when evaluating a scar that has both color (either red or brown) and elevation (hypertrophic or keloid), it is suggested to treat the texture before treating the color, because both vascular-targeting and pigment-targeting lasers penetrate best through scars that are flat and soft. This suggestion does not apply to scars with both color and depression, where order of treatment does not seem to affect outcome efficiency as greatly. In almost all cases, the author uses concomitant topical and intralesional corticosteroids, in addition to other modalities, to improve efforts to soften and flatten elevated scars.

Fractionated ablative laser treatment Fractionated ablative lasers of all kinds can be helpful in softening both hypertrophic and keloid scars by ablating channels of condensed collagen that contribute to the thickness and firmness of these types of scars.[11] Fractionated carbon dioxide lasers, and to a greater degree fractionated nonablative lasers, must be used with caution in softening elevated scars because collateral thermal damage caused by these lasers has the profibrotic potential to cause scars to become thicker and firmer.

The author has found that fractionated ablative laser treatment of elevated scars may be used to improve topical drug delivery via increased transepidermal penetration. For example, concomitant fractional laser resurfacing has been shown to improve the effects of topical corticosteroid home application to flatten and soften both keloid and hypertrophic scars (**Fig. 13**).

Confluent ablative laser treatment (with surgical excision) Surgical excision of both hypertrophic and keloid scars is challenging due to the propensity of these scars to recur, often larger and thicker than the initial scar. Confluent ablative laser treatment (Er:YAG, YSGG, and carbon dioxide) has been shown to decrease the size and thickness of scar recurrence postsurgery if laser treatment is performed at the base of the excised area immediately after surgical removal.[13] The author suggests repeated confluent ablative laser pulses to the base of the excised tissue to provide both hemostasis and a thin surface layer of eschar. Post-treatment wound care consists of 3 days of viscous topical moisturizer (eg, petrolatum) beneath an occlusive dressing, followed by nonviscous moisturizer until re-epithelialization has occurred. At the first sign of recurrent scar formation, topical corticosteroid preparations or topical imiquimod is suggested to prevent progression of fibrosis to control the new scar's thickness and firmness. This form of laser-assisted scar revision is particularly useful with keloid scars rather than hypertrophic scars, because the former often has a stalk or base that is of smaller diameter than the scar itself, making it easier to surgically remove and cauterize by laser.

Depressed (icepick and boxcar) scars
Confluent ablative laser treatment Resurfacing of depressed facial scars with Er:YAG, YSGG, and carbon dioxide laser vaporization has become popular in recent years.[14] Through selective ablation of water-containing tissue, the 3 laser systems offer predictable and reproducible ablation of tissue, yielding better control compared with traditional dermabrasion. During laser resurfacing, the epidermis and a variable portion of the dermis are thermally injured, resulting in vaporization and collagen injury, followed by re-epithelialization.

Pulsed Er:YAG lasers are approximately 12 times more selective for water than carbon dioxide lasers and twice as selective for water than their YSGG counterpart. Consequently, Er:YAG lasers result in maximal tissue vaporization and reduced residual thermal damage. This makes the Er:YAG safer for darker skin types and decreases post-treatment erythema, all with precise tissue depth of injury. The restricted photothermal effect on collateral tissue results in relatively decreased collagen stimulation and subsequently limited skin tightening, dermal thickening, and depressed scar improvement compared with that observed with YSGG and, more so, carbon dioxide laser treatment. With the use of the carbon dioxide laser, in particular, the production of increased dermal fibrotic elements is enhanced as a result of controlled collagen heating.

Overall, the Er:YAG laser is effective in resurfacing skin with shallow depressed scars, yielding similar results to that of the YSGG and carbon dioxide lasers. For these superficial scars, the Er:YAG laser may be the preferred method of treatment, offering comparable clinical effects with shorter recovery times. Deeper icepick and boxcar scars may be better treated with the YSGG or carbon dioxide lasers, which have greater collateral thermal heating capacity (**Fig. 14**). Many modern Er:YAG lasers, however, have the ability to produce longer pulse durations to create more collateral heating and simulate the effect of a YSGG and carbon dioxide laser.

Regardless of the confluent ablative laser system used, the goals in treating icepick and

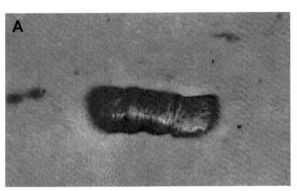 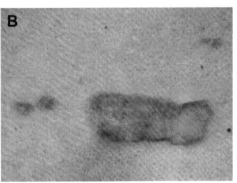

Fig. 13. Hypertrophic scar treated with a combination of fractionated ablative laser treatment and a potent topical corticosteroid preparation.

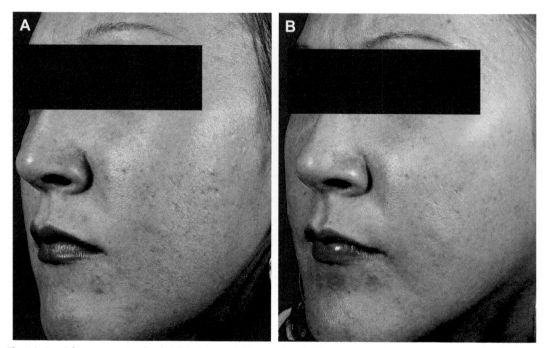

Fig. 14. Icepick acne scarring both (*A*) before and (*B*) 4 weeks after being treated with a one confluent YSGG laser treatment.

boxcar scars are (1) to soften the transition between the indentation and the normal skin surrounding it and (2) to stimulate collagen production within the depressed area. The entire cosmetic unit must be treated to minimize textural or color mismatch. If treating an isolated scar, the author advocates spot resurfacing and the use of a scanning hand piece, also known as a computer pattern generator when treating large areas, such as cheeks, forehead, and chin. Once ablation is achieved (typically requiring 1 pass with the carbon dioxide laser at 300 mJ, 1 to 2 passes with the YSGG laser at 3.5 J/cm^2, and 2 to 3 passes with the Er:YAG laser at 5 J/cm^2), the scar edges, or shoulders, can be further softened with additional vaporizing laser passes.

Historically with deep carbon dioxide laser resurfacing, it was recommended that skin eschar be wiped between laser passes. Today, however, pos–tlaser eschar wiping is not necessary because the depth of treatment is usually superficial and controlled, and the eschar itself can serve as a natural dressing, the wiping off of which can create excessive tissue damage. With Er:YAG and YSGG lasers, however, there is not much eschar to be wiped off, because these lasers have higher ablation potential. Deep treatment with the Er:YAG laser typically results in bleeding due to the poor ability of the Er:YAG laser to photocoagulate blood vessels.

Confluent nonablative laser treatment Warming of the dermis by nonablative laser treatment can provide mild-to-moderate improvement of all forms of depressed acne scarring by stimulating collagen production and remodeling. This modality of contour improvement where there is no vaporization of skin tissue is also called subsurfacing. Several different devices have been shown to have subsurfacing potential, including PDL, IPL, microsecond-pulsed and Q-switched Nd:YAG lasers, and a variety of lasers operating in the near infrared spectrum (eg, 1320 nm, 1440 nm, 1450 nm, 1540 nm, and 1550 nm). These infrared lasers target water within the deeper aspects of the dermis more efficiently, creating bulk heating and possibly more collagen stimulation.[15]

Although all of these devices have demonstrated improvement in depressed acne scarring, subsurfacing may take several months and multiple treatment sessions to appreciate the full benefits, given that collagen remodeling is a dynamic, slow process. Also, confluent subsurfacing can be painful, often requiring systemic analgesia. Consequently, ablative laser resurfacing is generally a more popular option for depressed scar improvement.

Fractionated ablative laser treatment Fractional resurfacing, both ablative and nonablative, can be effective in the treatment of depressed acne scarring of all kinds.[16,17] Fractionated ablative laser treatment is a minimally invasive procedure that creates microscopic zones or channels of thermal injury in a grid-like pattern on the skin (**Fig. 15**). Because only a small proportion of the skin surface is treated at one time, downtime is minimal and recovery is quick. A series of treatments, however, is usually required to demonstrate appreciable results compared with confluent ablative laser treatment. Ablative fractional resurfacing is gentler on the skin compared with confluent resurfacing and can thus be safer for darker skin types. The author suggests test spots on cosmetically insensitive areas before attempting any form of laser resurfacing on dark skin.

For icepick, boxcar, and rolled scars, fractional ablative resurfacing can successfully and predictably restore skin contour by causing skin tightening and smoothening via ablation and re-epithelialization (which occurs within 1 to 2 weeks) and elevation of the floor of depressed scars via collagen remodeling (which takes weeks to occur). Patients may prefer this treatment to nonablative confluent or fractional resurfacing, both of which operate on the principal of collagen remodeling alone and may take excessive time for results to be realized. Fractionated ablative laser treatment requires similar wound care to confluent ablative laser treatment, but the healing times may be significantly quicker.

The author prefers fractionated Er:YAG laser treatment for small diameter icepick and boxcar scars and for larger diameter scars in darker skin types. Because this laser has maximum water absorption and minimal collateral thermal injury,

treatments sessions often result in pinpoint bleeding due to poor blood vessel coagulation. Minor tissue bleeding is usually not problematic and typically self-coagulates within minutes.

Both fractionated YSGG and fractionated carbon dioxide lasers are the author's choice for icepick and boxcar scarring in white individuals. Both have excellent coagulation potential and sufficient nonspecific collateral thermal injury to stimulate adequate collagen remodeling and subsequently visible effects in a matter of weeks. Compared with the fractionated carbon dioxide laser, fractionated YSGG has slightly less downtime at the expense of less collagen remodeling over time. Fractionated carbon dioxide lasers also have greater parameter manipulation capability, which may be useful for advanced operators but can be intimidating for the novice user. Choice between these two ablative lasers depend on patient preference after consultation regarding downtime and time to achieve end results.

Fractionated nonablative laser treatment Unlike fractionated ablative laser treatment, nonablative fractional resurfacing does not create ablative air channels, rather only zones of microthermal skin injury. This is attractive to individuals who desire minimal to no downtime and who have the patience to experience the end result. Multiple treatment sessions are required, and these may be painful to the point of requiring oral analgesia. Fractional resurfacing sessions, however, are much more tolerable than confluent nonablative subsurfacing, because the latter represents far more heat being administered to nerve fiber-laden dermal tissue.[16]

Nonablative fractional resurfacing lasers currently in the market produce wavelengths in the midinfrared range and includes the fractionated 1440-nm, 1450-nm, 1540-nm, and 1550-nm lasers. These differ slightly in their depth of penetration due to their individual absorptive coefficients for tissue water as well as various individual ergonomic and electronic features.

Depressed (rolled) scars
With rolled acne scarring, treatment success depends on the degree to which the skin is bound down at the base of the scar. If the skin contour is tightly tethered, surgical subcision can be used before all other treatments to loosen the surface adhesion and dampen the tethering effect.[18] This preliminary and often repeated procedure ensures that other treatments, such as soft tissue filler placement and laser treatment, are more effective. Care should be taken not to perform fractionated ablative or nonablative laser treatment over the

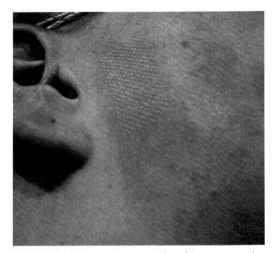

Fig. 15. Grid-like pattern on the skin representing microscopic channels as the result of fractionated ablative laser treatment.

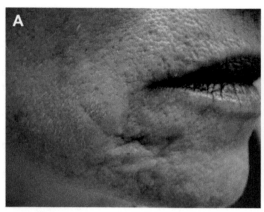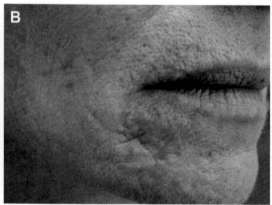

Fig. 16. Rolled acne scars both (*A*) before and (*B*) 4 weeks after 6 sessions with microsecond-pulsed Nd:YAG laser treatment.

site of recent filler treatment to avoid disruption of filler placement. The author usually waits at least 2 weeks post–filler placement before attempting any form of laser resurfacing over the site of a rolled scar.

Laser options for rolled scars include both confluent and fractionated nonablative laser treatment and fractionated ablative laser treatment. In all cases, it is important for laser energy to reach deeper components of the skin to stimulate collagen remodeling and possibly to weaken tethering adhesions (**Fig. 16**).

SUMMARY

Acne scarring is a complex and challenging problem with a variety of possible treatment modalities. By understanding the biologic and structural nature of acne and acne scarring, a simple yet practical classification schema has been presented. This conceptual framework can serve as the basis for organizing the many treatment options and assist in formulating a safe and effective management strategy for treating acne scarring.

Patients are blessed to be living in an era of comprehensive techniques and technology with capabilities of doing more than ever before. Although this article focuses on laser options, depending on specific patient factors, scar characteristics, and patient preferences, a combination of several treatment modalities may be appropriate. A thorough understanding of each treatment option is required to ensure patient safety, maintain predictable results, and construct the best possible individualized management strategy. Confidence and experience in assessing patients and formulating treatment plans greatly assist in developing therapeutic alliances with them. This is necessary to ensure compliance

and patience during the often long, and occasionally frustrating, treatment course of acne scarring.

It is important to explain treatment rationale and expectations to patients, particularly as they pertain to downtime and time course of results. In general, treatment of acne scarring is a multistep procedure. Caregivers must emphasize that the goal of treating acne scarring is improvement (ie, reduction in scar contrast to surrounding normal skin) and never entire reversal. If patients do not understand these concepts, the decision to embark on the treatment process should be reconsidered. If patients fully understand the goals, expectations, and principles outlined in this article, however, they gain an opportunity to reduce the physical and psychological effects of this condition as never before and substantially improve their quality of life. This can be tremendously rewarding for both patients and caregivers.

REFERENCES

1. Leyden JJ. A review of the use of combination therapies for the treatment of acne vulgaris. J Am Acad Dermatol 2003;49(Suppl 3):S200–10.
2. Rivera AE. Acne scarring: a review and current treatment modalities. J Am Acad Dermatol 2008;59(4):659–76.
3. Jacob CI, Dover JS, Kaminer MS. Acne scarring: a classification system and review of treatment options. J Am Acad Dermatol 2001;45(1):109–17.
4. Alster TS, McMeekin TO. Improvement of facial acne scars by the 585 nm flashlamp-pumped pulsed-dye laser. J Am Acad Dermatol 1996;35(1):79–81.
5. Baugh WP, Kucaba WD. Nonablative phototherapy for acne vulgaris using the KTP 532 nm laser. Dermatol Surg 2005;31(10):1290–6.
6. Choi YS, Suh HS, Yoon MY, et al. Intense pulsed light vsrsus pulsed-dye laser in the treatment of facial

acne: a randomized split-face trial. J Eur Acad Dermatol Venereol 2010;24(7):773–80.

7. Min SU, Choi YS, Lee DH, et al. Comparison of a long-pulse Nd:YAG laser and a combined 585/1,064-nm laser for the treatment of acne scars: a randomized split-face clinical study. Dermatol Surg 2009;35(11):1720–7.

8. Ho SG, Chan HH. The Asian dermatologic patient: review of common pigmentary disorders and cutaneous diseases. Am J Clin Dermatol 2009; 10(3):153–68.

9. Kim S, Cho KH. Treatment of facial postinflammatory hyperpigmentation with facial acne in Asian patients using a Q-switched neodymium-doped yttrium aluminum garnet laser. Dermatol Surg 2010; 36:1374–80.

10. Ross EV, Swann M, Soon S, et al. Full-face treatments with the 2790-nm erbium: YSGG laser system. J Drugs Dermatol 2009;8(3):248–52.

11. Tierney EP, Hanke CW. Review of the literature: treatment of dyspigmentation with fractionated resurfacing. Dermatol Surg 2010;36(10):1499–508.

12. Grema H, Raulin C. The excimer laser in dermatology and esthetic medicine. Hautarzt 2004;55(1): 48–57 [in German].

13. Morosolli AR, De Oliveira Moura Cardoso G, Murilo-Santos L, et al. Surgical treatment of earlobe keloid with CO2 laser radiation: case report and clinical standpoints. J Cosmet Laser Ther 2008; 10(4):226–30.

14. Batra RS, Jacob CI, Hobbs L, et al. A prospective survey of patient experiences after laser skin surfacing: results from 2½ years of follow-up. Arch Dermatol 2003;139(10):1295–9.

15. Bhatia AC, Dover JS, Arndt KA, et al. Patient satisfaction and reported long-term therapeutic efficacy associated with 1,320 nm Nd:YAG laser treatment of acne scarring and photoaging. Dermatol Surg 2006;32(3):346–52.

16. Geronemus RG. Fractional photothermolysis: current and future applications. Lasers Surg Med 2006;38(3):169–76.

17. Hedelund L, Moreau KE, Beyer DM, et al. Fractional nonablative 1,540-nm laser resurfacing of atrophic acne scars. A randomized controlled trial with blinded response evaluation. Lasers Med Sci 2010;25(5):749–54.

18. Alam M, Omura N, Kaminer MS. Subcision for acne scarring: technique and outcomes in 40 patients. Dermatol Surg 2005;31(3):310–7.

Laser Treatment of Skin Texture and Fine Line Etching

Lisa Danielle Grunebaum, MD[a],*, Jennifer Murdock, BS[b],
Gia E. Hoosien, MD[c], Ryan N. Heffelfinger, MD[d],
Wendy W. Lee, MD[e]

KEYWORDS

- Aging face • Skin texture • Facial lines • Rhytids

CAUSES OF CHANGES IN SKIN TEXTURE AND FINE LINES

Modern cosmetic medicine demands accurate recognition of all types of rhytids and their molecular causes to tailor treatment for improving aging skin appearance. This article examines the causes and treatment of fine rhytids. The underlying cause of fine lines, also known as *atrophic rhytids*, is dermal thinning. Myriad molecular mechanisms have been identified in the loss of dermal strength and architecture. Dermal thinning is caused by a loss of collagen and elastin in the dermis. After reviewing the histopathology of the role of dermal atrophy in the creation of fine rhytids, practitioners can better understand the prevention and treatment of fine lines. Although fine "crinkles" and lines appear superficial, the epidermis does not significantly contribute to wrinkle formation. In reality, the fine atrophic rhytids of the face are caused by molecular changes deeper in the underlying dermis. Therefore, laser rejuvenation therapies that penetrate the dermis and induce neocollagenesis and dermal remodeling are effective against the stigmata of mature skin.

As the skin ages, changes in the color, texture, and quality of the skin become apparent. Aged skin develops four different types of wrinkles: atrophic rhytids (fine lines), solar elastosis (permanent lines), dynamic expression lines, and gravitational folds. The skin becomes dry (asteatosis), yellow, rough, and leathery, with increased laxity and decreased turgor. Periorbital comedones often develop. A generalized decrease in the skin adnexal occurs, including sebaceous glands, sweat glands, and hair follicles. Changes in pigmentation may also occur, including irregular hyperpigmentation, such as sun spots or liver spots. Hypopigmentation may develop in the form of white macules called *pseudoscars* from excessive sun exposure. Vascular changes in the skin associated with aging include actinic purpura secondary to weak, leaky capillary beds in the dermis, and telangiectasias.[1]

The causes of cutaneous aging can be divided into intrinsic and extrinsic causes. The intrinsic causes are simply the passage of time and genetic programming that leads to thinning of the dermis from decreased collagen and elastic dermal support systems.[2] Normal skin aging is first noted as early as the third decade of life, with the first signs of skin fragility seen as fine shallow lines of epidermis draped over the thinning dermis.[3] These fine lines, or atrophic rhytids, are often the first

[a] Facial Plastic and Reconstructive Surgery and Dermatology, University of Miami Miller School of Medicine, 1450 NW 10th Avenue Suite 2044, Miami, FL 33136, USA
[b] University of Miami Miller School of Medicine, Miami, FL, USA
[c] Department of Otolaryngology/Head and Neck Surgery, University of Miami Miller School of Medicine, 1450 NW 10th Avenue Suite 2044, Miami, FL 33136, USA
[d] Director, Division of Facial Plastic and Reconstructive Surgery, Thomas Jefferson University Hospital, 925 Chestnut Street, 6th Floor, Philadelphia, PA 19107, USA
[e] Ophthalmic Plastic Surgery, Orbit and Oncology Bascom Palmer Eye Institute, University of Miami Miller School of Medicine, 900 NW 17th Street, Miami, FL 33136, USA
* Corresponding author.
E-mail address: lgrunebaum@med.miami.edu

Facial Plast Surg Clin N Am 19 (2011) 293–301
doi:10.1016/j.fsc.2011.05.006
1064-7406/11/$ – see front matter © 2011 Elsevier Inc. All rights reserved.

type of skin wrinkle to develop, and are a harbinger of further signs of aging skin.

Extrinsic causes of aging skin are multifactorial, and include the sequelae of environmental, behavioral, and general medical assaults on the skin. The worst offender is photoaging, also called *dermatoheliosis*. Signs of sun-induced skin damage may be visible as early as 15 years of age in cases of heavy childhood sun exposure. Photoaging, which certainly accelerates the normal aging process of dermal thinning and atrophic rhytid formation, is not analogous to normal aging.[3] Photoaging also leads to a host of additional molecular and histopathologic changes in the skin architecture. For example, photoaging leads to epidermal thickening, causing a rough, dry, leathery texture. The hallmark of dermatoheliosis is elastosis, a process of haphazard hypertrophy of elastic fibers that leads to heaped-up wrinkles with deep, crisscrossing, permanent furrows. Most mature skin pigment alterations, such as hyperpigmented macules and telangiectasias, are from photoaging.[1]

HISTOPATHOLOGY OF FINE LINES

Histologically, skin is a complex layered organ. The outermost layer is the epidermis, supported by the underlying dermis, which sits on subcutaneous fat that makes up the hypodermis. The epidermis is further divided into five layers, from superficial to deep: the stratum corneum, stratum lucidum, stratum granulosum, stratum spinosum, and stratum basale. The dermis has two main components. First are the papillary ridges that reach up to provide a sort of scaffolding under the epidermis. Deep to the papillary ridges lies the reticular dermis, an elastic bed supporting the skin.

The texture of the skin is largely because of the microrelief of fine furrows caused by the ridges of papillary dermis and the edges of corneocytes of the stratum corneum. Quatresooz and colleagues[2] studied the microrelief of youthful skin and aged skin. Although young skin is commonly regarded as smooth, it is perhaps more accurately described as velvety. Young skin is, in fact, not really smooth at all. Instead, the microrelief is a fine velvety polygonal crisscross of very fine furrows each measuring approximately 200 μm in depth. As the dermis atrophies with age and environmental insults, the papillary ridges become less polygonal and more parallel. The resulting appearance is that of atrophic rhytids, which are fine lines that smooth out easily when stretched but have poor elasticity to return to a taut position. These atrophic rhytids have the appearance of crumpled tissue paper or crepe paper, and are a pesky contributor to facial aging.

In summary, the causes of fine lines are

- Intrinsic (genetic) and extrinsic (environmental) dermal thinning
- Loss of oxytalan elastic fibers in the dermoepithelial junction and papillary dermis[4]
- Atrophy of the collagen VII bundles in the reticular dermis and hypodermis[2]
- Decrease in glucosaminoglycans surrounding dermal collagen bundles[2]
- Ultraviolet radiation–induced increase in cellular expression of matrix metalloproteinases that degrade dermal collagen, elastin, and the surrounding matrix at an accelerated rate.

Solar elastosis often occurs in conjunction with atrophic rhytids, because photoaging leads to both types of wrinkles. Other wrinkle types include dynamic expression lines, which are most successfully treated with botulinum toxin injection, and gravitational rhytids, which are best treated with surgical lifting.

IN-OFFICE EVALUATION OF FINE LINE– AND SKIN TEXTURE–RELATED COMPLAINTS

The in-office evaluation of patients seeking improvement of facial aesthetics should begin with a complete history and physical. This evaluation should include a detailed cosmetic history, including past cosmetic procedures, such as laser treatment, dermabrasion, chemical peels, botulinum toxin, and filler injections, and past facial plastic surgeries. Patient response and any unforeseen or undesirable outcomes should be noted. Any past medical problems that could impede wound healing, such as immunosuppression, cancer, smoking, or diabetes, must be noted and discussed with the patient as risk factors for a potentially suboptimal outcome. The (**Box 1**) indicates specialized elements of the medical history for patients considering laser treatment.

The patient encounter should then focus on the skin and cosmetic concerns. A general dermatologic examination begins with visual inspection in natural light, or artificial light that mimics natural light, to prevent color distortion. The color, moisture, temperature, mobility, and turgor of the skin must be evaluated. The hair and nails should be inspected, and any cutaneous lesions carefully noted.[1] Many factors contribute to skin color, such as melanin (genetic and environmental secondary to sun exposure), carotene (most visible on the palms and soles), oxyhemoglobin (arterial capillary beds), deoxyhemoglobin (venous

Box 1
Specialized elements of the medical history for patients considering laser treatment

- Past medical history for cosmetic patients

  ○ Diabetes
  ○ Hypothyroidism
  ○ Autoimmune disease
  ○ Immunosuppression (HIV/AIDS, corticosteroids, cancer, transplant)
  ○ Cancer, chemotherapy, radiation
  ○ Tendency to bleed/bruise
  ○ Complete cardiac, respiratory, gastrointestinal, renal, liver, musculoskeletal, neurologic history
  ○ Depression, mental health

- Past surgical history

  ○ Past surgeries, including cosmetic or other
  ○ Anesthetic history, including local and general
  ○ Gastroesophageal reflux disease

- Dermatologic history

  ○ Scar history
  ○ Previous skin cancers
  ○ Skin type

- Social history

  ○ Smoking
  ○ Alcohol
  ○ Drugs
  ○ Occupation
  ○ Hobbies and sun exposure

capillary beds), and the light scatter through the skin itself and opaque vessel walls.[1] Hyperpigmentation, hypopigmentation, scars, and telangiectasias should be recorded. The skin texture and moisture should be evaluated. The skin should be lifted gently to assess skin turgor, distensibility, and laxity. Fine lines tend to have a "crepe paper" appearance, disappear easily when the skin is stretched, and return to their crinkled appearance when released.

During the physical examination, a high index of suspicion should be maintained for potentially malignant lesions, such as malignant melanoma (caused by genetic predisposition and early childhood sunburns) and the common skin cancers of chronically sun-exposed areas, such as basal cell carcinoma (pearly, raised edges) and squamous cell carcinoma (erythematous, often pruritic patches).[1]

As part of the visit documentation, standardized digital photodocumentation of before and after assessments is recommended to track progress of treatments. Using consistent camera equipment, lighting, and background helps minimize variability of photos and increases the fidelity of the images.

Possibly the most important part of the in-office evaluation is the skin-type analysis. The time it takes to perform an in-depth dermatologic history will likely help the physician predict cosmetic outcomes and tailor treatments to each individual patient's skin. The Fitzpatrick scale remains the gold standard and classifies patients into six skin types based on the skin's reaction in the sun. Lasers are ideal for patients who have Fitzpatrick skin types I through III, although consideration for safe laser practices has been described for darker skin types.[5]

The cosmetic skin evaluation can be expanded to document wrinkles in a standardized fashion, such as using the Glogau Photoaging Classification (**Table 1**). This scale describes degrees of wrinkling and photoaging.

Topical treatments, such as retinoids, antioxidants, and sunscreen, are easy and low-risk interventions that certainly help reduce and prevent rhytids. However, given the aforementioned pathophysiology of skin aging and rhytid formation, laser therapy is an obvious choice for fine wrinkle reduction because of the ability of the laser to access the dermal layer of the skin and initiate rejuvenating changes at the dermal cellular layer. The authors advise all patients to begin a regimen of applying sun protection factor (SPF) 55 or greater sun screen to the treatment area for 2 weeks before treatment. The use of a retinoid may aid healing when used up to 5 to 7 days before treatment.[6] Patients at increased risk of hyperpigmentation, such as those of darker skin types or with a history of hyperpigmentation, may benefit from daily pretreatment with 4% hydroquinone.

Introduced in 1968, the fully ablative carbon dioxide (CO_2) laser was developed and became the original gold standard for improving photoaging. The CO_2 laser emits monochromatic light within the far-infrared wavelength range of 10,600 nm, which is highly absorbed by water and results in selective photothermolysis with rapid ablation of the epidermis and part of the dermis. As these skin layers reepithelialize, the treated areas heal with noticeable improvement in tone and texture. The erbium-doped yttrium aluminum garnet (Er:YAG) laser, with a wavelength of 2940 nm, was later introduced as another fully ablative option. The Er:YAG laser is similar to modern CO_2 lasers in that it is ablative with minimal heat dissipation.[7] However, because the Er:YAG emits light at a wavelength of 2940 nm, which is absorbed by water 10 times more than

Table 1
Glogau wrinkle scale

Type 1	No wrinkles	Mild photoaging	Mild pigmentary changes, no keratoses, minimal wrinkles Patient age: 20s or 30s Minimal or no makeup
Type 2	Wrinkles with motion	Moderate photoaging	Early senile lentigines visible, keratoses palpable but not visible, parallel smile lines beginning to appear Patient age: late 30s or 40s Usually wears some foundation
Type 3	Wrinkles at rest	Advanced photoaging	Advanced obvious dyschromia and telangiectasias, visible keratoses, wrinkles at rest Patient age: 50s or older Always wears heavy foundation
Type 4	Only wrinkles	Severe photoaging	Yellow-gray color of skin, prior skin malignancies, wrinkled throughout, no normal skin Patient age: 60s or 70s Do not wear makeup, "cakes and cracks"

Data from Glogau RG. Chemical peeling and aging skin. J Geriatr Dermatol 1994;2:5–10.

the CO_2 lasers, vaporization of the tissue occurs so rapidly that it limits the depth of ablation to only a superficial layer.[8] The efficacy of skin rejuvenation after fully ablative laser treatment perhaps remains unmatched, yet this aggressive treatment requires significant trade-off in long social downtime and the potential for difficult-to-treat and permanent complications, including dyspigmentation, infection, scarring, and prolonged erythema.[9]

The most recent laser literature supports the use of fractional photothermolysis as an alternate to traditional fully ablative technology, with a potentially improved efficacy-to-risk ratio for treatment of skin texture and rhytids. Traditional ablative lasers have been modified into fractional devices that minimize the risk of side effects by using fractional photothermolysis, which confines thermal injury to a precise pattern of narrow columns of dermis and epidermis—microthermal zones (MTZs). Because only a fraction of the skin has been thermally ablated, the intact surrounding tissue is able to enhance rapid reepithelialization and neocollagenesis.[10] Fractional devices are now available in a multitude of wavelengths.

The landmark prototype fractional device introduced by Manstein and colleagues[11] in 2004 was a 1550-nm erbium-doped fiber laser that showed histologic and clinical improvement in periorbital rhytids. This device is now commercially available (Fraxel re:store, Solta Medical, Inc Hayward, CA, USA) and delivers the best-studied nonablative wavelength for treating rhytids and texture. The depth of penetration of the MTZs can be modified and individualized to each patient and area, but this laser does not damage the epidermal barrier function; hence its characterization as a nonablative treatment.[12]

The histologic changes in the underlying skin that follow nonablative laser treatment and lead to rejuvenation have been described in forearm biopsy samples after treatment with 1550 nm at baseline and at defined times after treatment. Different energy levels were examined. An acute inflammatory response similar to wound healing is indicated by an increase in proinflammatory cytokines and several metalloproteinases. Heat shock protein 70 is also transiently expressed. Ultimately, the expected neocollagenesis and dermal remodeling are indicated by increased procollagen throughout the dermis. In this study, however, no difference in molecular changes was noted between low- and high-energy treatments.[13] Although 1550 nm may not be the optimal treatment for deep wrinkles, it is certainly proven to treat fine rhytids and skin texture with little or no downtime.[12] The 1550-nm nonablative wavelength has also improved upper lip rhytids,[14] hand skin wrinkling,[15] and general improvement in rhytids.[16] Only a fraction of the skin is treated during a single procedure, and therefore multiple passes are used during each treatment, and multiple treatments are usually necessary to achieve optimal results. The 1550-nm commercial device (Fraxel re:store) is now available in a dual-wavelength design using 1927 nm for added improvement in superficial pigmentation.[17] Further studies are needed to elucidate whether this additional wavelength might improve results in rhytids and texture in a synergistic manner. The authors find that results are usually apparent within 3 months of the first treatment (**Fig. 1**).

The authors note that the microsecond Q-switched 1064-nm nonablative treatment (Laser Genesis, Cutera, Brisbane, CA, USA) may be useful for mild rhytids if multiple treatments are used; however, further large-scale studies are needed.[18]

Nonablative lasers have a highly regarded safety record and few complications. As with any treatment, risks do exist but are generally minimal. Erythema after the procedure is expected but should subside within a few days. Darker-skinned patients or those with a history of pigment abnormalities should be treated cautiously, because they have a higher risk of dyspigmentation.[10] Although they have potentially lower risk and shorter downtime, the efficacy of nonablative lasers for treating rhytids and texture may not compare with the improvement seen with ablative lasers (**Fig. 2**).[9,15,19]

In 2007, Hantash and colleagues[20] introduced an ablative CO_2 fractional resurfacing device using multiple MTZs of customizable density and depth

that extend through the stratum corneum, epidermis, and dermis. Additionally, they showed immunohistochemistry with in vivo forearm skin, discovering that persistent collagen remodeling occurred for at least 3 months after treatment. Because the fractionated CO_2 elicits a greater degree of injury than traditional models, it has a potential for a greater and prolonged effect on new and remodeling dermal collagen.

Similar to other laser modalities, histologic and ultrastructural evidence suggest a wound repair mechanism for fractional laser healing along with increased deposition of new collagen.[21] Treatment with fractional CO_2 also induces mucin production in the papillary and superficial reticular dermis and an increased undulating rete (papillary) ridge pattern, which is normally decreased or absent in aging skin.[11,21] Reilly and colleagues[22] proposed similar molecular mechanisms of action for both fractional and fully ablative CO_2 laser resurfacing, showing statistically significant changes in the gene elucidated in fully ablative CO_2.

Further studies have shown that ablative fractional photothermolysis (AFP) using the CO_2 laser resulted in increased skin thickness and decreased subepidermal low-echogenic band (SLEB) thickness. The SLEB is the portion of the papillary dermis filled with solar elastosis. Tierney

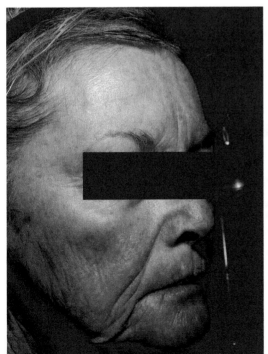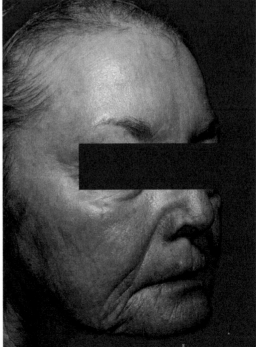

Fig. 1. Pre- and post treatment photos after non-ablative fractional resurfacing for rhytids with 1550 nm. (*Courtesy of* Joely Kaufman, MD, Miami, FL.)

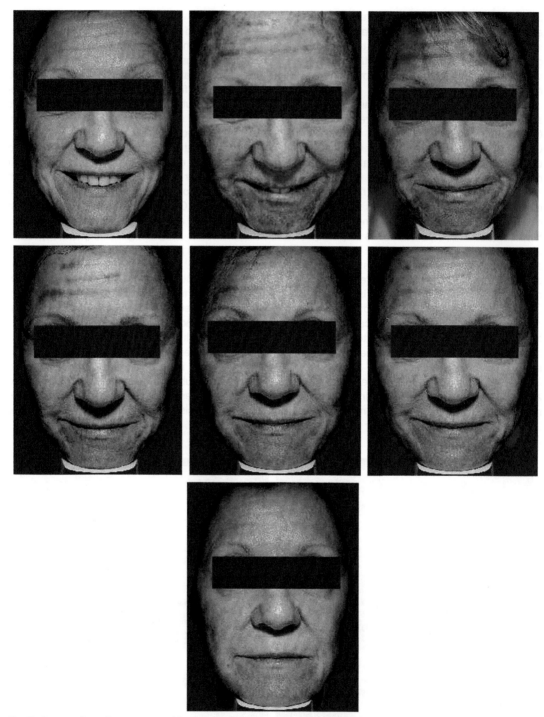

Fig. 2. Progression of treatment with CO_2 ablative fractional resurfacing from pre-treatment to 3 months post-treatment.

and colleagues[23] reported on a pilot study using CO_2 AFP that showed pigmentary and textural improvements in photoaged skin. Specifically, they saw mean score improvements in dyschromias, skin laxity, and rhytids of 61%, 54%, and 52%, respectively. The mean improvement in overall cosmetic outcome was 60%. Results were tallied using prelaser and postlaser photographs analyzed by a blinded physician. Others have confirmed that CO_2 ablative fractional resurfacing treatments are safe and very effective for periorbital and perioral rhytidosis. Kotlus[24] analyzed 6-month postlaser photographs and reported a 53% improvement in eyelid skin rhytidosis and a 42% improvement in eyelid skin redundancy. Patients underwent a dual-depth (one superficial pass and one deep pass) treatment (**Fig. 3**).

Although early split-face Er:YAG versus CO_2 fully ablative treatment comparisons indicate a slight trend in improved wrinkle reduction in the CO_2 treatments,[25] few comparison studies are available with fractional resurfacing. Weiss and colleagues[26] published a split-face trial, with one half treated with AFP (with CO_2) and the contralateral half treated with AFP (erbium). Results showed significantly better improvement in periocular rhytids in the AFP group.

Another ablative resurfacing laser available in both fractional and fully ablative delivery formats, the erbium:yttrium-scandium-gallium-garnet laser (Er:YSGG; Pearl, Cutera, Brisbane, CA, USA), produces a wavelength of 2790 nm that absorbs water less than an Er:YAG but more than a traditional CO_2 laser. A wavelength of 2790 nm has been shown to cause rapid vaporization but with deeper penetration than the 2940-nm Er:YAG laser. A pilot study of eight patients undergoing two treatments each with the Er:YSGG laser showed general safety and efficacy in wrinkle reduction, pigmentation, and tone and texture.[27] Lee and colleagues[28] reported overall safe clinical

improvement of periorbital wrinkles in 10 Korean patients using a 2790-nm Er:YSGG laser.

Another study evaluated outcomes and histologic findings from human and animal skin that underwent microfractional ablative skin resurfacing with both 2940-nm and 2790-nm lasers,[29] showing again overall safety and general efficacy in wrinkle reduction. This same study showed greater thermal damage with the 2790-nm handpiece, which might be useful for increased skin tightening.

Other investigators have shown results using 1440 nm for rhytid improvement. Lloyd[30] reported overall improvement in patients with rhytids, with 42% (5/12) of subjects experiencing good results using the 1440-nm laser with Combined Apex Pulse technology at moderate fluences. However, increasing the laser fluence did not improve efficacy. A later study supported these findings for both a 1440-nm and a 1320/1440-nm multiplex laser. Both lasers safely and effectively improved photodamage, and histopathology supported these findings.[31]

SPECIAL CONSIDERATION FOR TREATMENT OF PERIORBITAL FINE LINES

When performing laser treatments to the periorbital region of the face, the uniqueness of the skin in this area must be taken into consideration. The eyelid skin is the thinnest in the body, which contributes

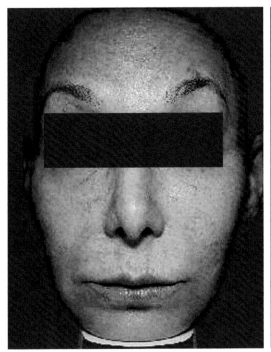
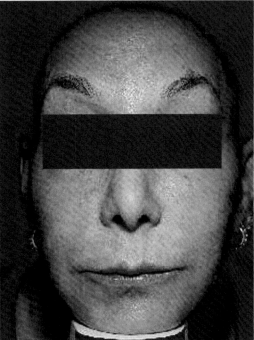

Fig. 3. Pre and post treatment photos after ablative fractional resurfacing with CO_2.

to early signs of aging in this area. Underlying contour defects and aging-related volume loss are also more apparent. Topical treatments, such as retinoids and chemical peels, are commonly used to treat periorbital fine lines, but often patients find consistent use of these treatments intolerable because of the sensitive skin in this area. Many patients experience burning, stinging, and eye irritation when treating the periocular area. Skin care companies rarely manufacture products with active ingredients in their eye creams because of fear of causing ocular irritation or damage. For these reasons, more permanent treatments such as laser rejuvenation have been sought.

Laser treatments are increasingly popular, because new technology allows long-lasting results and better safety with minimal downtime. The relative thinness of the periorbital skin also affects the water absorption by different laser wavelengths that target water as a chromophore. Rhytids in the periorbital region respond well to CO_2 lasers but, as with all treatments with CO_2 lasers, many patients decline this treatment because of the prolonged healing period and pronounced erythema that can last for months.[1] Similar to other areas affected by rhytids, wavelengths of 2790 nm and 1550 nm stimulate collagen, thereby reducing fine wrinkles and dark circles, and tightening the skin around the eyes. The authors believe that the 2790-nm Er:YSGG laser may be superior to the 1550-nm laser because fewer treatments are needed, but this has not yet been proven.[28] As with all laser and light treatments to the face, eye protection must be of the utmost concern during these procedures, especially when treating the periocular area. Stainless steel corneal eye shields for patients and eye goggles with the appropriate filter for the treating physician and personnel are highly recommended.

SUMMARY

Aging skin undergoes many changes. The texture roughens, the color yellows, small capillaries become visible (telangiectasias), and areas of irregular pigmentation may develop. Facial wrinkles reflect the passage of time and exposure to the sun. An important challenge faced by cosmetic physicians is the treatment of facial fine lines, or atrophic rhytids. These fine wrinkles are changes in the microrelief of the skin texture that lead to crinkled, fine, parallel lines that disappear when the skin is stretched. The underlying pathophysiology of fine line formation involves decreases in dermal collagen VII bundles, oxytalan elastin fibers, and glycosaminoglycans in the extracellular matrix. Photoaging is mediated largely by a family

of enzymes called matrix metalloproteinases that accelerate the normal aging process through degrading collagen, elastin, and extracellular matrix in the dermis. Solar elastosis is a photoaging process that causes thick wrinkles secondary to haphazard deposition of bulky, disorganized collagen, leading to deep permanent wrinkles. The clinical evaluation of these facial wrinkles begins with a full history and focused physical skin examination in natural lighting. Before and after photography helps document clinical outcomes. A complete history questionnaire should be used to uncover past medical and surgical history factors that may impede optimal healing. The Fitzpatrick skin type classification and the Glogau photoaging scales objectively describe skin types and help tailor therapies. The ideal laser skin rejuvenation candidate is a Fitzpatrick type III with mild to moderate wrinkles; however, indications for laser skin rejuvenation is expanding to include darker skin types. Successful laser treatment of facial fine lines starts with topical pretreatment of the skin with SPF 55 sunscreen, and possibly topical retinoids and hydroquinone.

Laser skin rejuvenation is effective in the treatment of facial atrophic rhytids and solar elastosis through causing dermal neocollagenesis and remodeling. Ablative laser treatments include the CO_2, Er:YAG, and Er:YSGG lasers. Nonablative laser resurfacing has decreased the "social downtime" and healing time through leaving behind MTZs that allow rapid epithelialization from intact, untreated areas of epidermis. Both fractional and ablative modalities have been successfully used to treat facial atrophic rhytids and solar elastosis, including periocular and perioral rhytids. The dermal response to both ablative and fractionated lasers leads to increases in proinflammatory cytokines, heat shock protein, and matrix metalloproteinases. These substances are released into the dermis and lead to neocollagenesis and dermal remodeling that continues histologically for at least 3 months. Further research on various laser modalities are needed to better elucidate the laser types and settings that best treat different kinds of wrinkles on varying skin types. With many laser technologies already available, cosmetic physicians can continue to improve cosmetic outcomes through future research and clinical experience.

REFERENCES

1. Bickley LS, Szilagyi PG. Bates' Guide to physical examination and history taking. 8th edition. Philadelphia: Lippincott Williams and Wilkins; 2003. p. 95–103.

2. Quatresooz P, Thirion L, Piérard-Franchimont C, et al. The riddle of genuine skin microrelief and wrinkles. Int J Cosmet Sci 2006;28(6):389–95.

3. Habif TP. Clinical dermatology. 5th edition. Philadelphia: Mosby; 2009.

4. Contet-Audonneau JL, Jeanmaire C, Pauly G. A histological study of human wrinkle structures: comparison between sun-exposed areas of the face, with or without wrinkles, and sun-protected areas. Br J Dermatol 1999;140(6):1038–47.

5. Shah S, Alster TS. Laser treatment of dark skin: an updated review. Am J Clin Dermatol 2010;11(6):389–97.

6. Alt TH. Technical aids for dermabrasion. J Dermatol Surg Oncol 1987;13(6):638–48.

7. Goldberg DJ. Facial rejuvenation. Berlin: Springer; 2007.

8. Brightman LA, Brauer JA, Anolik R, et al. Ablative and fractional ablative lasers. Dermatol Clin 2009; 27(4):478–89.

9. Alster TS, Tanze EL. Laser skin resurfacing: ablative and nonablative. In: Robinson J, Sengelman R, Siegel DM, et al, editors. Surgery of the skin. Philadelphia: Elseiver; 2005. p. 611–24.

10. Alexiades-Armenakas MR, Dover JS, Ardnt KA. The spectrum of laser skin resurfacing: nonablative, fractional, and ablative laser resurfacing. J Am Acad Dermatol 2007;58(5):719–37.

11. Manstein D, Herron GS, Sink RK, et al. Fractional photothermolysis: a new concept for cutaneous remodeling using microscopic patterns of thermal injury. Lasers Surg Med 2004;34:426–38.

12. Wanner M, Tanzi EL, Alster TS. Fractional thermolysis: treatment of facial and nonfacial cutaneous photodamage with a 1,550 nm erbium-doped fiber laser. Dermatol Surg 2007;33(1):23–8.

13. Orringer JS, Rittie L, Baker D, et al. Molecular mechanisms of nonablative fractionated laser resurfacing. Br J Dermatol 2010;163:757–68.

14. Geronemus R. Fractional photothermolysis: current and future applications. Lasers Surg Med 2006;38:169–76.

15. Jih MH, Goldberg LH, Kimyai-Asadi A. Fractional photothermolysis for photoaging of hands. Dermatol Surg 2008;34:73–8.

16. Rahman Z, Alam M, Dover JS. Fractional laser treatment for pigmentation and texture improvement. Skin Therapy Lett 2006;11:7–11.

17. Weiss E. Nonablative 1927 nm fractional resurfacing effective for facial actinic Keratoses. Presented at the American Society for Dermatologic Surgery (ASDS) National Meeting. Chicago (IL), 2010.

18. Schmults CD, Phelps R, Goldberg D. Erythema reduction and histologic evidence of new collagen formation using a 300-microsecond 1064-nm ND: YAG laser. Arch Dermatol 2004;140:1373–6.

19. Narurkar VA. Skin rejuvenation with microthermal fractional photothermolysis. Dermatol Ther 2007; 20(Suppl 1):S10–3.

20. Hantash BM, Bedi VP, Kapadia B, et al. In vivo histological evaluation of a novel ablative fractional resurfacing device. Lasers Surg Med 2007;39:96–107.

21. Berlin AL, Hussain M, Phelps R, et al. A prospective study of fractional scanned nonsequential carbon dioxide laser resurfacing: a clinical and histopathologic evaluation. Dermatol Surg 2009; 35(2):222–8.

22. Reilly M, Cohen M, Hokugo A, et al. Molecular effects of fractional carbon dioxide laser resurfacing on photodamaged human skin. Arch Facial Plast Surg 2010;12(5):321–5.

23. Tierney EP, Hanke CW, Petersen J, et al. Clinical and echographic analysis of ablative fractionated carbon dioxide laser in the treatment of photodamaged facial skin. Dermatol Surg 2010;36(12):2009–21.

24. Kotlus BS. Dual-depth fractional carbon dioxide laser resurfacing for periocular rhytidosis. Dermatol Surg 2009;35(7):1158–9.

25. Khatri K, Ross V, Grevelink J, et al. Comparison of erbium:YAG and carbon dioxide lasers in resurfacing of facial rhytides. Arch Dermatol 1999;135:391–7.

26. Weiss R, Weiss M, Beasley K. Prospective split-face trial of a fixed spacing array computed scanned fractional CO2 laser versus hand scanned 1,550 nm fractional for rhytids. Presented at American Society for Laser Medicine and Surgery Conference. Kissimee (FL), April 2008.

27. Ross EV, Swann M, Soon S, et al. Full-face treatments with the 2790-nm erbium:YSGG laser system. J Drugs Dermatol 2009;8(3):248–52.

28. Lee JW, Beom JK, Kim MN, et al. Treatment of periorbital wrinkles using a 2790-nm yttrium scandium gallium garnet laser. Dermatol Surg 2010;36: 1382–9.

29. Dierickx CC, Khatri KA, Tannous ZS, et al. Microfractional ablative skin resurfacing with two novel erbium laser systems. Lasers Surg Med 2008;40: 113–23.

30. Lloyd JR. Effect of fluence on efficacy using the 1440 nm laser with CAP technology for the treatment of rhytids. Lasers Surg Med 2008;40(6):387–9.

31. Geraghty LN, Beisman B. Clinical evaluation of a single-wavelength fractional laser and a novel multi-wavelength fractional laser in the treatment of photoaged skin. Lasers Surg Med 2009;41: 408–16.

Laser Treatment of Cutaneous Vascular Tumors and Malformations

S.M. Athavale, MD[a], W.R. Ries, MD[b], Paul J. Carniol, MD[c],*

KEYWORDS

• Vascular lesions • Hemangiomas • Laser treatment

The history of vascular lesions has origins in a variety of cultures, including ancient Greece, Rome, and Europe. Many vascular lesions are present in infancy, whereas other vascular lesions appear later in life. The latter group of vascular lesions includes, but is not limited to, telangiectasias, spider angiomas, pyogenic granulomas, and angiofibromas. The cutaneous vascular lesions that are present in infancy include vascular malformations and hemangiomas. These lesions are frequently called birthmarks. This term can imply a cause-and-effect relationship between a mother's behavior, cravings, or aversions, and the child's cutaneous lesion. This incorrect concept is referred to as maternal impression and has been present throughout the evolution of the understanding of these lesions.[1]

PEDIATRIC VASCULAR LESIONS

A child with a facial vascular lesion may be at a distinct disadvantage in terms of social, professional, and economic potential. Few prominent historical figures have had cutaneous vascular tumors or malformations. These figures include Marcus Tullius Cicero (106–43 BC), a Roman orator, and James II of Scotland (1403–1460), also known as James of the fiery face. James II of Scotland was depicted in one portrait as having what appears to be a hemifacial port-wine stain.[2]

A more recent historical figure to have a vascular malformation is Mikhail Gorbachev. The negative connotation associated with these lesions persists today, as pictures of Mr Gorbachev show. A review of 200 consecutive 1985 issues of Pravda (a leading newspaper of the Soviet Union and an official organ of the Central Committee of the Communist Party between 1912 and 1991) revealed that, in 24 pictures in which the vascular mark would be expected to show, it could not be discerned.[2] The pictures are believed to have been air brushed to eliminate the appearance of the vascular malformation.

This persistent misconception regarding vascular cutaneous lesions serves as a compelling inspiration for physicians to understand the classification of these lesions, the rationale for laser therapy, the various lasers available, and their respective strengths and weaknesses, and to use the information in treating patients with these lesions.[1]

CLASSIFICATION OF VASCULAR CUTANEOUS LESIONS

Vascular anomalies most frequently present at birth or in early childhood, and the craniofacial region is the most common site of involvement.[3] Pediatric vascular anomalies can be divided into 2 broad categories: vascular tumors and vascular malformations. First highlighted by Mulliken and

[a] Department of Otolaryngology, Vanderbilt University Medical Center, 1211 Medical Center Drive, Nashville, TN 37232, USA
[b] Department of Otolaryngology, Division of Facial Plastic Surgery, Vanderbilt University Medical Center, 1211 Medical Center Drive, Nashville, TN 37232, USA
[c] Department of Otolaryngology Head and Neck Surgery, New Jersey Medical School-UMDNJ, 185 South Orange Avenue, Newark, NJ 07103-2757, USA
* Corresponding author.
E-mail address: pjclaser@aol.com

Facial Plast Surg Clin N Am 19 (2011) 303–312
doi:10.1016/j.fsc.2011.05.009
1064-7406/11/$ – see front matter © 2011 Published by Elsevier Inc

Glowacki[4] in 1982, this biologic classification is based on differences in natural history, cellular turnover, and histology. In 1996, an updated classification was introduced by the International Society for the Study of Vascular Anomalies (ISSVA), which simplified and further categorized vascular tumors and malformations. Vascular tumors include idiopathic hemangiomas (IH); congenital hemangiomas, including noninvoluting and rapidly involuting variants dubbed noninvoluting congenital hemangiomas (NICH) and rapidly involuting congenital hemangiomas (RICH), respectively; as well as kaposiform hemangioendotheliomas and tufted angiomas. Vascular malformations can be further subdivided into low-flow lesions (capillary, lymphatic, and venous malformations) and high-flow lesions (arteriovenous malformations and arteriovenous fistulae). Mixed lesions are common (**Table 1**).[5]

This article focuses on 4 specific types of vascular tumors/malformations that are amenable to laser therapy: (1) infantile hemangiomas, (2) capillary malformations, (3) venous malformations, and (4) lymphatic malformations.

TREATMENT OPTIONS

Treatment options for pediatric vascular cutaneous lesions include both laser and nonlaser techniques. Nonlaser methods include watchful waiting and allowance of time for involution (infantile hemangiomas), ligation and excision, artificial ulceration, electrolysis and thermal cautery, sclerosant therapy, radiation, steroids (local injection or systemic administration), chemotherapy, embolic therapy, and, most recently, systemic therapy with β-blockers. This article focuses on laser treatment options, but this modality is just one part of an otolaryngologist's armamentarium in treating pediatric vascular lesions.

This article is presented in 2 parts: (1) a discussion of specific lasers and their physical characteristics; (2) a discussion of each type of vascular tumor or malformation and the optimal laser treatment modality, focusing specifically on the optimal laser, when to treat, and outcomes. Our goal is for the reader to understand why a specific laser is useful for the treatment of a given lesion. By understanding the histologic characteristics of the lesion and the physical properties of the laser, we hope that the reader will understand when and how to use lasers in the treatment of vascular tumors and malformations.

LASER BASICS

A Google search for lasers demonstrates that advances in laser technology and its applications to various skin conditions have expanded rapidly in the past 40 years, with an even greater acceleration in the past 15 years. With an exceptional diversity in laser options, matching the specific

Table 1
Classification of vascular anomalies (simplified and adapted from the ISSVA 1996 classification)

Vascular Tumors		Vascular Malformations	
Infantile hemangioma	Superficial Deep Mixed	Low flow	Capillary Venous Lymphatic
Congenital hemangioma	RICH NICH	High flow —	Arteriovenous malformation Arteriovenous fistula
Kaposiform hemangioendothelioma	± Kasabach-Merritt phenomenon	Combined	Capillary-lymphatic-venous (Klippel-Trenaunay)
Tufted angioma	± Kasabach-Merritt phenomenon	—	Capillary-venous (mild eases of Klippel-Trenaunay)
Pyogenic granuloma	—	—	Capillary-venous with arteriovenous shunting (Parkes-Weber syndrome)
Spindle cell hemangioendothelioma	—	—	Capillary-arteriovenous malformation
More rare hemangioendotheliomas (eg, Dabska tumor, lymphangioendotheliomatosis)	—	—	Arteriovenous malformation-lymphatic malformation

From Puttgen KB, Pearl M, Tekes A, et al. Update on pediatric extracranial vascular anomalies of the head and neck. Childs Nerv Syst 2010;26(10):1417–33; with permission.

laser to the specific problem is critical for optimizing results and minimizing morbidity. Effective treatment starts with fully understanding laser physics, which allows appropriate application. A high priority must also be placed on laser safety, with appropriate eye protection for the patient and all personnel involved.

Laser Mechanics

The word laser is an acronym for light amplification by stimulated emission of radiation. This acronym has elements of a misnomer because light is significantly different than the energies that are traditionally considered to be radiation. Absorption of light by the tissue provides an effect, which is most often photothermal. Selective photothermolysis is the process by which controlled thermal injury is induced in a selected tissue target that absorbs light at a specific emitted wavelength.[6] This selected target tissue is called a chromophore.

Lasers are designed to target chromophores such as hemoglobin, water, or melanin. Some laser wavelengths are absorbed by the primary chromophore and by a competing chromophore. The issue of competing chromophore absorption should be considered in the design and use of the laser. The light that is absorbed by the chromophore is converted to heat. Tissues heated to 60° to 70°C coagulate, and structural proteins, including collagen, are denatured. At more than 100°C, tissue vaporization occurs.[7] The pulse duration of this laser energy is important in achieving the goals of treatment and minimizing undesirable effects.

To limit collateral damage, the laser wavelength usually should approximate the absorption peak of the targeted chromophore in relation to other optically absorbing molecules in the surrounding skin. This specific targeting is a key element to efficacy, but safety is further enhanced by limiting the exposure times of absorption and the resultant heating (pulse width) so that the tissue effect is further limited to the specific target.[7] Appropriate protective cooling of adjacent structures adds another element of safety to nontargeted tissue.[7] Thus, proper use of the laser depends on matching the wavelength, spot size, energy density, power, and duration of action (pulse width) to the specific target.[7]

Wavelength is directly proportional to the depth of penetration within the visible wavelength spectrum (approximately 400–700 nm). Longer wavelengths effect deeper penetration, whereas shorter wavelengths exhibit greater scatter and less tissue penetration.[7] It is also key to remember that the larger the spot size, the deeper the penetration. The pulse width is a measure of the time that the target tissues are exposed to the laser. Ideally, it should approximate the target thermal relaxation time, defined as the time it takes for a specific volume of tissue to dissipate 51% of the energy absorbed.[6] A pulse width that is shorter than the thermal relaxation time of a blood vessel results in inadequate photocoagulation. However, a significantly longer pulse width can lead to heat dispersion to surrounding nontarget tissue. This dispersion can decrease laser effectiveness. Therefore, optimizing pulse width is critical to safety and efficacy.[7]

TYPES OF LASERS

The flashlamp pumped dye laser (PDL) was introduced in 1989 and revolutionized the treatment of cutaneous vascular lesions.[8] The PDL uses a flashlamp to energize rhodamine dye and subsequently generates a pulse of yellow light. The original PDL emitted light at 577 nm and was later increased to 585 nm to allow deeper tissue penetration without losing its ability to selectively target oxyhemoglobin.[9–12] Today, the most commonly used PDL systems emit wavelengths of 585 or 595 nm and are generally considered the first treatment of choice for hemangiomas and port-wine stains in the pediatric population. In addition to the excellent clinical efficacy of PDLs, the dynamic cooling devices included in certain PDL systems have also led to an outstanding safety profile by reducing the risk for epidermal injury.[13–15] The more recently developed PDLs have longer wavelengths (595 and 600 nm), larger spot sizes (7–12 mm), and higher peak fluence potential, thereby allowing for better treatment of more deeply situated vessels in hemangiomas and port-wine stains.[16–18]

After treatment with the PDL, most patients experience varying degrees of erythema and/or purpura, potentially lasting up to 7 to 10 days. Less common side effects of the PDL include hyperpigmentation and hypopigmentation. Atrophic scarring has been documented but is exceedingly rare.[8]

Intense Pulsed Light Laser

Intense pulsed light laser (IPL) systems emit polychromatic light in a broad wavelength spectrum. Attached to these devices are filters designed to allow a defined wavelength band to penetrate the skin and target specific structures.[19] Depending on the attached filter, which results in the application of wavelength bands in the range of 500 to 1400 nm, superficial or deeper vessels may be treated.

Within the pediatric population, many different vascular lesions have been treated with IPL, including port-wine stains and hemangiomas.[20]

Neodymium:Yttrium-Aluminum-Garnet Laser

The wavelength of the neodymium:yttrium-aluminum-garnet laser is 1064 nm and in the near-infrared spectral region. As is true for the CO_2 laser, the Nd:YAG requires a helium-neon aiming beam because the near-infrared spectral region is not visible to the human eye. Although most tissues in the body do not absorb this wavelength well, pigmented tissues absorb it better than do nonpigmented tissues. Laser energy is transmitted through the superficial layers of most tissues and is scattered into the deeper layers.

In comparison with the CO_2 laser, the scatter of the Nd:YAG laser is considerably greater. The depth of penetration is therefore greater, and thus the Nd:YAG laser is well suited for coagulating deeper vessels. Experimentally, the depth of maximum coagulation is about 3 mm (coagulant temperature, 60°C).[21]

Nd:YAG lasers can penetrate deeply (4–6 mm) and have been used for years for the treatment of port-wine stains.[22,23] With the deeper penetration and nonselective destruction, pain and scarring become factors during treatments. Therefore, anesthesia is usually required to help with pain control and conservative power settings, a pointillistic approach to the lesion, and avoidance of treatment in areas of thin skin are necessary to prevent posttreatment scarring.[1] One benefit of the 1064-nm wavelength is the inherently lower absorption coefficient for melanin. With this wavelength, there is less concern for coincident pigment-induced epidermal damage and it can be used more safely in patients with higher Fitzpatrick skin types.[8] Nevertheless, epidermal pigment must be protected in darkly pigmented individuals by using cooling and/or adjusting pulse duration. Cooling options common to 1064-nm devices include cryogen spray cooling (Dynamic Cooling Device, Candela Corporation), forced cold air, or contact cooling via chilled sapphire windows or conductive metal plates.[20]

TREATMENT OF SPECIFIC LESIONS
Infantile Hemangiomas

With the expanding role of β-blockers for the treatment of infantile hemangiomas, the indications for laser therapy for these lesions is changing.[24] However, a 2003 article by Vlachakis and colleagues[25] discussed the indications for laser therapy for infantile hemangiomas. In that article, the indications for treatment were as follows: in 72 (65.5%) patients, the hemangioma had affected a vital function such as vision, respiration, hearing, or feeding; in 25 (22.7%) patients there was recurrent ulceration and hemorrhage; and 13 (11.8%) patients had significant cosmetic disfigurement and psychological problems related to appearance.

The laser treatment of infantile hemangiomas can be classified as superficial lesions and deep lesions. In the past 10 years, laser treatment of infantile hemangiomas has focused mainly on the use of PDLs to lighten the lesions (**Fig. 1**), induce regression, or stop growth. Because of its limited depth of penetration (approximately 1 mm), PDL is less effective in deep hemangiomas that extend into the subcutaneous tissue, and is primarily used for superficial lesions.[7] Batta and colleagues[26] reported that PDL treatment of hemangiomas at the early macular stage induced early complete clearance but posed a greater risk of skin atrophy and hypopigmentation. Similarly, Garden and colleagues[27] observed an average lightening of 93.9% in superficial hemangiomas after 4 treatments with the flashlamp/PDL. Ashinoff and Geronemus[28] reported similar favorable results. However, expectations must be clearly defined, because most parents want elimination, not just lightening, of the lesion.[7] In addition, PDLs can be used to treat ulcerated hemangiomas both acutely and early to hasten healing of the troublesome and painful ulceration.[29]

PDLs are less effective for deeper hemangiomas because of their shallow depth of penetration. In a study of 33 cutaneous hemangiomas, Garden and colleagues[27] reported that PDL is less effective in lesions more than 3 mm thick. There are other articles that contend that hemangiomas responding to PDL treatment might have resolved without treatment.[7] One report by Batta and colleagues[26] details that the number of children whose lesions showed complete clearance or minimum residual signs at 1 year was not significantly different in the PDL-treated and observation groups. For these reasons, it is advisable to reserve PDL treatment of hemangiomas for thinner lesions.

The 1064-nm Nd:YAG laser is effective in treating deeper and larger vascular lesions. Clymer and colleagues[30] treated 8 children with hemangiomas with the interstitial laser and reported a reduction in size between 67% and 100% in 5 patients and 50% in another after 4.7 treatments. Because the Nd:YAG is a more powerful laser, morbidity such as blistering, nonspecific tissue heating, and scarring is more of a possibility than with the PDL. Treatment should proceed with a respect for both the potential treatment value and potential morbidity.[7]

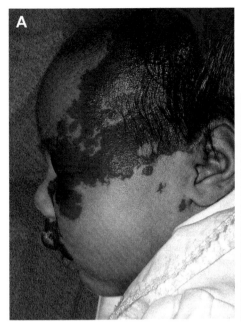

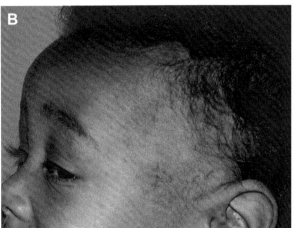

Fig. 1. (A, B) Superficial hemangioma treated with a PDL. (A) Before treatment. (B) After laser treatment. (*Courtesy of* W.R. Ries, MD, Nashville, TN.)

Currently, most practitioners use both the PDL and the Nd:YAG laser in the treatment of combined superficial/deep hemangiomas. Each laser surgeon should decide what is most appropriate for a given patient. Generally, practitioners start with the Nd:YAG laser to treat the deep component of the hemangioma in a percutaneous manner. The superficial component and residual telangiectatic vessels of the hemangioma are then treated with the PDL. After surgery, swelling can be significant for several days and should be expected. Again, warning parents of this expected sequelae is mandatory.

In summary, careful application of both PDL and Nd:YAG laser can provide significant improvement in promoting involution and reduction in size of superficial/deep hemangiomas.

Venous Malformations

Although cosmetic concerns are real, and facial lesions are an important concern to parents and patients alike, pain or functional deficiencies are the 2 most common indications for treatment of a venous malformation. Traditionally, treatment has included surgical resection, sclerotherapy, elastic compression, or a combination.[7]

Thankfully, in the past 15 years, Nd:YAG laser treatment has surfaced as an effective treatment of superficial venous malformations. Historically, the literature reports mainly intralesional treatments through a flexible optic fiber.[31–34] However,

more recently, individuals have found that treatment with direct laser stimulation offers an effective method for treating the superficial venous malformation component.[7] The wavelength emitted is 1064 nm, near the infrared range, which allows for penetration up to 10 mm, resulting in deep coagulation of vessels. The goal of treatment is to reduce bulk and improve contour without scarring. Small venous malformations can be obliterated completely, and the volume of large venous malformations can be reduced to a point at which they are acceptable or more amenable to surgery, providing an environment for less blood loss and smaller scars.[7]

The 1064-nm Nd:YAG laser can cause dermal damage but, if delivered prudently, the skin surface can be protected. Skin protection is achieved both by superficial cooling and by the fact that the 1064-nm wavelength is absorbed only minimally by melanin. The laser can effectively coagulate vessels up to 3 mm in diameter.[7]

The 1064-nm Nd:YAG laser demands extreme safety precautions and should only be used by well-trained personnel. Misuse can lead to tissue necrosis and blindness if appropriate eye protection is not used. Eye safety should be a priority for both the patient and the practitioner. All safety and wavelength-specific eye precautions should be used.[7]

As a general rule, the initial treatment should be applied with less aggressiveness to determine the endpoint and individualized tissue reaction. The residual tissue can be treated during subsequent visits. Multiple treatments are anticipated and discussed with the parents in advance. The treatment is repeated no sooner than every 8 to 12 weeks, depending on the response and size of the lesion.[7] In a group of 5 patients, Ulrich and colleagues[33] reported that 40% showed an excellent response with a more than 90% reduction in size, and 1 patient showed a 25% to 50% clearance. Chang and colleagues[35] reported a mean size reduction of 87% with a mean follow-up of 9.5 months in 10 patients with venous malformations of the tongue using the intralesional Nd:YAG laser. Some larger, thicker hemangiomas do not respond to laser therapy alone. These hemangiomas require combined sequential laser and surgical treatment (**Fig. 2**).

Complications are rare but can include hypopigmentation, scarring, blistering, and burns. When used appropriately, the Nd:YAG laser can serve as a valuable tool for the improvement of venous malformations as a stand-alone treatment of superficial lesions or as an adjunct following sclerotherapy or surgery.[7]

Capillary Malformations (Port-wine Stain)

Although not life threatening, untreated capillary malformations can lead to long-lasting emotional disturbances. In a group of 231 patients aged 9 to 20 years, Troilius and colleagues[36] reported that 47% suffered from low self-esteem, 73% were disturbed by their port-wine stains, and 62% were convinced that their life would change radically if their port-wine stains could be eliminated.

The principle of selective photothermolysis plays a critical role in optimizing the treatment of capillary malformations. Oxyhemoglobin serves as the target chromophore, exhibiting 3 absorption peaks (418, 542, and 577 nm).[7] The 418-nm wavelength has the highest peak, and the first laser designed to treat capillary malformations, the argon laser (488–514 nm), was developed with this concept in mind. Although absorption was excellent, the problem was that depth of penetration was limited to 0.1 mm and significant melanin absorption occurs at these wavelengths.[7] The superficial delivery of the energy, coupled with the fact that the energy was delivered in a continuous, nonpulsed beam, resulted in an intolerable rate of scabbing, blistering, and scarring. Pain was also a problem, because healing involved open wounds.

A better understanding of thermal relaxation time led to pulsed lasers. In the visible light spectrum, longer wavelengths penetrate more deeply, so focus shifted to the 532-nm (potassium-titanyl-phosphate) and 577-nm wavelengths. Currently, the 585-nm and 595-nm PDLs seem to be the most popular choices and most effective because of their proximity to an absorption peak and even deeper penetration.[10]

Clinically, the response of port-wine stains to PDLs is dependent on several factors including,

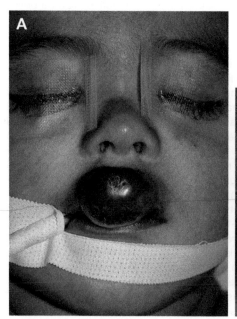
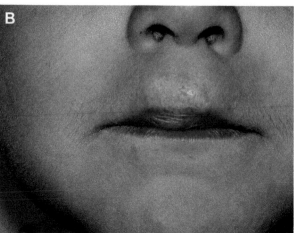

Fig. 2. (*A, B*) A child with a large, thick hemangioma of the upper lip. It was treated with the Nd:YAG laser to reduce vascularity, followed by surgical excision. (*Courtesy of* W.R. Ries, MD, Nashville, TN.)

but not limited to, anatomic location, color of lesion, Fitzpatrick criteria, and patient age. Histologically, the depth and diameter of the ectatic vessels play a significant role in the response as well. Smaller vessels found deeper in the dermis respond more poorly.[7] Using video microscopy, Motley and colleagues[37] revealed 2 abnormal microvascular patterns in port-wine stains. Type 1 showed ectasia localized to the capillary loops, and type 2 was composed of dilated ectatic vessels in the superficial horizontal plexus in a ring pattern. They reported that patients treated with type 1 abnormality had an excellent response to PDLs compared with a poor response to type 2.[37]

Anatomically, Renfro and Geronemus[16] reported that lesions in the V1, V3, and C2 to C3 revealed an excellent response, whereas the central facial region of the V2 distribution dermatome responded less favorably. Fitzpatrick and colleagues[12] reported favorable results in patients younger than 10 years with skin type I to III. With an increase in skin melanin chromophore content there is an increased risk for side effects.[7] Otherwise, PDL treatment in the pediatric population is safe, with few side effects. Purpura usually develops immediately after laser treatment and resolves within 1 to 2 weeks; this is an expected occurrence and therefore not considered a side effect. Considering that, in some patients, the ecchymosis and swelling can be notable, this should be discussed with the patient and/or parents before treatment.

Postinflammatory hyperpigmentation is uncommon but it can develop. This hyperpigmentation can develop from the laser treatment or, if appropriate, from the cooling spray. Hyperpigmentation is more common in patients with higher Fitzpatrick skin types. Hypopigmentation is uncommon. It usually resolves in time but can be permanent. Scarring is even more rare, but can occur, even in experienced hands.[7]

Kauvar and Geronemus[38] reported greater than 75% fading of port-wine stains after more than 10 treatments in 69 patients. In a study by Nguyen and colleagues[39] of 91 patients aged 18 years or younger, patients younger than 1 year with port-wine stains smaller than 20 cm^2 in areas of the face achieved maximal improvement in the first 5 treatments.[38] It is important to discuss with the patient and parents in the preoperative consultation that few patients achieve 100% port-wine stain clearance (**Fig. 3**).[7]

Lymphatic Malformations

Lymphatic malformations can present as small, superficial cutaneous/mucosal blebs or large multilocular lesions. Between 80% and 90% of these lesions present by age 2 years.[7] Any ablative laser, such as the carbon dioxide or erbium laser used in cosmetic procedures, can be used to palliate lymphatic malformations. Good results can also be achieved with the PDL. They are not definitive with this treatment.

For unresectable lesions that have cutaneous blebs that are draining, ablative lasers can eliminate the cutaneous blebs and purposely lay down a sheet of scar tissue, thus eliminating external exposure and subsequent infections.[7]

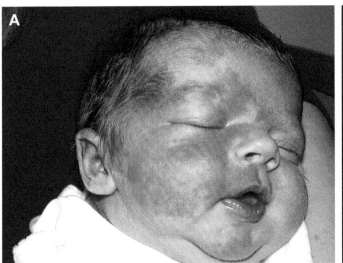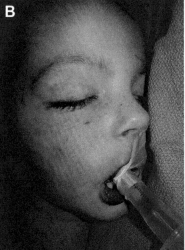

Fig. 3. (*A, B*) Vascular malformation treated with a PDL. Although the lesion has not cleared completely, there is significant lightening. (*Courtesy of* W.R. Ries, MD, Nashville, TN.)

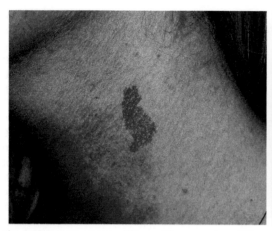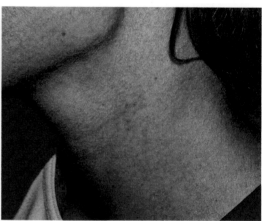

Fig. 4. A young woman with a capillary vascular malformation on her neck, which had a good response to 2 treatments with a flashlamp dye laser. (*Courtesy of* Paul J. Carniol, MD, Summit, NJ.)

TREATMENT OF VASCULAR LESIONS IN ADULTS

Adults usually present with cutaneous vascular malformations when they are unhappy with the appearance of the lesions. Treatment of these lesions varies depending on the specific disorder.

Capillary vascular malformations (port-wine stains) can be a significant source of embarrassment for patients. They can affect the lives of patients in work and other social interactions. If left untreated, they usually darken and thicken, placing them at greater risk for bleeding. With this darkening and thickening, they become less responsive to treatment with vascular lasers. One of the mechanisms that contribute to this process is gradual dilatation of the blood vessels in the malformation.

Most of these lesions respond to treatment with the flashlamp PDL. The initial versions of these lasers had a pulse duration of 0.45 milliseconds. Flashlamp PDL with short pulse duration has significant associated purpura. This purpura typically required at least a week to fully resolve. More recent versions of these lasers with longer pulse durations and/or pulse chains often have less purpura than is found with the earlier shorter pulse lasers. This difference is important for patients because most adults have significant obligations, such as work or family, and do not want to lose time from their regular activities because of swelling and purpura. The patient in **Fig. 4** had a vascular malformation on her neck, which had significant improvement after 2 treatments with a flashlamp PDL. The laser was used at a longer pulse duration (10 milliseconds) to minimize associated purpura.

More commonly, adults present with facial telangiectasia and/or diffuse pinkness, sometimes in association with rosacea. Patients with rosacea who present for laser/light treatment may have been on prior medical therapy and may still have some persistent facial pinkness. This facial pinkness can be improved with laser or intense pulse light therapy. For facial telangiectasias, the third author prefers to use a vascular laser. It is important to explain to patients that vascular lasers treat the results of the underlying condition but do not treat the condition. Thus, in time, new telangiectasias will develop and facial pinkness will increase.

Frequently, the third author uses a 532-nm laser to treat smaller, more superficial facial telangiectasia, and reserves longer wavelength vascular lasers for resistant, larger or deeper telangiectasias. There is visible immediate lightening after treatment with a 532-nm laser. Typically, there is no associated purpura. The treated area is usually light pink in color after treatment. This light pink color usually resolves within 30 minutes to 4 hours.

SUMMARY

Both pediatric and adult patients can present with vascular lesions. Although not effective for all lesions, most respond to laser treatments. However, no single laser is best suited for the treatment of all lesions. The surgeon must understand the physical characteristics of each laser, including the wavelength of the laser and laser-tissue interactions. A thorough understanding of cutaneous vascular lesions is also paramount in delivering optimal care. When equipped with a solid foundation in laser mechanics and an understanding of the various vascular tumors and malformations, facial plastic surgeons can adeptly use laser therapy to help properly treat their patient populations.

REFERENCES

1. Ries RWM, Clymer MA, Charous SJ. Laser treatment of cutaneous vascular lesions. Facial Plast Surg Clin North Am 1995;3(3):307–18.
2. Mulliken JB, Young AE. Vascular birthmarks in folklore, history, art, and literature. Hemangiomas and Malformations. Philadelphia: WB Saunders; 1988.
3. Werner J, Dünne A-A, Folz BJ, et al. Current concepts in the classification, diagnosis and treatment of hemangiomas and vascular malformations of the head and neck. Eur Arch Otorhinolaryngol 2001;258:141–9.
4. Mulliken JB, Glowacki J. Hemangiomas and vascular malformations in infants and children: a classification based on endothelial characteristics. Plast Reconstr Surg 1982;69(3):412–22.
5. Puttgen KB, Pearl M, Tekes A, et al. Update on pediatric extracranial vascular anomalies of the head and neck. Childs Nerv Syst 2010;26(10):1417–33.
6. Anderson RR, Parrish JA. Selective photothermolysis: precise microsurgery by selective absorption of pulsed irradiation. Science 1983;220:524–9.
7. Burns AJ, Navarro JA. Role of laser therapy in pediatric patients. Plast Reconstr Surg 2009;124(Suppl 1): 82e–92e.
8. Railan D, Parlette EC, Uebelhoer NS, et al. Laser treatment of vascular lesions. Clin Dermatol 2006; 24:8–15.
9. Garden JM, Polla LL, Tan OT. The treatment of port wine stains by the pulsed dye laser: analysis of pulse duration and long-term therapy. Arch Dermatol 1998;124:889–96.
10. Tan OT, Sherwood K, Gilchrest BA. Treatment of children with portwine stains using the flashlamp-pumped pulsed dye laser. N Engl J Med 1989;320:416–21.
11. Alster TS, Wilson F. Treatment of port-wine stains with the flashlamp-pumped pulsed dye laser. Ann Plast Surg 1994;32:478–84.
12. Fitzpatrick RE, Lowe NJ, Goldman MP, et al. Flashlamp-pumped pulsed dye laser treatment of port-wine stains. J Dermatol Surg Oncol 1994;20:743–8.
13. Sommer S, Sheehan-Dave RA. Pulsed dye laser treatment of port-wine stains in pigmented skin. J Am Acad Dermatol 2000;42:667–71.
14. Chang C, Nelson JS. Cryogen spray cooling and higher fluence pulsed dye laser treatment improve port-wine stain clearance while minimizing epidermal damage. Dermatol Surg 1999;25:767–72.
15. Waldorf HA, Alster TS, McMillan K, et al. Effect of dynamic cooling on 585-nm pulsed dye laser treatment of port-wine stain birthmarks. Dermatol Surg 1997;23:657–62.
16. Renfro L, Geronemus RG. Anatomical differences of port-wine stains in response to treatment with the pulsed dye laser. Arch Dermatol 1993;129: 182–8.
17. Lou WW, Geronemus RG. Treatment of port-wine stains by variable pulsed width pulsed dye laser with cryogen spray: a preliminary study. Dermatol Surg 2001;27:963–5.
18. Dierickx CC, Casparian JM, Vengopalan V, et al. Thermal relaxation of port-wine stain vessels probed in vivo: the need for 1–10 millisecond laser pulse treatment. J Invest Dermatol 1995;105:709–14.
19. Ross EV, Smirnov M, Pankratov M, et al. Intense pulsed light and laser treatment of facial telangiectases and dyspigmentation: some theoretical and practical comparisons. Dermatol Surg 2005;31:1188–98.
20. Galeckas KJ. Update on lasers and light devices for the treatment of vascular lesions. Semin Cutan Med Surg 2008;27(4):276–84.
21. Brackett KA, Sankar MY, Joffe S. Effects of Nd:YAG laser photoradiation on intra-abdominal tissues: a histological study of tissue damage versus power density applied. Lasers Surg Med 1986;6:123.
22. Rogachefsky S, Silapunt S, Goldberg DJ. Nd:YAG (1064nm) irradiation for lower extremity telangiectases and small reticular veins: efficacy as measured by vessel color size. Dermatol Surg 2002;28: 220–3.
23. Ross EV, Domankevitz Y. Laser treatment of leg veins: physical mechanisms and theoretical considerations. Lasers Surg Med 2005;36:105–16.
24. Guo S, Hunt MG, Superstein R. Treatment of infantile hemangiomas. J Pediatr Ophthalmol Strabismus 2010;47(4):198–201.
25. Vlachakis I, Gardikis S, Michailoudi E, et al. Treatment of hemangiomas in children using a Nd:YAG laser in conjunction with ice cooling of the epidermis: techniques and results. BMC Pediatr 2003;3:2.
26. Batta K, Goodyear HM, Moss C, et al. Randomised controlled study of early pulsed dye laser treatment of uncomplicated childhood haemangiomas: results of a 1-year analysis. Lancet 2002;360:521–7.
27. Garden JM, Bakus AD, Paller AS. Treatment of cutaneous hemangiomas by the flashlamp pumped pulsed dye laser: prospective analysis. J Pediatr 1992;120:555–60.
28. Ashinoff R, Geronemus RG. Capillary hemangiomas and treatment with the flashlamp-pumped pulsed dye laser. Arch Dermatol 1991;127:202–5.
29. David LR, Malek MM, Argenta LC. Efficacy of pulse dye laser therapy for the treatment of ulcerated haemangiomas: a review of 78 patients. Br J Plast Surg 2003;56:317–27.
30. Clymer MA, Fortune DS, Reinisch L, et al. Interstitial Nd:YAG photocoagulation for vascular malformations and hemangiomas in childhood. Arch Otolaryngol Head Neck Surg 1998;124:431–6.
31. Rebeiz E, April MM, Bohigian RK, et al. Nd-YAG laser treatment of venous malformations of the head and neck: an update. Otolaryngol Head Neck Surg 1991;105:655–61.

32. Derby LD, Low DW. Laser treatment of facial venous vascular malformations. Ann Plast Surg 1997;38:371–9.

33. Ulrich H, Gaumler W, Hohenleutner U, et al. Neodymium-YAG laser for hemangiomas and vascular malformations: long term results. J Dtsch Dermatol Ges 2005;3:436–40.

34. Bradley PF. A review of the use of the neodymium YAG laser in oral and maxillofacial surgery. Br J Oral Maxillofac Surg 1997;35:26–35.

35. Chang CJ, Fisher DM, Chen YR. Intralesional photo-coagulation of vascular anomalies of the tongue. Br J Plast Surg 1999;52:178–81.

36. Troilius A, Wrangsjo B, Ljunggren B. Potential psychological benefits from early treatment of port-wine stains in children. Br J Dermatol 1998; 139:59–65.

37. Motley RJ, Lanigan SW, Katugampola GA. Videomicroscopy predicts outcome in treatment of port-wine stains. Arch Dermatol 1997;133:921–2.

38. Kauvar AN, Geronemus RG. Repetitive pulsed dye laser treatments improve persistent port-wine stains. Dermatol Surg 1995;21:515–21.

39. Nguyen CM, Yohn JJ, Huff C, et al. Facial port wine stains in childhood: prediction of the rate of improvement as a function of the age of the patient, size and location of the port wine stain and the number of treatments with the pulsed dye (585 nm) laser. Br J Dermatol 1998;138(5):821–5.

Treatment of Hyperpigmentation

Anthony M. Rossi, MD, Maritza I. Perez, MD*

KEYWORDS

- Hyperpigmentation • Melasma
- Postinflammatory hyperpigmentation • Laser therapy

Disorders of hyperpigmentation are as common as they as are distressing. The color of the skin is the cumulative addition of not only the amount but also the distribution of melanin within the epidermis and dermis. The color of the skin that is portrayed is the result of melanin's light absorption and subsequent reflection. Therefore, disorders of hyperpigmentation are the result of an increase in melanin production and even a change in density of activated melanocytes. In addition, the skin can become discolored as a result of deposition of medications as well as elements such as heavy metals. Labile melanocyte responses to injury or inflammation in skin of color can result in an increased prevalence of pigmentary disorders. Hyperpigmentation can be diffuse, circumscribed, linear, or reticulated, and such patterns can aid in a specific diagnosis. Two prevalent disorders of hyperpigmentation are melasma and postinflammatory hyperpigmentation (PIH). These disorders can be very concerning for patients and therefore treatment is greatly sought after. The treatment of hyperpigmentation is multifactorial, and can require multiple modalities as well as time and patience. These disorders also affect skin-of-color patients preferentially and therefore there is an added component of concern when treating skin of color patients, as one does not wish to depigment the skin in the treatment process. Both melasma and PIH can be very problematic and distressing for patients. The treatment of both can pose a challenge for the physician. Both disorders are discussed in this article, with a focus on a multimodality approach to treating pigmentary disorders. Often one treatment option is not enough, and a multifocus approach needs to be used.

DISORDERS OF HYPERPIGMENTATION
Melasma

Melasma, also called chloasma or the mask of pregnancy, is a common disorder of hyperpigmentation that preferentially affects women. It is a circumscribed hypermelanosis with characteristic symmetric hyperpigmented patches occurring most frequently on the face, but can occur on the extensor arms. Melasma develops and progresses slowly and is often associated with hormonal changes, underlying genetic factors, and exposure to ultraviolet (UV) light as well as heat.[1] In the United States melasma affects about 5 to 6 million individuals, and in one study the incidence of melasma in males was about 5% to 10%. It is more common among the Hispanic, Asian, African, and Middle Eastern populations, and tends to persist longer in those of darker phototypes. Melasma is an extremely prevalent and concerning problem in the Latino population. Sanchez and colleagues[2] reported that melasma constitutes 8.2% of the diagnosis encountered in a Latino private practice population. Known exacerbating factors include pregnancy, oral contraceptives, and sun exposure. The pathogenesis, while not completely elucidated, is thought to involve UV exposure, or another exacerbating factor, in conjunction with hyperfunctional melanocytes that produce increased amounts of melanin.[3] UV irradiation is thought to play the central role, and this is supported by the

Disclosure: Dr Mariza Perez is a consultant for Cutera. Dr Rossi has nothing to disclose.
There was no outside funding for this project.
St Luke's Roosevelt Hospital, 1090 Amsterdam Avenue Floor 11, New York, NY 10025, USA
* Corresponding author. Advanced DermCare, 25 Tamarack Avenue, Danbury, CT 06811-4829.
E-mail address: miptulla@aol.com

facialplastic.theclinics.com

observation that melasma tends to improve during the winter months and by involvement of sun-exposed areas. Documented exacerbating factors are hormonal estrogen and possibly progesterone, medications such as phenytoin-related anticonvulsants and phototoxic medications, as well as increased expression of c-kit and stem cell factor within lesion skin. Perez and colleagues[4] reported that fertile women who developed melasma without ever having been pregnant or on oral contraceptive medications may show a mild ovarian dysfunction consistent with polycystic ovarian syndrome. The melanocytes of melasma-affected skin have been shown to be highly dendritic, exhibit rapid DNA synthesis on UV sun exposure, and multiply rapidly.[2] On histologic examination melanin deposition is seen in all layers of the epidermis, as well as an increased number of dermal melanophages.

In clinical terms facial melasma is divided into 3 patterns: 1) Centrofacial; 2) Malar; 3) Mandible. The centrofacial area is the most commonly affected area, seen in about two-thirds of patients. The malar area is the second most common, occurring in about 20% of patients, followed by the mandible area in about 16% of patients.[5] Melasma is also subclassified into 4 subtypes based on illumination by Wood's lamp: epidermal, dermal, epidermal and dermal (mixed), or intermediate. Lesions composed of epidermal pigment deposition are said to accentuate on Wood's lamp illumination and those that are composed mainly of dermal pigmentation become less conspicuous or blend in on Wood's lamp illumination. Melasma can be very disturbing for patients, and frustration can set in on recalcitrance to treatment. Factors that contribute to the severity of melasma are the surface area affected, intensity of pigmentation relative to the surrounding skim, and homogeneity of the lesions, with more surface area, 3 or more shade differences, and more homogeneous lesions all considered to be more severe.

Postinflammatory Hypermelanosis (PIH)

PIH, or postinflammatory hypermelanosis, is another frequently encountered, cosmetically concerning disorder of hyperpigmentation. As the name implies, PIH is an acquired hyperpigmentation that involves areas of prior cutaneous inflammation, allergic contact, irritant reactions, or trauma such as burns and friction. It can also occur after medication reactions or at sites of vesiculobullous diseases. Of course, cosmetic procedures such as chemical peeling, cryosurgery, laser therapy, intense pulse light therapy, and fillers can

all produce PIH and therefore patients should be informed about the risk of such a development. PIH can affect all skin phototypes and is prevalent among the skin-of-color population. PIH can occur anywhere on the skin surface including the mucous membranes, and becomes apparent in the areas of inflammation once the initial erythema resolves. Patients of any age can be affected, and the incidence is equal in men and women. Although it occurs in all skin types, PIH may be more apparent in phototypes III to VI. Moreover, in these skin types the hypermelanosis may last longer and sometimes never fades completely.[6] Halder and colleagues[7] reported in 1983 that pigmentary disorders, other than vitiligo, were the third most common dermatoses among African American patients but were the seventh most common dermatoses among Caucasian patients. In 2007 Alexis and colleagues[8] confirmed this observation by reporting that dyschromias was the second most common diagnosis among African American patients, whereas dyschromias did not make the top 10 most common diagnoses among Caucasian patients.

The pathogenesis of PIH depends on where the pigment resides. In the epidermal form there is an increase in melanin production and dendritic transfer to keratinocytes. In mice and possibly humans, mediators of inflammation such as prostaglandins E2 and D2 may enhance pigment production. In dermal hypermelanosis, melanin enters or "drops" into the dermis via a damaged epidermal basement membrane secondarily to the inflammatory process. This pigment incontinence is phagocytosed by the dermal melanophages where it resides.[9] Some investigators report that patients with skin of color are more apt to develop postinflammatory pigmentation because of the large amount of melanin contained with the melanosomes within the epidermis. Others believe that the amount of PIH is related more to the individual's type of melanocyte categorized as normal, weak, or strong. The difference is that weak melanocytes, after an inflammatory insult, lead to a decreased production of melanin, giving rise to clinical hypopigmentation, whereas strong melanocytes produce increased amounts of melanin after an inflammatory response, resulting in hyperpigmentation. Normal melanocytes remain unaltered, producing appropriate quantities of melanin.[10] Although melanin is increased in this disorder, the number of melanocytes remains the same. On dermatopathologic examination, the epidermal form of PIH shows increased pigment in epidermal keratinocytes whereas the dermal form is characterized by melanin deposition within dermal macrophages. Although a biopsy is not routinely needed to make the diagnosis, if the diagnosis is questioned a biopsy is sometimes helpful. Included in the differential diagnosis of PIH are disorders such as melasma, exogenous ochronosis, amyloidosis, lichen planus, acanthosis nigricans, erythema dyschromicum perstans, morphea, and tinea versicolor. It is important to check for signs and symptoms and to rule out underlying Addison disease and systemic lupus erythematosus.

PIH presents clinically as asymptomatic macules or patches that range in color from tan to dark brown when there is epidermal melanin, and from blue-gray to gray-brown when there is dermal melanin. Wood's lamp examination may be helpful when trying to distinguish between epidermal and dermal melanin deposition, with the epidermal melanin becoming accentuated under Wood's lamp. Epidermal pigment will show fluorescence under Wood's lamp illumination whereas dermal pigment should not. Mixed and intermediate level pigmentation will show a gradation between the former two. The deeper the pigment, the less fluorescence will occur on Wood's lamp examination. Often the borders of these lesions are not distinct, due to the distribution in areas of prior inflammation. Often the areas of the hyperpigmentation are clues to the underlying inflammatory etiology. In acne vulgaris the resultant hyperpigmented lesions occur on the head, neck, and upper trunk area, are usually less than 1 cm, and tend to be perifollicular. In lesions resulting from lichen simplex chronicus, areas favored include the ankle and antecubital/popliteal fossae. For lesions due to an atopic dermatitis, in infants the face and forearms are affected whereas older children usually have involvement of the flexural areas. In suspected fixed drug eruptions, circular or nummular lesions are observed usually at a perioral, acral, or genital site. Epidermal hypermelanosis is more responsive to treatment than the dermal counterpart. Postinflammatory epidermal hyperpigmentation should resolve with time once the underlying inflammatory disorder is treated, which may take anywhere from 6 to 12 months. Conversely, dermal hypermelanosis is sometimes permanent.

Both melasma and PIH can be distressing for the patient, and the physician should not minimize the psychosocial impact that these disorders may have on the patient's social and professional life. These conditions can have major detrimental effects on a patient's quality of life. Patients may experience feelings of depression and social isolation. Often a feeling of frustration regarding multiple failed treatments as well as frustration with one's self can arise from experience of both pigmentary disorders.

Explanation and discussion of the pathogenesis, clinical course, and treatment options before embarking on treatment can help to manage expectations and set realistic goals for the patient. Because there is no "quick fix," patients must be counseled on the time that is required for treatments to take effect so that they themselves do not become discouraged. Because both disorders are characterized by increased epidermal and dermal melanin, production and deposition treatments for both are discussed together. The theme of a stepwise approach combining multiple modalities is emphasized, and prevention especially against ultraviolet radiation exposure is paramount. When approaching both clinical entities a stepwise approach to treatment is recommended while always assessing the patient's clinical progress, satisfaction, and any adverse events that may occur. It is recommended to start with medical therapy, including topical bleaching agents, retinoids, and low-potency corticosteroids, with treatment durations described in the next section. If adequate resolution is not achieved, treatment can progress to chemical peels and laser therapies, although these should only be done by those who have extensive experience in treating disorders of hyperpigmentation, especially in skin of color. Due to the adverse effects of chemical peeling and laser therapy, including further hyperpigmentation and scarring, one should exercise caution when initiating such therapies.

MEDICAL THERAPY

For the treatment of PIH specifically the first aspect to be addressed is the treatment of the underlying inflammatory etiology, if still active; this will help halt any further pigmentary alteration. It is acceptable to initiate treatment of the postinflammatory pigmentation concurrently with treatment of the underlying cause; however, the physician must be cognizant that the treatment of the hypermelanosis can exacerbate or cause PIH itself by causing further inflammation. The patient's assessment of the treatment should always be included at each stage of treatment.

Photoprotection

For both melasma and PIH, photoprotection should be initiated early and throughout the treatment process. Photoprotection is an integral part of the pathogenesis and persistence of melasma and PIH, as continued UV radiation exposure causes melanocyte activation and continued melanin deposition. Broad-spectrum sun protection that covers the UVB and UVA range should be initiated and should be used year-round because daily sun exposure even in winter months, while nominal in some areas, may be a contributory factor. Because the action spectrum of melanogenesis is considered to be in the longer-wavelength UVA range, UVA protection is indispensable. UV protection is of particular importance for those with skin of color and darker phototypes who many not routinely consider that sun protection is necessary—a common misconception among those with darker phenotypes. In fact when data from the 1992 National Health Interview Survey was analyzed, it was found that only a minority of the 1583 African American responders were likely to use sunscreen, wear protective clothing, or stay in the shade.[11] Vitamin D levels may be of concern in people who are using daily sunscreen, especially for patients with darker skin types who are already at risk for vitamin D deficiency. The American Academy of Dermatology has released a consensus statement regarding the use of daily supplementation for people with darker skin phototypes who are at risk for vitamin D deficiency. Through diet and supplementation a total daily dose of 1000 IU for adults is recommended.[12]

Hydroquinone

The next step, and one of the mainstays of the treatment of melasma and PIH, is use of the phenolic compound hydroquinone. This skin-lightening medication acts by blocking the conversion of dihydroxyphenylalanine (DOPA) to melanin through inhibiting the enzyme tyrosinase, the essential step in melanin synthesis.[13] Hydroquinone may also work through inhibiting DNA and RNA synthesis, selective cytotoxicity toward melanocytes, and melanosome degradation by autooxidation and phenol oxidases leading to highly reactive oxygen radicals. These reactive substances prevent melanin production within melanosomes and increase degradation of melanosome packages after transfer to adjacent keratinocytes. Hydroquinone produces a gradual reduction of the dyschromia by melanocyte downregulation through prevention of production of melanosomes in the actual transfer of melanin to the keratinocytes. Hydroquinone is most commonly prescribed at a concentration of 4%, but is available up to 10% by prescription and over the counter at 2% concentration. The 4% concentration is the standard therapy for melasma and PIH, and has been used for more than 5 decades. For milder forms of pigment deposition the lower 2% concentration may be effective. Higher 10% concentrations are used for more severe clinical phenotypes. It must be noted though that chronic use of topical hydroquinone, even at 2%, can be associated with the risk of exogenous ochronosis, especially with the darker phototypes. Higher concentrations are also more likely to induce irritation and exogenous ochronosis.[14] This condition is most commonly reported in blacks in South Africa, and there have been a few reports of exogenous ochronosis in the United States. However, there has been an increase in the selling of illicit higher concentrations of hydroquinone at ethnic stores in the United States.[15] When used as a monotherapy, hydroquinone's effectiveness is seen around 20 weeks of treatment and the efficacy plateaus after 6 months. It is effective when applied twice daily and should be applied to the entire facial area, as excessive lightening of skin not affected by melasma has not been documented. In actuality, localized or so-called spot treatment can lead to "bull's eye" areas of discoloration.[16]

Hydroquinone and Topical Retinoid

For more moderate to severe melasma topical hydroquinone is combined with a topical retinoid, such as 0.1% tretinoin. The retinol product can be used at night, and this combination can be used for 3 months. Tretinoin and retinol (the precursor to tretinoin) have been shown to be effective in prevention and reversal of photodamage at the molecular level. Pathak and colleagues[17] conducted clinical trials involving 300 Hispanic women with melasma who were treated with various concentrations of hydroquinone formulations. It was concluded that 2% hydroquinone and 0.05% to 0.1% retinoic acid produced the most favorable results. When hydroquinone is combined with a topical retinoid the risk of irritation is increased, and this possibility should be monitored for.[18] If after 3 months the patient does not see improvement than a triple therapy can be initiated. Kligman and colleagues[19] created an early triple-therapy formulation that included 5% hydroquinone, 0.1% tretinoin, and 0.1% dexamethasone, which was highly effective but had inherent problems due to the high concentrations of tretinoin and the fluorinated steroid. Of note, Kligman and colleagues noted poor results when each ingredient was used as monotherapy. A less irritating formulation is that of TriLuma (Galderma, Fort Worth, TX, USA), which contains 4% hydroquinone, 0.05% tretinoin, and 0.01% fluocinolone acetonide. This formulation has been used to treat both melasma and PIH, with successful results. This cream should be tried once a day for 2 months, then treatment should continue with the hydroquinone and retinol product daily for 6 months. After 1 year with no recurrence, maintenance therapy should be initiated with the use of the tretinoin cream at night. If recurrence does occur, the patient should resume the original therapy. Patients with severe melasma who are using the triple therapy should be monitored. Due to the steroid, after 8 weeks of therapy steroid-related side effects such as telangiectasias and steroid acne have been observed.[20]

Mequinol

If hydroquinone is too irritating to the patient, a derivative and alternative is 4-hydroxyanisole or mequinol. Mequinol has been found to be less irritating than hydroquinone. The mechanism of action, while not completely elucidated, is thought to involve a competitive inhibition of tyrosinase. Mequinol is available as a 2% concentration and can be formulated with 0.01% tretinoin. Multiple clinical trials have shown that mequinol can effectively treat solar lentigos in a broad range of skin phototypes; one study compared mequinol 2%/tretinoin 0.01% with hydroquinone 4% and showed that both were equally effective.[21]

Nonphenolic Compounds

Nonphenolic compounds that are used in both melasma and PIH include retinoids, azelaic acid, kojic acid, arbutin, niacinamide, N-acetylglucosamine, ascorbic acid, licorice, and soy.

Retinoids are a widely used medication, and are structural and functional analogues of vitamin A. These agents are effective alone or in combination for both conditions, and can be used as maintenance therapy. Retinoids act via modulation of cell proliferation, differentiation, induction of apoptosis, and expression of anti-inflammatory properties. Tretinoin is all-*trans* retinoic acid and a first-generation retinoid; its concentration ranges from 0.01% to 0.1% and is often formulated with hydroquinone to act synergistically on aberrant pigment. Callender and colleagues[22] conducted a clinical trial with black patients to test the efficacy and safety of tretinoin 0.1% in the treatment of PIH. Tretinoin was significantly more effective in treating PIH than the control; however, 50% of patients developed retinoid dermatitis. To combat tretinoid dermatitis one can titrate the dosage, use alternate-day dosing, and dilute the tretinoin with a moisturizer base. Griffiths and colleagues[23] reported significant improvement in 68% of melasma patients treated with 0.1% tretinoin in a 40-week trial. The newer, third-generation retinoids,

adapalene and tazarotene, have both been shown in clinical trials to effectively treat PIH. Tazarotene is category X.

Azelaic acid is a dicarboxylic acid (1.7-heptanedicarboxylic acid) that occurs naturally and is isolated from *Pityriasis versicolor*. Azelaic acid inhibits tyrosinase, and inhibits DNA synthesis and mitochondrial enzymes in abnormal and hyperactive melanocytes. This process may be mediated via the inhibition of mitochondrial oxidoreductase activity. Azelaic acid is formulated as a 15% gel normally prescribed for rosacea and a 20% cream commonly used for melasma, PIH, and acne vulgaris. Lowe and colleagues[24] tested azelaic acid in skin types IV to VI with facial PIH or melasma, and demonstrated that it was safe and effective for the treatment of both conditions in these darker skin types. Allergic sensitization and phototoxic reactions are rare, and more common side effects include mild erythema, scaling, and burning.[25]

Kojic acid is another nonphenolic treatment of both melasma and PIH. It is a fungal metabolite of the fungi *Acetobacter*, *Aspergillus*, and *Penicillium*. Kojic acid inhibits tyrosinase and is available in 1% to 4% concentrations, and can also be formulated with other skin-lightening medications such as hydroquinone. Lim and colleagues[26] studied the use of 2% kojic acid combined with hydroquinone for the treatment of melasma, with results showing improvement and efficacy. Therefore, those patients not seeing results from hydroquinone may benefit from the addition of kojic acid to the regime. Kojic acid is becoming a frequent added ingredient in over-the-counter cosmeceutical formulations and thus is becoming an increasing offender for allergic contact dermatitis; therefore, one should not overlook its sensitizing potential.

Arbutin is another naturally derived compound used for hyperpigmentation. It is formulated from the dried leaves of the bearberry shrub, cranberry, pear, or blueberry plants. Arbutin is a derivative of hydroquinone but does not have the same melanotoxic effects. It also inhibits tyrosinase activity but also inhibits melanosome maturation. The effects of arbutin are dose dependent but higher concentrations can cause hyperpigmentation, so this should be monitored for. Synthetic forms have been produced, which show greater tyrosinase inhibition. One study showed that arbutin was effective in treating solar lentigenes in lighter phototypes but failed to have an effect in darker-skinned patients.[27]

Niacinamide is the active derivative of vitamin B3 (niacin), and has been shown in vitro to decrease melanosome transfer from melanocytes to keratinocytes without inhibiting tyrosinase or cell proliferation. It may also interfere with cell signaling pathways.[28] Niacinamide is stable in an array of compounds and is not inactivated by light. It is formulated as 2% to 5% preparations, but its efficacy has not been shown in darker phototypes. Niacinamide has been shown to have efficacy in treating melasma and hyperpigmentation when combined with N-acetylglucosamine, which is a precursor to hyaluronic acid. N-Acetylglucosamine inhibits tyrosinase glycosylation, which is one step in melanin production. It is usually formulated as a 2% compound combined with niacinamide in cosmeceuticals.[29]

Ascorbic acid, or vitamin C, is another compound that has been tried for treatment of hyperpigmentation. It is an antioxidant found in various fruits and foods. The mechanism of action in pigment alteration involves interaction with copper ions at the tyrosinase active site as well as reduction of oxidized dopaquinone, which is a substrate in melanin synthesis. There are also some documented anti-inflammatory and photoprotective properties.[30] Ascorbic acid is unstable in many topical preparations so the esterified derivatives, such as ascorbyl-6-palmitate and magnesium ascorbyl phosphate, are used in compounds. There are reports of its efficacy in Latino and Asian patients in the treatment of melasma.[31] Iontophoresis has also been employed to increase the penetration of ascorbic acid into the skin.

Recent studies have shown that **flavonoids from licorice roots,** such as glabrene and isliquiritigenin, are effective tyrosinase inhibitors and can therefore be used to treat hyperpigmentation. Liquiritin is also a flavonoid available in a 2% cream, which has the ability to cause depigmentation through melanin dispersibility. A study of women with melasma showed efficacy of liquiritin in 80% of patients tested. Mild irritation was seen in only 20% of patients.[32]

Soy proteins are other naturally occurring compounds that have garnered much attention regarding their medicinal purposes. Soy proteins include soybean trypsin inhibitor and Bowman-Birk inhibitor, and act by inhibiting the activation of protease-activated receptor 2 cell receptors on keratinocytes. These keratinocyte receptors mediate the transfer of melanosomes from melanocytes to keratinocytes. Therefore, the action of these soy proteins in the phagocytosis of melanosomes into keratinocytes is reduced and depigmentation occurs. Soy is currently being formulated alone or in combination with retinol and other products in cosmeceuticals, not only for hyperpigmentation but also photodamage.[33]

SURGICAL THERAPY

The next step in the treatment of hyperpigmentation is the employment of surgical therapy, which includes the use of chemical peels. There is a variety of chemical peels in an array of strengths, and careful selection should be made of the type of acid used and for which skin phototype. Chemical peels are a good adjuvant treatment to topical therapy for the treatment of hyperpigmentation, and can work very well. It is important to take a detailed medical history including medication history, a history of herpes simplex infection, prior reactions to cosmetic procedures, and a history of other dermatologic conditions. It is important to remember that while chemical peels can ameliorate dyspigmentation, they also have the ability to induce new areas of hyperpigmentation, and in susceptible persons can induce keloid formation and hypertrophic scars. Therefore chemical peeling in darker phototypes IV to VI should be considered with caution. The mechanism of action involves the removal of melanin rather than that of previous treatments, which inhibited the melanocytes or the process of melanogenesis. The risk of complications seen from peels increases with the depth of the insult created. Superficial peels therefore impart the lowest risk of complications, though resultant hyperpigmentation can still be seen. Glycolic acid peels are the most common type used but salicylic acid, trichloroacetic acid (TCA), lactic acid, tretinoin, and resorcinol peels are also available.

Glycolic Acid Peels

Glycolic acid (GA) is an α-hydroxy acid that acts via epidermolysis as well as by dispersing basal layer melanin. It also increases dermal collagen synthesis. The available concentrations range from 20% to 70%. GA is often used as an ingredient in skin-lightening creams in a 10% concentration as well. As a peel it requires neutralization with water of sodium bicarbonate. Multiple studies have been preformed that document the efficacy of GA peels in melasma and PIH. Such peels have also been shown to be safely used in skin types IV to VI. Burns and colleagues[34] showed that the addition of GA peels to topical treatment in patients with skin types IV to VI lead to a more rapid and greater improvement compared with controls and topical treatment alone.

Salicylic Acid Peels

Salicylic acid is another type of superficial peeling agent. It is a β-hydroxy acid that is derived from willow tree bark and induces keratolysis through breaking intercellular lipid linkages. Superficial salicylic acid peels have concentrations from 20% to 30% and are considered self-neutralizing peels, which can be seen as a frost once the peel neutralizes. Grimes[35] reported in 25 patients with pigmentary disorders the effects of a series of 5 salicylic acid peels ranging from 20% to 30%. The peels were well tolerated in skin types V and VI and side effects were absent in 84% of his patients. Moreover, of those who were treated for melasma, 66% showed improvement with a combination of the salicylic acid peels and hydroquinone 4%.

Trichloracetic Acid Peels

Superficial TCA peels as well as lactic acid (a mild α-hydroxy acid) peels are also used as treatments. All peels should start out at low concentrations and be slowly increased continually while monitoring for side effects including erythema, burning, PIH, and reactivation of herpes simplex, superficial desquamation, and vesiculation. Also, patients again should be educated on the continual use of photoprotection.

Peels for Different Skin Types

In patients with oily skin and a tendency toward acne, salicylic acid peels are preferred. Patients should be started out at the lowest strength 4 weeks after topical therapy is initiated. The potency is increased on a monthly basis, as tolerated. In patients with dry skin types, GA is preferred.

Individualized Approach

These superficial peels can accelerate improvement as adjuvant therapy and as maintenance. In the hands of experienced physicians, a medium-depth peel as described by Perez and colleagues[1] can be performed for severe melasma by using 70% GA for 3 to 4 minutes followed by a 35% TCA peel. This procedure should not be done as an initial peel because such a medium-depth peel can induce postpeel pigmentary alteration. After the skin recovers, the patient should return to topical therapy with hydroquinone 4%/retinol twice a day for 6 weeks. The use of these medium-depth combination peels can be used on select type IV and V skin types but should never be used on patients with skin type VI. A higher level of experience with these types of peels is needed before treating patients with skin types IV or V. When treating these darker skin types with chemical peeling therapy the physician must anticipate hyperpigmentation before it occurs, therefore skin-lightening therapy should be initiated before hyperpigmentation develops. An individualized

approach should always be used, as every patient will not react in the same way to chemical peels.

LASER THERAPY

A newer and advanced part of the armamentarium in hyperpigmentation treatment is the use of laser therapy. The use of lasers and light sources has become an increasing treatment modality for melasma and PIH. Laser therapy is based on the concept of selective photothermolysis, which states that a specific spectrum of light will be selectively absorbed by specific chromophores. Pulses of light that are shorter in duration than a target's thermal relaxation time are preferentially absorbed by said structure, and causes selective heating and destruction with minimal surrounding thermal damage. Melanin has a wide absorption spectrum ranging from 250 to 1200 nm. The choice of wavelength of the laser determines the depth of penetration, with longer wavelengths penetrating deeper into dermal skin. In the 400 to 600 nm wavelength there is strong competition for absorption by oxyhemoglobin, another chromophore in skin. It will compete with melanin in this wavelength range and therefore vascular damage will occur more than will melanin destruction. At longer wavelengths greater than 600 nm, absorption by oxyhemoglobin is significantly reduced and absorption by melanin over blood pigment is favored, with resultant destruction of the melanin-containing structures.

Many lasers of varying wavelengths to treat hyperpigmentation have been studied. However, they should be used only by trained physicians experienced with laser therapy, because both laser light and intense pulsed light (IPL) therapies have the ability to produce even greater hyperpigmentation and exacerbate conditions such as melasma when aggressive fluences or incorrect wavelengths are used, especially in darker phototypes IV to VI. As always, test spots should be used before commencing full treatment. For the treatment of hyperpigmentation the 1064-nm neodymium:yttrium aluminum garnet (Nd:YAG) laser, IPL system, 2790-nm erbium:yttrium-scandium-gallium-garnet (Er:YSGG) laser (Pearl Laser; Cutera, Brisbane, CA, USA), and the 1550-nm mid infrared erbium doped laser (Fraxel SR, Solta Medical, Hayward, CA, USA; Mosaic, Lutronic, San Jose, CA, USA) are discussed here (**Fig. 1**).

Intense Pulsed Light (IPL) Lasers

The IPL system has been employed to treat melasma and hyperpigmentation in a variety of skin types, and has been used in skin types IV and V. Want and colleagues[36] documented improvement

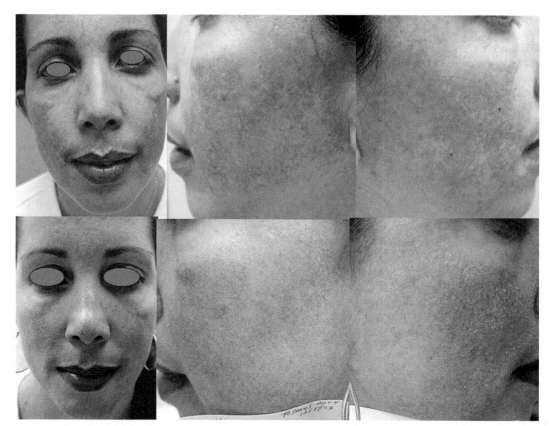

Fig. 1. Combined treatments for melasma. Intense pulsed light and Pearl Laser (Cutera) combination followed by 6 treatments of the 1064-nm Nd:YAG (Genesis; Cutera) laser.

in patients with refractory melasma who were phototypes III and IV. These patients were treated with 4 sessions of the IPL system as well as hydroquinone. There was on average a 40% improvement on the relative melanin index compared with controls. A majority of patients experienced posttreatment microcrust formation 2 to 3 days later. As stated earlier, the longer wavelengths greater than 600 nm should be used because of decreased competition from oxyhemoglobin with less vascular damage. IPL has been reported to exacerbate subclinical melasma when aggressive fluences are used. Negishi and colleagues[37] reported that lower IPL parameters should be used in patients who have subclinical melasma detected by UV photography. As a guide the IPL-induced erythema should last only a few minutes, not hours. The longer the erythema lasts, the greater the risk of melasma-like posttreatment hyperpigmentation.

Nonablative Lasers

Nonablative lasers are also useful in treating melasma and PIH, especially in patients with skin types IV to VI. The nonablative 1064-nm Nd:YAG is often used for treatment of these disorders. The longer wavelength and longer pulse duration are able to target deeper into the dermis, targeting dermal melanin which is often a component of both disorders. This targeting also protects the epidermis from incidental damage that can exacerbate both melasma and PIH. The exact mechanism of action has not been fully elucidated, but there is dermal remodeling from the release of cytokines that can enhance the texture of the skin. Often Q-switched lasers are used in skin-of-color patients, and there is reported success in using these for pigmented lesions; however, for melasma there are mixed reviews. Q-switched lasers have the ability to produce very short pulses with higher energy in comparison with continuous wave mode lasers. The "Q" refers to a quality factor of energy storage in the lasing medium. Q-switched lasers have pulse durations in the 10- to 100-nanosecond range as well as fluences in the 2- to 10-J/cm^2 range. The Q-switched ruby laser emits at 694 nm and is suitable for phototypes IV or less; the Q-switched alexandrite at 755 nm is useful for phototypes V or less; and the Q-switched Nd:YAG laser at 1064 nm is useful for all skin types. Treatments should be kept 1 to 2 months apart, and a total of 4 to 8 sessions may be needed to achieve clinical response. Chan and colleagues[38] have reported that the Q-switched Nd:YAG laser was more effective than the Q-switched alexandrite laser after 3 treatment sessions when treating nevi of Ito and Ota. Chan and colleagues[39] have recently reported a case series of facial depigmentation after treatment with low-fluence Q-switched 1064-nm Nd:YAG laser for skin rejuvenation and melasma in Asian patients. Polnikorn[40] reported two case treatments of refractory dermal melasma using 10 weekly treatments with the 1064-nm Q-switched Nd:YAG laser at subthreshold photothermolytic fluences (<5 J/cm^2), resulting in reduction of epidermal and dermal pigmentation with no recurrences at 1-year and 6-month follow-up. Wattanakrai and colleagues[41] reported that 5 weekly treatments of low-fluence 1064-nm Q-switched Nd:YAG laser is an effective treatment for dermal and mixed melasma.

Fractional Photothermolysis

Fractional photothermolysis is another nonablative laser technique that has been used for melasma and postinflammatory pigmentation in a range of skin phototypes. This process creates microscopic treatment zones of thermal injury that have a 5:1 depth-to-width ratio without extensive cutaneous damage, and are small enough to repair themselves. The thermal injury zones are on average 100 µm in diameter and the depth can be adjusted up to 1 mm. The density of the thermal injury zones can be adjusted for greater or less thermal injury. Manstein and colleagues[42] published guidelines regarding the use of fractional photothermolysis. These investigators used the 1550-nm mid infrared erbium doped laser (Fraxel SR, Mosaic). For melasma in skin phototypes I to II they recommend an energy/MTZ parameter of 6 mJ, a density of 250 MTZ/cm^2, and 12 passes for a total treatment density of 3000 MTZ/cm^2. For skin types III to VI they recommend the same parameters except that the number of passes is decreased to 8 for a total treatment density of 2000 MTZ/cm^2.

When treating melasma and PIH in skin-of-color patients or those with skin types IV to V, it is advised to pretreat with hydroquinone for about 1 month before. Prophylaxis with an antiviral medication for herpes simplex also is routine. Starting at a low energy and low density is advised, and of course a test spot with reevaluation in 1 month is suitable. Topical anesthesia is necessary and

multiple treatments, 3 to 5, are needed spaced about 4 to 8 weeks apart. PIH can be observed and is often transitory, but there is a risk of permanent pigmentary alteration. Therefore, proper precounseling should be done with an emphasis on possible hyperpigmentation as well as treatment failure.

Ablative Skin Resurfacing

Ablative skin resurfacing is a very useful treatment for hyperpigmentation. Resurfacing removes the old epidermis via the process of ablation while stimulating contraction and remodeling the dermis posttreatment via the process of coagulation. The heat generated under the ablative layer of tissue denatures and shrinks collagen, causing a visible tightening of the skin. Ablative resurfacing produces a controlled partial-thickness burn of the epidermis and partially of the dermis, so its use in phototypes V and VI is not indicated because of the risk of scarring, hyperpigmentation, and delayed-onset hypopigmentation.

The main ablative lasers are the 10,600-nm CO_2 laser, the 2940-nm Er:YAG laser, and the newer 2790-nm Er:YSGG laser. Interaction between laser light and tissue in the ablative regime is dominated by water absorption; therefore, the water absorption coefficient is a major factor in wavelength selection. The water absorption coefficients for the 3 aforementioned wavelengths differ by an order of magnitude (103 cm^{-1} for CO_2 laser at 10,600 nm, 104 cm^{-1} for Er:YAG laser at 2940 nm, and 102 cm^{-1} for Er:YSGG laser at 2790 nm). The newer 2790-nm Er:YSGG laser (Pearl Laser) is at a wavelength slightly below the 2940-nm Er:YAG. The 2940-nm Er:YAG laser emits a wavelength of 2940 nm that is close to the absorption peak of water, and yields an absorption coefficient 16 times that of the CO_2 laser. The 2790-nm Er:YSGG has a slightly shorter wavelength and is thought to ablate the top 10 to 30 µm of the epidermis, and below that the epidermis is coagulated. Moreover, the residual thermal damage is thought to stimulate new dermal collagen synthesis.

The concept of fractional therapy has also been applied to the ablative wavelength lasers, and fractional ablation is becoming an increasingly used modality for resurfacing. As in ablative laser resurfacing, the areas of thermal ablation are repopulated by fibroblast collagen production and epidermal proliferation. However, compared with total ablative resurfacing, fractional ablative lasers do not produce full epidermal ablation because the ablation is confined to the microscopic treatment zones.

In fractional ablation the laser is used to produce microscopic, thermal wounds in the skin while the intact, undamaged skin around each wound acts as a reservoir, allowing relatively rapid reepithelialization of the treatment zone with, consequently, little risk of infection and scarring. Fractional ablative CO_2 lasers have been shown to reduce downtime and result in more rapid wound healing.[43]

Case Study: Patient with Type IV Phototype with Melasma

Here the authors review and provide pretreatment and posttreatment results for a patient with type IV phototype with melasma. This patient has had melasma for 16 years, which started as isolated lesions but then progressed to larger patches. The patient was currently using TriLuma, triple-combination, therapy every fourth night because of irritation, but still with residual melasma (see online Video 1: Initial Evaluation of the Melasma Patient; www.facialplastic.theclinics.com). The patient decided to undergo laser treatment for the treatment of her melasma. Combination laser therapy is used first with IPL (LimeLight; Cutera), followed by ablation with the 2790-nm Er:YSGG laser (Pearl Laser). The patient is anesthetized with a lidocaine 23% and tetracaine 7% compound for 1 hour while not under occlusion. The IPL (LimeLight) is used on mode C, which is at a wavelength greater than 800 nm and with a longer pulse duration suitable for melasma and this phototype. The fluence is at 16 J and 1 Hz, and one pass is preformed (see online Video 2: IPL Settings Discussed and Video 3: IPL Treatment; www.facialplastic.theclinics.com). The patient is cooled with cold compresses after the IPL treatment. After the initial IPL treatment the patches of melasma appear darker than the surrounding normal skin, which is exploited by the following ablative procedure with the 2790-nm Er:YSGG (Pearl) laser (see online Video 4: Post IPL Treatment Cooling; www.facial-plastic.theclinics.com). Before the Pearl laser treatment is commenced an acetone scrub is done to defatten the epidermis so that the ablative laser will be more effective (see online Video 5: Acetone Scrub Pre Pearl Laser Treatment; www.facialplastic.theclinics.com). The Er:YSGG 2790-nm laser is set at 3.5 J/cm^2, with a 20% overlap, 0.4-millisecond pulse duration, and the largest pattern grid (see online Video 6: 2790 Settings; www.facialplastic.theclinics.com). After one pass the patient is cooled again with cold compresses (see online Video 7: Pearl Laser and Video 8: Post 2790; www.facialplastic.theclinics.com). This action concludes the treatment. The patient is instructed to start acetic acid compresses 4 to 5 times per day followed by Vaseline ointment application. The acetic acid soaks help to prevent superficial wound infection. By day 3 after treatment the patient is told to expect that the epidermis will slough (see online Video 9: Post Treatment Day 3; www.facialplastic.theclinics.com). On day 3 the patient is slightly erythematous but no burns are noted, as expected. The hyperpigmentation from the melasma is already gone. One week after treatment (see Video 10: 1 Week Post Treatment Final Evaluation; www.facialplastic.theclinics.com) the patient is completely healed and the melasma patches are not visible. Postprocedure the patient continues maintenance treatment with hydroquinone 4% and tazarotene, a topical retinoid, nightly.

SUMMARY AND LIMITATIONS

This article provides an overview of the treatment of hyperpigmentation, mainly melasma and PIH, that uses medical, surgical, and laser technologies. Emphasized is the use of combination therapy. Not only are topical medical combinations frequently used, but in experienced hands combinational laser procedures can also be used to combat hyperpigmentation. Again, an individualized approach is stressed, as not every patient will respond in the same way to similar treatments. The use of test spots not only for lasers but also for medical therapies is warranted. Caution must be exercised because patients with melasma and PIH are already prone to hyperpigmentation, so any insult to the epidermis or dermis can result in further dyspigmentation. Also, when treating skin types IV and greater, less aggressive modalities should be employed. Limitations are encountered not only because of the increase of adverse effects seen in darker phototypes but also because these procedures can be costly and time consuming.

Notes to early users

- Melasma and PIH are two prevalent disorders of hyperpigmentation that can be difficult to treat
- These disorders are more prevalent in patients of darker phototype, therefore possible adverse effects limit the treatment of these patients
- A combined therapeutic and individual patient approach is best suited for treatment
- Sun protection should always be used during the treatment and maintenance process
- Triple-combination therapy with topical hydroquinone, a topical retinoid, and

- a low-potency corticosteroid is a suitable initial approach
- Chemical peeling and laser therapies should be done by experienced physicians who have undergone training with these modalities.

SUPPLEMENTARY DATA

Supplementary videos related to this article can be found at doi:10.1016/j.fsc.2011.05.010.

REFERENCES

1. Perez MI. The stepwise approach to the treatment of melasma. Cutis 2005;75:217–22.
2. Sanchez NP, Pathak MA, Sato S, et al. Melasma: a clinical light microscopy, ultrastructural, and immunofluorescence study. J Am Acad Dermatol 1981;4:698–710.
3. Grimes PE. Melasma: etiologic and therapeutic considerations. Arch Dermatol 1995;131:1453–7.
4. Perez MI, Sanchez JL, Aguilo F. Endocrinologic profile of patients with idiopathic melasma. J Invest Dermatol 1983;81:543–5.
5. McDonald RR, Georgouras KE. Skin disorders in Indo-Chinese immigrants. Med J Aust 1992;156: 847–53.
6. Taylor SC, Burgess CM, Callender VD, et al. Postinflammatory hyperpigmentation: evolving combination treatment strategies. Cutis 2006;78:1–25.
7. Halder RM, Grimes PE, McLaurin CI, et al. Incidence of common dermatoses in a predominately black dermatologic practice. Cutis 1983;32:388–90.
8. Alexis AF, Sergay AB, Taylor SC. Common dermatologic disorders in skin of color: a comparative practice survey. Cutis 2007;80:387–94.
9. Masu S, Seiji M. Pigmentary incontinence in fixed drug eruptions. Histologic and electron microscopic findings. J Am Acad Dermatol 1983;8:525–32.
10. Ruiz-Maldonado R, Orozco-Covarrubias ML. Postsinflammatory hypopigmentation and hyperpigmentation. Semin Cutan Med Surg 1996;16:36–43.
11. Hall HI, Rogers JD. Sun protection behaviors among African Americans. Ethn Dis 1999;9:126–31.
12. James WD. Position statement on Vitamin D. American Academy of Dermatology; 2009.
13. Grimes PE. Management of hyperpigmentation in darker racial ethnic groups. Semin Cutan Med Surg 2009;28:77–85.
14. Burke P. Exogenous ochronosis: an overview. J Dermatol Treat 1997;8:21–6.
15. Halder RM. Pigmentary disorders in pigmented skins. In: Halder RM, editor. Dermatology and dermatological therapy of pigmented skins. Boca Raton (FL): CRC/Taylor and Francis; 2006. p. 91–114.
16. Draelos Z. Hydroquinone: optimizing therapeutic outcomes in the clinical setting of melanin-related hyperpigmentation. Today's Therapeutic Trends 2001; 19:191–203.
17. Pathak MA, Fitzpatrick TB, Kraus EW. Usefulness of retinoic acid in the treatment of melasma. J Am Acad Dermatol 1986;15:894–9.
18. Nordlund JJ. Mechanisms for post-inflammatory hyperpigmentation and hypopigmentation. Advances in Pigment Cell Research: proceedings of Symposia and Lectures from the Thirteenth International Pigment Cell Conference. Tucson (AZ): Lissl; 1988:219–39.
19. Kligman AM, Willis I. A new formula for depigmenting human skin. Arch Dermatol 1975;111:40–8.
20. Taylor SC, Torok H, Jones T, et al. Efficacy and safety of new triple-combination agent for the treatment of facial melasma. Cutis 2003;72:67–72.
21. Piacquadio D. Mequinol 2%/tretinoin 0.01% solution monotherapy and combination treatment of solar lentigines and postinflammatory hyperpigmentation. J Am Acad Dermatol 2004;52(Suppl):P175.
22. Callender VD. Acne in ethnic skin: special considerations for therapy. Dermatol Ther 2004;17:184–95.
23. Griffiths CE, Finkel LJ, Ditre CM, et al. Topical tretinoin (retinoic acid) improves melasma: a vehicle-controlled, clinical trial. Br J Dermatol 1993;129:415–21.
24. Lowe NJ, Rizk D, Grimes P, et al. Azelaic acid 20% cream in the treatment of facial hyperpigmentation in darker skinned patients. Clin Ther 1998;20:945–59.
25. Fitton A, Goa KL. Axelaic acid. Drugs 1991;41:780–98.
26. Lim JT. Treatment of melasma using kojic acid in a gel containing hydroquinone and glycolic acid. Dermatol Surg 1999;25:282–4.
27. Boissy RE, Visscher M, DeLong MA. DeoxyArbutin: a novel reversible tyrosinase inhibitor with effective in-vivo skin lightening potency. Exp Dermatol 2005; 12:601–8.
28. Hakozaki T, Minwalla L, Zhuang J, et al. The effect of niacinamide on reducing cutaneous pigmentation and suppression of melanosome transfer. Br J Dermatol 2002;147:20–31.
29. Bisset DL, Miyamoto K, Sun P, et al. Topical niacinamide produces yellowing, wrinkling, red blotchiness, and hyperpigmented spots in aging facial skin. Int J Cosmet Sci 2004;26:231–8.
30. Farris PK. Topical vitamin C: a useful agent for treating photoaging and other dermatologic conditions. Dermatol Surg 2005;31:814–8.
31. Espinal-Perez LE, Moncada B, Castanedo-Cazares JP. A double blind randomized trial of 5% ascorbic acid vs. 4% hydroquinone in melasma. Int J Dermatol 2004;43:604–7.
32. Amer M, Metwalli M. Topical liquiritin improves melasma. Int J Dermatol 2000;39:299–301.
33. Wallo W, Nebus J, Leyden JJ. Efficacy of a soy moisturizer in photoaging: a double blind, vehicle

controlled, 12 week study. J Drugs Dermatol 2007;6: 917–22.

34. Burns RL, Prevost-Blank PL, Lawry MA, et al. Glycolic acid peels for postinflammatory hyperpigmentation in black patients: a comparative study. Dermatol Surg 1997;23:171–4.

35. Grimes PE. The safety and efficacy of salicylic acid chemical peels in darker racial-ethnic groups. Dermatol Surg 1999;25:18–22.

36. Wang CC, Hui CY, Sue YM, et al. Intense pulsed light for the treatment of refractory melasma in Asians persons. Dermatol Surg 2004;30:1196–200.

37. Negishi K, Kushikata N, Tezuka Y, et al. Study of the incidence and nature of "very subtle epidermal melasma" in relation to intense pulsed light treatment. Dermatol Surg 2004;30:881–6.

38. Chan HH, Ying SY, Ho WS, et al. An in vivo trial comparing the clinical efficacy and complications of Q-switched alexandrite and Q-switched Nd:YAG lasers in the treatment of nevus of Ota. Dermatol Surg 2000;26:919–22.

39. Chan NP, Ho SG, Shek SY, et al. A case series of facial depigmentation associated with low fluence Q-switched 1,064 nm Nd:YAG laser for skin rejuvenation and melasma. Lasers Surg Med 2010;42: 712–9.

40. Polnikorn N. Treatment of refractory dermal melasma with the MedLite C6 Q-switched Nd:YAG laser: two case reports. J Cosmet Laser Ther 2008;10:167–73.

41. Wattanakrai P, Mornchan R, Eimpunth S. Low-fluence Q-Switched neodymium-doped yttrium aluminum garnet (1,064 nm) laser for the treatment of facial melasma in Asians. Dermatol Surg 2001; 36(1):76–87.

42. Manstein D, Herron GS, Sink RK, et al. Fractional photothermolysis: a new concept for cutaneous remodeling using microscopic patterns of thermal injury. Lasers Surg Med 2004;34:426–38.

43. Hantash BM, Bedi VP, Chan KF, et al. Ex vivo histological characterization of a novel ablative fractional resurfacing device. Lasers Surg Med 2007;39(2): 87–95.

Laser Hair Reduction and Removal

Whitney Hovenic, MD[a],*, John DeSpain, MD[b]

KEYWORDS

- Laser • Hirsutism • Hypertrichosis • Electrolysis • Removal

Dermatologists and plastic surgeons, as well as other aesthetically oriented physicians and licensed aestheticians, provide services for both temporary and permanent forms of hair reduction in a variety of clinical settings. According to the American Society of Plastic Surgeons, laser hair removal alone accounts for $406 million in revenue annually and is the third most popular cosmetic nonsurgical procedure, with 1,280,031 cases done in 2009.[1] Hair removal or reduction methods can be used on any hair-bearing body site, but are most popular in sites of secondary sexual hair areas including the axillae, the pubic area, face, and chest.

Cosmetically disturbing, unwanted hair growth is separated into hirsutism and hypertrichosis and defined as increased hair growth in male secondary sexual areas in a woman, including the mustache, beard, chest, escutcheon, and inner thigh. Hair growth in these areas is restricted to strongly androgen-responsive hair follicles. Hypertrichosis refers to increased growth of terminal hairs in areas normally rich in vellus hairs. This hair growth is beyond the length or density of normally accepted growth in any age, sex, or group. The excess hair may be generalized or localized. Terminal hairs are produced by large hair follicles located in the subcutis. The diameter of individual hairs is greater than 0.03 mm. Vellus hairs are produced by small, fully cycling hair follicles that reside in the dermis and do not extend to the subcutaneous tissue. These hairs are less than 0.03 mm in diameter, depigmented, short, and lacking a medullated hair shaft.[2]

Terminal hair growth in women is under hormonal effect and, in some women, may be associated with increased circulating levels of androgens. However, in many women, androgen levels are normal, suggesting a hyperresponsiveness of the hair follicle to androgen stimulation. Other features of hyperandrogenism that support investigation by the practitioner into potential reversible causes of hyperandrogenism include oligorrhea or amenorrhea, infertility, acne, acanthosis nigricans, female pattern hair loss, virility, and clitoromegaly.[3] Polycystic ovarian syndrome is the most common cause of hyperandrogenism; rapid onset of symptoms and testosterone levels greater than 200 ng/mL warrants an investigation for an androgen-secreting tumor. Patients with long-standing normal menses, normal fertility, and mild hirsutism may not need any systemic work-up for hirsutism. Sudden onset of generalized hypertrichosis lanuginosa should prompt work-up for malignancy; acquired hypertrichosis may be seen in porphyria cutanea tarda, variegate porphyria, and erythropoietic porphyria and with the use of multiple medications including cyclosporine, minoxidil, and phenytoin.[4]

Techniques for removal of unwanted hair are discussed later. Hair can be reduced by temporary means that delay hair growth and have an effect for approximately 1 to 3 months, consistent with induction of the telogen phase of the hair cycle: the period of relative quiescence. Hair cycle duration is site dependent and varies from patient to patient. Permanent hair reduction techniques lead to a significant reduction in the number of terminal hairs after a given treatment. By definition, this reduction is stable for a period of time longer than the complete growth cycle of hair follicles at a given site. **Table 1** may be useful when considering the timing of treating actively growing

[a] Department of Dermatology, University of Missouri, 1 Hospital Drive, MA111, Columbia, MO 65212, USA
[b] DeSpain Cayce Dermatology Center, 2011 Corona Road, Suite 207, Columbia, MO 65203, USA
* Corresponding author.
E-mail address: hovenicw@health.missouri.edu

Facial Plast Surg Clin N Am 19 (2011) 325–333
doi:10.1016/j.fsc.2011.04.002
1064-7406/11/$ – see front matter © 2011 Elsevier Inc. All rights reserved.

Table 1
Hair growth

Hair Growth Chart

Body Area	% Anagen	Duration of Telogen	Duration of Anagen	Daily Growth Rate (mm)	Approx Depth of Anagen Follicle (mm)
Scalp	85	3–4 mo	2–6 y	0.35	3–5
Eyebrows	10	3 mo	4–8 wk	0.16	2–2.5
Ear	15	3 mo	4–8 wk	—	—
Cheeks	50–70	—	—	0.32	2–4
Beard/chin	70	10 wk	1 y	0.38	2–4
Mustache	65	6 wk	16 wk	—	1–2.5
Axillae	30	3 mo	4 mo	0.3	3.5–4.75
Trunk	—	—	—	0.3	2–4.5
Pubic area	30	12 wk	Months	—	3.5–4.75
Arms	20	18 wk	13 wk	0.3	—
Legs and thighs	20	24 wk	16 wk	0.21	2.5–4
Breasts	30	—	—	0.35	3–4.5

Data from Dierickx CC. Hair removal by lasers and intense pulsed light sources. In: Fitzpatrick RE, Goldman MP, editors. Cosmetic laser surgery. St Louis (MO): Mosby; 2000.

follicles (anagen) as well as considering efficacy of permanent hair reduction at a given site.

A BRIEF HISTORY OF HAIR REMOVAL

Though hair has long served its purpose in ultraviolet protection and thermal regulation, humans have a long history of desiring to remove excess hair. Hair removal techniques, including razors and depilatories, date back to ancient times. Ancient Egyptian men were known to shave both their heads and beards; not for vanity but for survival, given that a smooth head and beard reduced the enemy's ability to use the hair as a handhold grip for decapitation in combat. In the Roman world, a clean-shaven man became the symbol of civilization and progress.[5] The current trend in hair removal in the United States was sparked nearly a century ago with a 1914 Harper's Bazaar advertisement campaign depicting underarm hair as unhygienic and unfeminine with the emerging trend of more revealing female fashion. Following the lead of the fashion world and cultural trends, those involved in hair loss noted several additions to the field of hair removal that had otherwise remained stagnant, depending solely on razors and depilatories that had been unchanged for several centuries. In 1916 came the invention of electrolysis, and in the 1940s came the invention of Nair, the most effective depilatory cream to date.

Laser hair removal devices were first developed in the 1970s; however, techniques were ineffective and painful, limiting use. In 1995, the US Food and Drug Administration approved the neodymium yttrium aluminum garnet (Nd:YAG) as the first laser for hair removal and, soon after, the first article on laser hair removal was published in the New England Journal of Medicine.[6] Subsequently, dozens of different brands of hair removal lasers/lights have become available using several different wavelengths to induce reduction.

TECHNIQUES FOR HAIR REMOVAL/ REDUCTION

Physical methods to temporarily reduce unwanted hair include plucking, shaving, waxing, and electrolysis. These techniques are best used on limited body surfaces, because the side effects of irritation and pain are common. Hair loss is not permanent and frequent treatments are required to produce desired results.

Topically applied eflornithine 13.9% (Vaniqa) cream inhibits ornithine decarboxylase. It is approved for reduction of unwanted facial hair in women when applied twice daily. Hair growth is slowed but not eliminated. Patients must be appropriately counseled on medication compliance and slow onset of results.

Electrolysis uses electricity for the removal of unwanted hair. This removal is performed by passing low-flow direct current (DC) through tissue between 2 electrodes, resulting in tissue damage and destruction of hair follicles by the creation of a chemical reaction at the tip of the electrode.[7]

Electrons are released at the negatively charged electrode, producing hydrogen gas and hydroxide ions from water; the resultant hydroxides then chemically destroy the adjacent hair follicle.[8] Nonphysician personnel performing electrolysis use pure galvanic or blended galvanic and high-frequency electrolysis, whereas medical professionals tend to prefer high-frequency electro-epilation, which achieves faster results. Galvanic electrolysis is safer, less likely to scar, and less painful than high-frequency electrolysis but works slower.[9] In order for hair removal to be permanent, the hair follicle root must be destroyed. To minimize risk of scarring, the superficial portion of the hair follicle is not treated. Good lighting and clean skin are required for best results, as is correct placement of the electrolysis needle. Use of an insulated needle limits heat generation to the base of the follicle only, minimizing damage to the upper perifollicular dermis and, therefore, decreasing risk of scarring.[10] Use of timers allows for safe use of both insulating and noninsulating needles. Home-use, hand-held electrolysis devices are available and may be used for minimal areas of hypertrichosis and hirsutism.

LASER/LIGHTS: OVERVIEW

Laser epilation of unwanted hair is currently the most popular and effective way to achieve permanent to semipermanent reduction of hair. Laser hair removal is 60 times more effective, less painful, and requires fewer sessions than electrolysis.[11]

The mechanism of action of laser epilation is dependent on selective photothermolysis of melanized hair through the absorption of light energy.[12] The principal of selective photothermolysis was conceived by Anderson and Parrish[13] in 1983. Selection of preferentially absorbed wavelength and delivery at appropriate fluence and pulse duration allows for destruction of target tissue with limited damage to surrounding tissues. **Fig. 1** shows the absorption spectrum of hemoglobin and melanin and the corresponding wavelengths of commonly used lasers.

To maximize damage to the desired chromophore (melanin), light sources are chosen based on the wavelength(s) best penetrating into the dermis to the hair follicle where melanin is present, and using pulse duration shorter than or equal to the thermal relaxation time (the time required for heated tissue to lose 50% of its heat). Clean ablation of tissue is defined as the ability to ablate faster than the heat is conducted to surrounding tissue.[14] Terminal hair follicles with a diameter of 300 μm have a thermal relaxation time of 100 milliseconds. Permanent hair removal requires damage to follicular stem cells in the bulge region of the hair follicle, whereas temporary hair loss is achieved through damage causing induction of catagen. Follicular stem cells are nonpigmented targets located at a distance from melanin chromophores in a pigmented hair shaft. To damage nonpigmented targets, heat must diffuse from the target chromophore to the nonpigmented

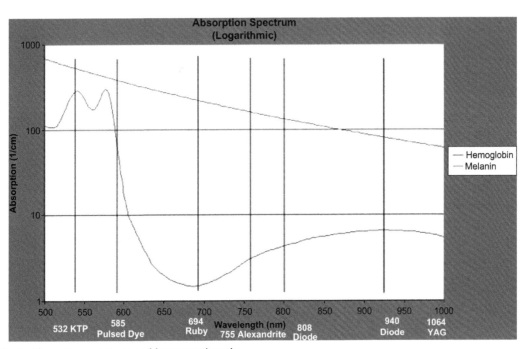

Fig. 1. Absorption spectrum and laser wavelengths.

desired portion. Miniaturization of terminal hairs results in vellus hair formation but not complete removal. Typical laser pulse durations range from 3 to 100 milliseconds. Complete degeneration of the hair follicle with fibrosis occurs with pulses of high energy greater than 20 milliseconds in the red to near infrared spectrum. Super-long pulse heating (>100 milliseconds) seems to allow for long-term hair removal. If the pulse width is too long, there is insufficient time for heat to dissipate, and an undesirable temperature increase occurs with resulting thermal injury to nonfollicular structures that may lead to scarring or pigment irregularities.[9] The ideal pulse duration in laser hair removal is approximately 10 to 50 milliseconds, which is between the thermal relaxation time for the epidermis (3–10 milliseconds) and that for the hair follicle (40–100 milliseconds); this varies based on terminal follicle diameter.[15]

Another variable that can be adjusted in laser technique is spot size. Spot size, the width of the laser beam, is approximately 4 times the width of the target depth, because larger spot sizes allow for less effect of scatter as the laser interacts with the tissue. Hair removal lasers/lights have spot sizes of 8 mm up to several centimeters. Assuming other factors are stable, a larger spot size penetrates more deeply and may improve efficacy by targeting terminal hair follicles located deep in the dermis and subcutis.

Given that melanin is the chromophore, or target, for selective photothermolysis, hair shafts lacking melanin (blond or white hair) respond poorly to laser hair removal[16] and this technique is therefore inappropriate. The best candidates for laser hair removal are dark-haired, fair-skinned patients. Laser hair removal can be performed on tan or darkly pigmented skin but with an increased risk of postinflammatory hyperpigmentation or hypopigmentation. Certain wavelengths or devices, such as Nd:YAG devices, are safer in dark skin types (see later discussion). Because only anagen follicles are susceptible to thermal injury, all protocols for laser/light hair reduction call for multiple sessions in a period of months to attain successful outcomes. Properly timed and dosed treatments to a given area generally result in incremental reduction in hair density after each treatment, but, even after many treatments, an area will continue to grow at least some hair.

The best results with long-term laser hair removal have been shown to correlate with the amount of eumelanin pigment in the hair follicle.[17] To improve results in fair-haired individuals, additional exogenous chromophores including dyes, photosensitizers, and carbon particles have been used. Most recently, studies have been with the use of liposome technology to deliver melanin to the hair follicle. Liposomes are phospholipids (the biologic lipids of cell membranes) that spontaneously adopt bilayers in water.[18] Melanin-encapsulated liposomes have been shown to selectively deliver melanin to the hair follicle and shaft.[19] The studies published to date of liposomal melanin spray have been mixed.[18,20]

PRACTICAL TREATMENT CONSIDERATIONS

Before starting laser treatment on any patients, several important components of patient history should be addressed (**Box 1**). Patients with excessive or sudden onset of hirsutism or hypertrichosis must be worked up appropriately for underlying causes. This requirement is especially important in the nonclinical settings in which underlying conditions may not be recognized or properly addressed. Laboratory evaluation for underlying causes of hirsutism may include total and free testosterone and serum dehydroepiandrosterone (DHEA-S). If polycystic ovarian syndrome is suspected, a serum luteinizing hormone level should be checked as the luteinizing hormone/follicle-stimulating hormone ratio in polycystic ovarian syndrome is commonly increased to greater than 2. Rapid onset of hirsutism warrants the addition of a serum androstenedione level. Androstenedione can originate in the ovaries or adrenals; a level of greater than 100 ng/mL suggests the presence of an ovarian or adrenal neoplasm. Patients should also be questioned on history of

---

> **Box 1**
> **Contraindications/precautions in laser hair removal treatment**
>
> - Contraindications:
>   - Sudden onset of hirsutism or hypertrichosis without appropriate work-up
>   - Active infection with HSV in area to be treated
>   - Pregnancy
>   - Use of gold salts
>   - Recent use of isotretinoin
>
> - Precautions:
>   - History of keloids
>   - History of vitiligo
>   - Diabetic patients
>   - Use of photosensitizing agents (ie, tetracyclines)
>   - Concurrent use of topical retinoids, hydroquinone
>   - Use of nonsteroidal antiinflammatory drugs, aspirin, anticoagulants

hyperpigmentation or hypopigmentation following trauma and inflammation and identified for herpes simplex virus (HSV) prophylaxis if necessary. Areas that are currently infected should not be treated. Most authorities agree that pregnancy is a contraindication to any elective laser treatments.

Patients with a history of keloids need to be warned about risk of increased scarring, and more conservative settings may need to be selected. Ideally, patients should not tan a treatment area for several months before treatment, or for several weeks after each session. For this reason, many laser treatment centers specialize in treating facial or leg areas in winter months, and axillae/bikini in summer months. Pretreatment of areas with hydroquinones may be appropriate for some skin types, as well as diligent use of sunblocks. Patients with vitiligo may need to be warned that pigment loss may increase with laser treatments. Diabetic patients may have delayed wound healing if any sort of epidermal burn occurs. Topical tretinoin as well as hydroquinone products should be withheld for about 2 weeks before treatments. Patients are generally instructed not to remove hair by any method other than shaving for at least 6 weeks before laser treatment to avoid removing the desired chromophore from the tissue.

The use of photosensitizing medications such as tetracycline derivatives needs to be considered. Recent treatment with isotretinoin may increase the risk of scarring. Patients who have taken gold salts must not be treated with lasers because the metal particles in tissue may react with many wavelengths. Patients taking anticoagulants or nonsteroidal antiinflammatory agents may experience bruising after treatments.

After thorough discussion and consideration of all risks, as well as confirming realistic patient expectations, a signed informed consent should be obtained before treatment. Side effects of laser hair treatment must be addressed and minimized. Because melanin chromophores in the epidermis and hair follicle have nearly identical absorption spectrums, there is great potential for damage to epidermal structures resulting in hyperpigmentation or hypopigmentation, because light must travel through the pigmented epidermis to reach hair follicles. As noted previously, the greatest risk is in treating darkly pigmented skin. Skin cooling is a means of minimizing epidermal damage by cooling the superficial structures but sparing deeper, desired targets. Most cooling methods involve extraction of heat by conduction at the skin surface. Three different mechanisms of skin cooling exist, which include precooling, parallel cooling, and postcooling. Some devices have built-in cooling; some use an external cryogen. Many clinics supplement with ice gel packs or the commercially available Zimmer Chiller.

Typically, the area to be treated with laser is shaved before treatment, either at home by the patient shortly before the session or by the treating technician. Failure to do so increases the risk of surface skin burns and interferes with absorption of laser energy at the preferred target, the hair bulb and not surface hair, as well as creating an unpleasant odor.

As with the use of lasers for all conditions, care must be taken to protect from iris or retinal damage in both the user and the recipient of the treatment. This warning is especially true in laser hair removal devices because these lasers are designed to target deeply pigmented structures. Both the retina and uveal tract are highly pigmented. Anterior eye injury usually involves inexperienced personnel trying to remove lower eyebrow hairs without an eye shield in place.[21] Blindness occurs rapidly and painlessly even by experienced dermatologists when only 1% of the beam is reflected into the eye from glossy metal, glass, or plastic surfaces. Eyewear is rated by optical density (OD) at wavelengths corresponding to the laser in use. OD = log (I/T) where I is the wavelength and T is the transmittance of light through the laser. Use of OD 4 or greater is recommended.

Equipment settings vary greatly depending on equipment wavelength, spot size, patient skin type, hair color and density, and the patient's response to previous sessions. During and shortly after treatment, desirable treatment end points of perifollicular edema and/or erythema are observed. Before treating an entire area, it may be desirable to treat a small test area and check for these end points after about 15 minutes. With appropriate cooling, the treatment should not be perceived as painful. Intense erythema or complaints of pain should prompt immediate reduction of energy settings and/or abandoning of treatment. Topical anesthetic creams are not often recommended for this procedure because they increase the patient's pain threshold and increase the risk of epidermal burns.

Further treatments are scheduled carefully to coincide with anagen hair growth, usually 1 to 3 months apart (see **Table 1**). Many protocols indicate that treatments should be repeated when the patient notes any regrowth in a treatment area. After an area of skin is exposed to laser, dormant follicles often are pushed into anagen phase (see **Table 1**) and patients may experience increased hair growth after the first session or two, hence they should be warned about this side effect.

Patients may note skin erythema and a sunburn sensation for up to 2 to 3 hours after a treatment session. Posttreatment instructions vary, and generally include not to tan for several weeks, to keep the areas clean and moist, and to report any skin burns or irritation promptly. Complications include skin erosions or blisters that may result in areas of hypopigmentation or hyperpigmentation or even scarring. Any of these issues relate to treating tan skin, using excess fluence for skin type, or lack of appropriate cooling methods during treatment. Patients who experience any complications should be seen immediately and receive careful guidance to optimize wound healing and minimize the risk of scarring. Note that laser-induced pigment changes may take up to a year to resolve.

Paradoxic hair growth has been noted in areas treated by laser hair removal. This effect tends to occur more often in patients with skin type III or higher, more commonly after intense pulsed light (IPL) treatment, and may occur in areas of adjacent untreated skin.[22] In addition, paradoxic hair growth may be more common in patients with undiagnosed hormonal conditions, emphasizing the need for thorough history before onset of treatment (see later discussion). The effect of paradoxic hair growth is unclear; it is speculated that lower-range fluences of light in darker skin types paradoxically stimulate hair growth.[23] In some cases, changing equipment or settings obviates this side effect, but, in some cases, these patients should abandon hair removal by laser or light methods.

CURRENT LASER TECHNIQUES BY WAVELENGTH

Deep and selective heating of the hair shaft, the hair follicle epithelium, and the heavily pigmented matrix is possible in the 600-nm to 1100-nm region. Several laser devices that emit in this spectrum:

- Ruby (694 nm)
- Alexandrite (795 nm)
- Diode (800 nm)
- ND:YAG (1064 nm)
- Pulsed light devices (770–1100 nm).

RUBY LASERS

Ruby lasers have a wavelength of 694 nm and emit light in the deep red spectrum. Laser hair removal was first introduced with the use of a normal-mode ruby laser in 1996. This first study showed promise in reduction of hair density in light-skinned and dark-haired individuals. Biopsies from subjects showed selective thermal damage to pigmented hair follicles, vaporization of hair shafts, and perifollicular injury. Four of the 13 treated patients

had less than 50% hair regrowth at 6 months.[24] Follow-up study at 1 to 2 years showed that 4 of 7 patients had persistent hair loss.[6] Despite confirmed efficacy of ruby lasers ranging from 30% hair reduction after a single treatment[25] to 60% after multiple treatments,[26] use of ruby lasers for hair reduction/removal has slowed with the advent of new wavelengths and devices.

ALEXANDRITE LASERS

Alexandrite lasers emit light at 755 nm and penetrate deeper in the dermis than the ruby laser discussed earlier. This action allows for improved penetration to deeper dermal structures with less damage to epidermal structures, allowing for treatment of skin types I to IV. Hair reduction rates of 40% to 56% 6 months after a single treatment with a variable-pulsed alexandrite laser have been reported.[27] The 2 long-pulsed alexandrite lasers currently available for use are the Apogee System from Cynosure (Cynosure, Westford, MA, USA) and the Gentlelase System from Candela (Candela, Wayland, MA, USA).

DIODE LASERS

Diode lasers are solid-state laser devices ranging in wavelength from 800 to 855 nm. These devices penetrate even deeper into the dermis and use sophisticated epidermal cooling devices to minimize epidermal and superficial dermal damage. There are several diode lasers currently available on the market, the most popular being the Light Sheer produced by Lumenis (Santa Clara, CA, USA), an 810-nm diode laser with contact cooling device. Diode lasers have shown effectiveness in permanent hair removal studies with efficacy rates of up to 90% with minimal side effects and successful treatment of darker-skinned individuals.[28,29]

ND:YAG LASERS

Nd:YAG 1064-nm lasers are available as Q-switched and long-pulsed lasers. Long-pulsed Nd:YAG lasers are popular for their efficacy in hair reduction and ability to be used in skin type VI. Longer wavelengths have the advantage of increased dermal penetration and reduced scatter of epidermal light; however, absorption by melanin-containing structures is reduced, which is advantageous for epidermal melanin-containing structures and allows for treatment of a wider range of skin types. To effectively damage the hair follicle, higher fluences (power) and larger spot size are used to compensate for reduced melanin absorption. In addition, the incorporation of epidermal cooling devices into the laser devices minimizes epidermal injury and adds to the increased efficacy in darker skin types.[30] Hair reduction has been shown with the long-pulsed Nd:YAG. After 3 treatments, hair reduction rates from 58% to 62% were achieved on facial sites 1 month after the last treatment; for nonfacial sites, reduction rates of 66% to 69% were seen.[31] Reduction rates of 70% are achieved with 5 treatments with the long-pulsed Nd:YAG.[32] Given the high rates of success with this laser and the range of skin types for which it can be safely used, it is of little surprise that the long-pulsed Nd:YAG is popular among those who perform laser hair removal. Several long-pulsed Nd:YAG lasers are currently available on the market. Q-switched Nd:YAG lasers are capable of delaying hair growth but do not cause permanent hair reduction and are more suitable for tattoo removal and other pigmentation issues.[33]

IPL AND OTHER LIGHT METHODS

Intense pulsed nonlaser light sources emit noncoherent multiwavelengths ranging from 590 to 1200 nm with pulse durations in the milliseconds range. These wavelengths are sufficient to penetrate dermal and subcutis structures, showing benefits comparable with laser hair removal. Cutoff filters are used to eliminate short wavelengths so only longer, deeper-penetrating wavelengths (770–1100 nm) are emitted, which are preferentially absorbed by melanin, especially by combining long pulse durations and large spot size. Some devices allow variable programming of wavelength and pulse duration as well as built-in cooling depending on skin type, and have been effective and safe in all skin types from I to VI (Prowave by Cutera, Brisbane, CA, USA).

Several studies illustrate comparable efficacy of IPL against the ruby, diode, alexandrite, and Nd:YAG lasers. Amin and Goldberg[34] compared the decrease in hair count with 4 devices: an IPL with a red filter (Palomar, Starlux RS 65 J/cm^2), IPL with yellow filter (Palomar, Starlux Y, 35 J/cm^2), an 810-nm diode (Lumenis Light Sheer, 28 J/cm^2) and a 755-nm alexandrite (Candela, Gentlelase 18 J/cm^2) and, although all 4 devices showed a decrease in hair coverage after 2 treatments, there was no statistical difference between devices. IPL was superior to normal-mode ruby laser after 3 treatments and patients previously treated with ruby laser who subsequently were treated with IPL achieved a further reduction in hair density.[35] Long-pulsed Nd:YAG showed greater proportion of hair reduction in hypertrichosis of the face, axillae, and legs compared with IPL in darker-skinned individuals.[36]

HOME LASERS/LIGHT TREATMENTS

Home laser/light treatments have sparked much consumer enthusiasm. Currently, an 810-diode laser source reliably induces temporary reduction of pigmented hair when used at home by consumers.[37] However, such devices harness less energy than office-based equipment and hence are less effective; they would have to be used much more frequently than professional devices. In addition, there are serious safety concerns about do-it-yourself laser devices.

WHAT IS ON THE HORIZON?

Because removal of unwanted hair remains popular among consumers, new techniques for achieving the best cosmetic results are developing. Among these techniques is the use of photochemical destruction of hair follicles. Photodynamic therapy is the use of a light and photo-sensitizer to produce therapeutic effects. Aminolevulinic acid (ALA) is a precursor in porphyrin synthesis that is rapidly and selectively converted to protoporphyrin IX by cells derived from the epidermis and follicular epithelium. On absorption of a photon, protoporphyrin IX efficiently crosses into an excited triplet state. Excited triplet states generate singlet oxygen by collision with ground-state oxygen. These singlet oxygen molecules are potent oxidizers that damage cell membranes and proteins. Hair removal with topical ALA has been reported in a pilot study. Mean hair loss of 40% was reported in 12 volunteer subjects after single exposure to 630-nm light 3 hours after an application of 20% ALA to the skin.[38] Goldberg and colleagues[39] combined pulsed light bipolar radiofrequency device with and without topical ALA in the removal of nonpigmented hair. An average terminal white hair removal of 35% was observed at 6 months. With pretreatment with topical ALA, the average hair removal of terminal white hairs increased to 48%. Other porphyrins, chlorins, phthalocyanines, purpurins, and phenothiazine dyes can act as photodynamic agents and are being developed as drugs for photodynamic therapy. ALA or one of these other drugs will likely prove useful for hair removal. Photosensitizers tend to localize in the follicular epithelium, facilitating photochemical destruction of all hair follicles independent of size or color. This approach will potentially provide an effective means of treating nonpigmented hair, which is a limitation with lasers.[40]

SUMMARY

Hair removal by any means is unlikely to decrease in popularity, especially with the advent of laser technology allowing for effective treatment of hypertrichosis and hirsutism. There are many effective laser and intense light sources. Although virtually all skin types can be treated, the ideal target is a dark hair on light colored skin, and, to date, treatment of nonpigmented or vellus hairs has been disappointing with this method. Therefore, the physical hair removal methods will continue to be popular options as well. The practice of aesthetic medicine should include consideration of offering hair reduction using lasers or light sources.

REFERENCES

1. American Society of Aesthetic Plastic Surgery. Top 5 surgical and non surgical cosmetic procedures. Available at: http://www.surgery.org/sites/default/files/2009Top5_Surg_NonSurg.pdf. Accessed August 1, 2010.
2. Paus R, Olsen EA, Messenger AG. Hair growth disorders. In: Wolff, Goldsmith, Katz, et al, editors. Fitzpatrick dermatology in general medicine. 7th edition. New York: McGraw-Hill; 2008. p. 753–4.
3. Rosenfield RL. Hirsutism. N Engl J Med 2005;353:2578.
4. Olsen EA. Hypertrichosis. In: Olsen EA, editor. Disorders of hair growth: diagnosis and treatment. New York: McGraw-Hill; 2003. p. 400–23.
5. Spange JP. Look Sharp! Feel Sharp! Be Sharp! Gillette Safety Razor Company for Fifty Years!, vol. 1. New York: The Newcomen Society in North America; 1951. p. 9.
6. Dierickx CC, Grossman MC, Farinelli WA, et al. Permanent hair removal by normal-mode ruby laser. Arch Dermatol 1998;134(7):837–42.
7. Kalkworf KL, Krejci RF, Edison AR, et al. Subjacent heat production during tissue excision with electrosurgery. J Oral Maxillofac Surg 1983;41:653.
8. Kligman AM. Histologic changes in human hair follicles after electrolysis: a comparison of two methods. Cutis 1984;34:169.
9. Wheeland RG. Laser assisted hair removal. Dermatol Clin 1997;15(3):469–77.
10. Koybashi T. Electrosurgery using insulated needles: epilation. J Dermatol Surg Oncol 1985;11:993.
11. Görgü M, Aslan G, Aköz T, et al. Comparison of alexandrite laser and electrolysis for hair removal. Dermatol Surg 2000;26(1):37–41.
12. Haedersdal M, Wulf HC. Evidence-based review of hair removal using laser and light sources. J Eur Acad Dermatol Venereol 2006;10:9.
13. Anderson R, Parrish JA. Selective photothermolysis: precise microsurgery by selective absorption of pulsed radiation. Science 1983;220(4596):524–6.
14. Hruza GJ, Geronemus RG, Dover JS, et al. Lasers in dermatology. Arch Dermatol 1993;129:1026–33.
15. Lask G, Eckhouse S, Slatkine M, et al. The role of laser and intense light sources in photo-epilation: a comparative evaluation. J Cutan Laser Ther 1999;1:3–13.
16. Hirsh R, Wall T, Avram M, et al. Principles of laser-skin interactions. In: Bolognia J, Llorizzo J, Rapini R, editors. Dermatology. 2nd edition. Elsevier; 2008. p. 2089–97.
17. Liew SH, Ladhani K, Grobbelaar AO, et al. Ruby laser-assisted hair removal success in relation to anatomic factors and melanin content in hair follicle. Plast Reconstr Surg 1999;103:1736–43.
18. De Leeuw J, Van der Beek N, Neugebauer D. Permanent hair removal of white, gray and light blond hair after laser treatment combined with melanin encapsulated liposomes. Available at: www.lipoxom.nl. Accessed August 1, 2010.
19. Hoffman RM. Topical liposome targeting of dyes, melanin's, genes, and proteins selectively to hair follicles. J Drug Target 1998;5:67–74.
20. Sand M, Bechara FG, Sand D, et al. A randomized controlled double blind study evaluating melanin encapsulated liposomes as a chromophore for laser hair removal of blond, white and gray hair. Ann Plast Surg 2007;58:551–4.
21. Hamme S, Augustin A, Raulin C, et al. Pupil damage after periorbital treatment of port wine stain. Arch Dermatol 2007;143:392–4.
22. Goldberg DJ. Lasers and light based hair removal: an update. Expert Rev Med Devices 2007;4:253–60.
23. Tierney EP, Goldberg DJ. Laser hair removal pearls. J Cosmet Laser Ther 2008;10:17–23.
24. Grossman MC, Dierickx CC, Farinelli W, et al. Damage to hair follicles by normal mode lasers pulses. J Am Acad Dermatol 1996;35(6):889–94.
25. Lask G, Elman M, Noren P, et al. Hair removal with the EpiTouch ruby laser: a multicenter study. Lasers Surg Med 1997;(Suppl 9):32.
26. Sommer S, Render C, Burd R, et al. Ruby laser treatment for hirsutism: clinical response and patient tolerance. Br J Dermatol 1998;138(6):1009–14.
27. McDaniel DH, Lord J, Ask K, et al. Laser hair removal: a review and report on the use of the long pulsed alexandrite laser for hair reduction on the upper lip, leg, back and bikini region. Dermatol Surg 1999;25(6):425–30.
28. Dierickx CC, Grossman MC, Farinelli W, et al. Hair removal by a pulsed infrared laser system. Lasers Surg Med 1998;(10):198.
29. Handrick C, Alster TS. Comparison of a long pulsed diode and long pulsed alexandrite lasers for hair removal: a long term clinical and histologic study. Dermatol Surg 2001;27(7):622–6.
30. Gold MH. Lasers and light treatments for the removal of unwanted hair. Clin Dermatol 2007;25:443–53.
31. Tanzi EL, Alster TS. Long-pulsed 1064n, Nd:YAG laser-assisted hair removal in all skin types. Dermatol Surg 2004;30:13–7.

32. Lorenz S, Brunnberg S, Landthaler M, et al. Hair removal with the long pulsed Nd:YAG laser: a prospective study with one year follow-up. Lasers Surg Med 2002; 30:127–34.

33. Kilmer SL, Chotzen VA, Calkin J. Hair removal study comparing the Q-switched Nd:YAG and long pulse ruby and alexandrite lasers. Lasers Surg Med 1998;(12):203.

34. Amin SP, Goldberg DJ. Clinical comparison of four hair laser removal lights and light sources. J Cosmet Laser Ther 2006;8:65–8.

35. Bjerrring P, Cramers M, Egekvist H, et al. Hair reduction using a new intense pulsed light irradiator and a normal mode Ruby laser. J Cutan Laser Ther 2006;8:65–8.

36. Goh CL. Comparative study on a single treatment response to long pulsed Nd:YAG lasers and intense pulsed light therapy for hair removal on skin type IV to VI–is longer wavelengths lasers preferred over shorter wavelengths lights for assisted hair removal. J Dermatolog Treat 2003;14:243–7.

37. Wheeland RG. Simulated consumer use of a battery powered, hand held portable diode laser (810 nm) for hair removal: a safety, efficacy and ease of use study. Lasers Surg Med 2007;39:476–93.

38. Grossman MC, Dwyer P, Wimberley J, et al. PDT for hirsutism. Lasers Surg Med 1995;7(Suppl):44.

39. Goldberg DJ, Marmur ES, Hussain M. Treatment of terminal and vellus non-pigmented hairs with an optical/bipolar radiofrequency energy source–with and without pretreatment using topical aminolevulinic acid. J Cosmet Laser Ther 2005;7:25–8.

40. Weishaupt KR, Gomer CJ, Dougherty TJ. Identification of singlet oxygen as the cytotoxic agent in photoinactivation of a murine tumor. Cancer Res 1976; 36(7 PT 1):2326–9.

The Pelleve Procedure: an Effective Method for Facial Wrinkle Reduction and Skin Tightening

Michael Stampar, DO

KEYWORDS

- Pelleve procedure • Monopolar radiofrequency
- Dermal heating • Facial wrinkle reduction • Skin tightening
- Cosmetic procedures

The use of thermal injury to rejuvenate and repair aging facial skin has been part of the nonsurgical skin treatment for decades.[1] Ablative light-based energies, the gold standard being full carbon dioxide laser resurfacing, offered the potential for remarkable smoothing and moderate tightening at a superficial level but came with significant pain, downtime, healing complications, and unwanted pigment-related changes.[2] To reduce the downtime and complications, lesser-ablative and nonablative wavelengths were devised, but consistent results were still dependent on having the proper skin type, dosing, and healing response. The advent of the use of radiofrequency (RF) energy represented a change away from light-based energy, dependant on generating heat by absorption of energy by a target chromophore.

High-frequency electron flow, RF, generates heat because of the differences in impedance between tissue types (**Fig. 1**).

Streaming electrons flow through the low resistance of the epidermis and dermis and meet the highly resistant fat at the dermal-subdermal junction. The sudden change in impedance turns kinetic energy into thermal energy, and the surrounding tissues are heated. This method not only eliminates the problem of heating unwanted target chromophores in the skin, such as melanin, as seen with light-based lasers, but also allows the heat to be generated in the deep dermis where existing residual collagen bundles are most plentiful. Also present at the dermal-subdermal junction are the connections of subdermal connective tissue bands that run through the subdermal fat to the underlying fascia. A controlled thermal injury reaching the threshold temperature for denaturing collagen of 60°C to 65°C can cause contraction of the thinned collagen in the deep dermis immediately and trigger an inflammatory response that generates new collagen bundle reorganization and thickening evident at 12 weeks as seen on electron microscopy.[3,4] Controlled thermal contraction down the deep connective tissue bands causes a vertical and 3-dimensional tissue contraction, compacting the fatty globules without injuring the fat itself (**Fig. 2**).

This mechanism is in contrast to that of uncontrolled thermal injury in which temperatures obtained in deep tissue can reach or exceed 70°C, causing a necrotic injury, irregular wound contraction, fat loss, and atrophy, which has been reported with pulsed devices.[5] Despite the potential benefits of deep RF dermal heating, the pain associated with the treatments and the inability to generate consistently predictable results continue to plague this technology.[6]

The shortcomings of pulsed RF-based devices include the need to deliver a safe dose without crossing the heat threshold that results in tissue

Disclosures: The author is a paid trainer of new users of the Ellman device. Training travel expenses are paid by Ellman. The author neither holds equity in Ellman nor profit sharing in company sales.
Private Practice, 115 Taylor Street, Punta Gorda, FL 33950, USA
E-mail address: mchstam@aol.com

Facial Plast Surg Clin N Am 19 (2011) 335–345
doi:10.1016/j.fsc.2011.05.012
1064-7406/11/$ – see front matter © 2011 Elsevier Inc. All rights reserved.

- Thermal characteristics of the tissue energy interaction are determined by tissue type and waveform and frequency

- At 4.0 MHz, fat is ~12 times as resistive as wet skin; therefore, broad application of moderate continuous energy allows the energy to penetrate and cause a concentration of heat in the dermal tissue centered at the dermal/subdermal junction

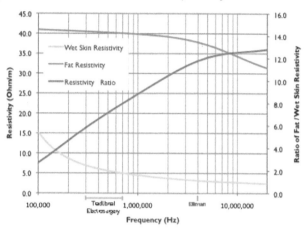

➢ Tissue resistance values are from calculations based upon data and models presented by S. Gabriel, R.W. Lau and C. Gabriel in "The dielectric properties of biological tissues" Parts II & III in Phys. Med. Biol. 41 (1996) and discussed at http://niremf.ifac.cnr.it/tissprop/

Fig. 1. Principles of RF energy.

necrosis.[7] To assure this safety, the treatment protocols are typically the same for all patients, not allowing customization of the dosing to improve treatment outcomes. However, it is obvious that not all skins respond equally to the same amount of energy, thus, the reputation for unpredictable results. Pulsed devices also raise the temperatures rapidly, which can cause pain and necessitates surface cooling to prevent superficial burns. However, without the control of the actual depth of cooling, favorable thermal effects on the dermis, such as wrinkle reduction, horizontal contraction, and shrinkage of pores, can be limited in thinned-skin individuals because of the excessive cooling of the middle to upper dermis. The need to optimize these treatment parameters of the myriad of devices available has been emphasized by many investigators who have evaluated the devices that have come into the market.[8,9]

MECHANISM OF CONTROLLED THERMAL INJURY

The Pelleve procedure, performed using the 4.0 S5 Surgitron (Ellman International, Oceanside, NY, USA), differs from other methods of delivering RF energy because it delivers a progressive but controlled thermal injury to the dermis and subdermis and overcomes many of the shortcomings associated with pulsed and fixed dosed methods.

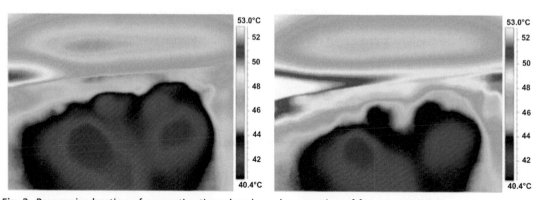

Fig. 2. Progressive heating of connective tissue bands, and contraction of fat compartment.

A 4.0-MHz high-frequency energy is used, so the difference in resistance between the dermal skin and underlying fat is maximal and results in heat generation and diffusion only from the dermal-subdermal junction. The energy delivery is continuous, but because of the constant movement of the electrode over the treatment area, heating is gradual, rather than sudden, allowing the procedure to be painless but thorough when performed properly. A dispersion gel is used on the skin to allow smooth movement of the electrode and immediate dispersion of the energy of the otherwise-focused flow of electrons. Because all the heat generated emanates from deep at the dermal-subdermal junction as seen on infrared images (**Fig. 3**), no direct surface cooling is required and potentially beneficial effects to the middle and upper dermis are not compromised. In addition, because the heat conducted down connective tissue bands is also gradual and progressive, it has been demonstrated that the fat compartments are contracted, giving 3-dimensional deep tissue contraction without the fat cells reaching temperatures that could cause atrophy or necrosis.

This process has been demonstrated in vivo (**Fig. 4**). With progressive heating, the "cloud" of thermal energy rises up into the dermis and down the connective bands. Temperature levels at the surface have been documented to be approximately 20° cooler than those at the dermal-subdermal junction as seen in **Fig. 3**.

The optimal threshold temperatures at, and adjacent to, the dermal-subdermal junction can be reached repeatedly in a controlled manner by monitoring the surface temperature and staying aware of the patient's pain response, which correlates nicely with temperature levels and seems to be consistent from patient to patient.

It has been shown with the Thermage device (Solta Medical, Hayward, CA, USA) that multiple passes at lower energy levels produce more collagen contraction and new collagen production than single passes at higher energy levels.[10,11]

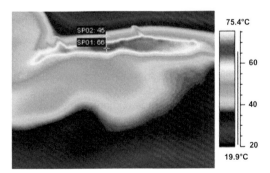

Fig. 3. Sagittal infrared imaging of monopolar heating from the dermal-subdermal junction.

With the gradual heating characteristic of the Pelleve procedure, the patient's response to a threshold temperature of 40°C to 45°C at the surface correlates with a heat sensation of "just getting hot" or a heat perception level of 7 to 8 out of 10. An infrared surface temperature monitor can be used in addition to the patient's feedback so that repeated passes can be preformed to the therapeutic threshold until clinically significant smoothing or tightening is seen in every patient without pain or unforeseeable jumps in temperature to dangerous levels. This subjective goal of repeating passes to threshold temperature until no additional contraction or smoothing is seen in each treatment session can be objectively stated to be 1 pass per decade of age plus or minus one pass depending on the anatomic area and the skin's age and condition. In the case of the Pelleve procedure, a pass is defined as reaching threshold temperature confluently over the entire section being treated, not just covering the area with the probe passing over it, followed by forced cooling for 10 to 20 seconds. This procedure may take 30 seconds to a minute or more of persistently going over an area to bring it to the threshold temperature depending on energy output settings, the speed of the operator's hand movement, and how much area is being treated at once. With experience, higher settings can be used comfortably and passes can be completed more efficiently, which reduces the overall treatment time. So again, a pass is defined as bringing the selected treatment area, that is, half the forehead, cheek, and periocular area, confluently to a threshold temperature of 40°C to 45°C and then cooling for 10 to 20 seconds, maximal 3-dimensional contraction is desired. One pass per decade of age plus or minus one pass in each area seems to be the amount of treatment in a given session to achieve clinically reliable and lasting results. One to 3 sessions may be required to achieve the desired degree of improvement that depends on multiple factors. These factors include age, degree of collagen loss, degree of volume loss, stage of volume loss, and genetic factors. Therefore, a session, single complete procedure, is the completion of the appropriate number of passes to all planned treatment areas. Clinically, it seems that each additional pass generates progressively greater contraction to a point to which no further benefit is seen or palpated, and this technique is what yields predictable results painlessly.

COOLING CONTROVERSY

After several months' experience, using multiple passes from 40°C to 45°C, going on to an adjacent

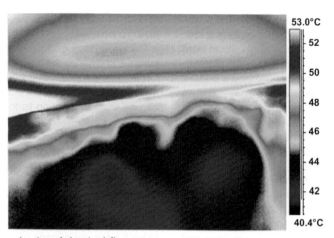

53.0°C
52
50
48
46
44
42
40.4°C

Fig. 4. Infrared images: in vivo abdominal flap.

area to allow spontaneous cooling of the treated area, and then returning to the treatment area, the possibility that the progressive swelling occurring with each pass might overcome the ability for acute tissue contraction became apparent. At that time, I began cooling the treated area directly with frozen reusable cold packs to force contraction of the solid proteins that were being heated and, at the same time, minimized the acute swelling associated with repeated heating. The immediate contraction and firming of the treated area was apparent, and it allowed repeated passes of continuing RF energy on the same areas until maximal contraction was seen without having to go to adjacent areas to allow passive cooling to occur. After only 20 to 30 seconds of cooling, the subsequent passes seemed to trigger an even more significant contraction without the swelling seen when letting the tissue cool passively. The distance between a point on the nasolabial fold and the tragus, for instance, increases after a pass of heat solely but decreases after a pass followed by cooling. The principle of physics governing cooling solids is that all solids, except water, contract with cooling. If application of cold causes even a fraction of a millimeter of additional contraction of the denatured collagen, then each subsequent pass would reach that much deeper and cause greater contraction and increase the density of the layers of deep dermal collagen. This occurrence is apparent on pinching the skin after each pass of hot and cold application.

Some investigators have suggested that heat shock proteins triggered by the injury could be adversely affected.[12] It was shown that only cooling at or less than 5°C adversely affected the tissue's response to injury, and cooling to that level is not advocated here.

To document what I have observed over the past several years, 10 consecutive patients were treated with one side heated to threshold temperature and then cooled for 30 seconds using an iced stainless steel roller and the other side of the face heated to threshold but left to cool passively while an adjacent area was treated. The midface was treated at a setting of 80 for 5 passes; the forced cooling for 30 seconds reduced the temperature to 20°C to 24°C. The opposite midface was treated at the same level for 5 passes but allowed to come to baseline temperature of approximately 33°C passively while an adjacent area was treated. The acute evaluation at the end of the treatment session and an evaluation 1 month later revealed significantly more contraction and lift on the side with cold applied for forced contraction at both end points. All 10 patients felt that the side with cold applied for forced contraction felt tighter at rest and felt denser when pinched relative to the passively cooled side. All patients were then treated the opposite way, and, at the end of the second month, all felt equally tight. The acute response at the end session was the same, the cooled side felt tighter and denser. All 10 patients also felt that the 2 treatments gave significant firmness and tightening to their skin, greater with the second treatment, and each could see an obvious contraction through the midface relative to their pretreatment photos.

INDICATIONS

The ideal candidates for the Pelleve procedure are from their late 30s to mid-40s showing some visible lines at rest, some midface laxity and upper face volume loss, and early neck softening. At this stage, with firm dermal support, all these signs of aging can be significantly reduced or erased with a single treatment or with a second treatment if complete improvement is not seen 4 to 6 months later. The typical Pelleve patients in Southwest

Florida are in their early 50s to mid-60s and have significant wrinkles at rest, nasolabial and melolabial folds, neck laxity, and midface ptosis. The degree of severity of these findings relative to the patient's chronologic age helps predict the success of the procedure outcome and how many sessions will be required to achieve a clinically obvious and satisfactory result. Most patients respond to 2 sessions delivering a pass per decade to each treated area, but fuller faces, extremely thick dermis, and male faces require 3 sessions. Regardless of the chronologic age, the skin responds more promptly with generous dermal density; those with a greater overall volume loss and loss of dermal collagen integrity respond less favorably. However, all skins become more smooth and firm when enough passes to threshold temperature are delivered in a single session. Long-term observations allow patients to be told in the middle of their aging process that the procedure typically needs to be repeated every 12 to 18 months. The youngest and oldest patients are told that it may last for 2 years or more, always relative to how fast they are losing volume. Treatment sessions 4 to 6 weeks apart allow the acute response to the thermal injury to subside. Several experienced physicians from Japan and Russia treat every 2 weeks for a total of 3 sessions and feel no detriment to this schedule. Some patients have been treated as soon as 3 weeks and have seen significant additional smoothing and tightening at that time. In fuller faces, less dramatic changes should be expected with the first procedure because much of the initial contraction is in the anteroposterior dimension, which is more difficult for the patient to appreciate. Once this slack is

taken up, further contraction results in more obvious horizontal contraction. One patient considered a failure after 4 sessions returned after 2 years and showed a remarkable and persistent improvement in skin laxity and the depth of several facial folds (**Figs. 5** and **6**).

In the United States, the Pelleve procedure has received the Food and Drug Administration (FDA) clearance for the treatment of mild to moderate facial wrinkles for skin types I to IV with a duration claim of 6 months. In their submission to the FDA, 87% of the patients receiving a single treatment showed persistent results at 6 months (**Fig. 7**).

In my experience since April 2007, I have seen results last 18 months or more and as long as 4 years in a case of sculpting the midface. Most patients older than 50 years, having no other cosmetic treatment other than 1 to 2 treatment sessions with the Pelleve procedure, return 18 to 24 months later with complaints of progressive aging. Examination of the treated areas usually reveals volume loss resulting in recurring skin laxity. No patient failed to respond to a single additional Pelleve procedure at the time of retreatment, with improved skin tightness, density, and smoothing.

Given that the process of denaturing and contracting the collagen proteins is irreversible, persistence of the result depends on the degree of improvement achieved, the degree of volume loss, and the rate of aging, which includes further loss of collagen, native or newly developed with the procedure. Obviously, the younger the patient and thicker the dermal collagen at the time of the procedure, the longer the result remains visibly apparent. From the perspective of an acute response, no patient has failed to respond to 1 to

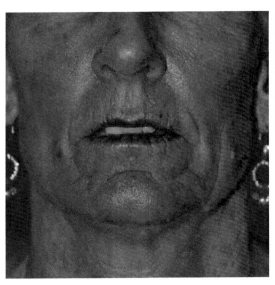 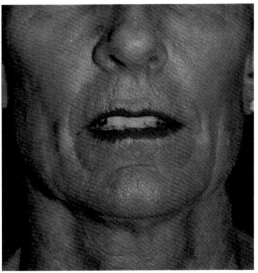

Fig. 5. Two years after failure after 4 treatments.

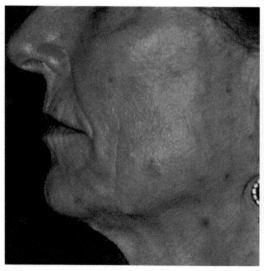
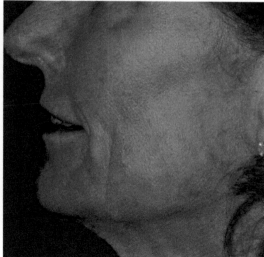

Fig. 6. Two years after failure after 4 treatments.

3 sessions of Pelleve procedure performed as described.

In the process of developing a reliable method to truly "iron" the skin, providing significant and lasting wrinkle reduction and skin tightening, the procedure has been used in almost all patients presenting with aging concerns alone or as an adjunct to neurotoxin therapy, fillers, volume replacement, or surgery for more than 3 years. All patients seeking reversal of visibly aging aspects of their appearance have a loss of collagen integrity, thickness, and facial volume to some extent. Therefore, all patients need a modality that can contract and firm existing collagen and trigger new collagen formation to slow or reverse, to some degree, the process of facial aging.

WRINKLE REDUCTION WITH OR WITHOUT FILLER OR NEUROTOXIN

Surgeons encounter the dense adhesion of the base of wrinkles every time they undermine

a neck and struggle with elevating the adherent base from the underlying soft tissue. The "valley" of any wrinkle is made of dense collagen, and the "shoulders" are made of less-dense collagen, creating the depth discrepancy to be lessened with neurotoxin or effaced with dermal fillers. Most experienced injectors know that some degree of subcision improves filler results by facilitating the migration of the filler material under the deepest aspect of the valley of the wrinkle. Previously, only ablative surface treatments could reduce the shoulder height of wrinkle reduction, but this is not practical for immediate wrinkle manipulation before injecting filler.

Using the Pelleve procedure as a modality to reduce the height discrepancy, reliably, painlessly, and with no added downtime before injection, has created a new treatment paradigm for true wrinkle reduction. This method addresses the cause and then restores the local soft tissue volume loss with the filler material. Vertical contraction of the high sides of a wrinkle or fold is achieved by repeatedly heating and cooling the shoulders of the wrinkle or fold, as well as the adjacent tissue, to flatten and redistribute the associated excess skin (**Fig. 8**). Heating the base of the wrinkle to therapeutic temperatures denatures and softens the collagenous scar, making it pliable, capable of being flattened manually, or more easily manipulated during filler insertion. This deep thermal injury in the therapeutic temperature range, meaning that which triggers neocollagenesis, is synergistic with the filler therapy and should leave the patient with an improved appearance relative to baseline, even after the filler itself is reabsorbed (see **Fig. 8**).

Similarly, using a neurotoxin to immobilize a wrinkled area, so that new collagen formation

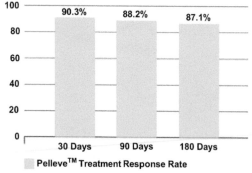

*Response rate of total study population after one treatment with Pelleve (n=93)[1]

Fig. 7. Continued results over time.

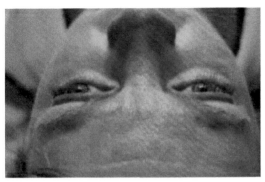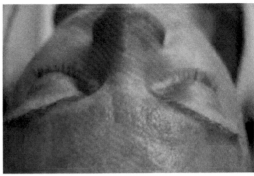

Fig. 8. Rf treatment of glabellar lines and the forehead prior to filler injection.

after the Pelleve procedure can be generated without the repetitive crush-inducing movement that caused the wrinkle, should lead to more effective flattening of the wrinkle. The denatured collagen is softened and flattened, and new collagen can be laid down to restore some of the loss that led to the wrinkle being visible at rest. These expected results have now been observed routinely. Patients who underwent filler therapy returning 1 year after filler placement pretreated with Pelleve procedure persist to have an improvement over baseline, despite the need to augment the soft volume deficit. Although the Pelleve procedure can reduce the resting depth of wrinkles when used alone, patients who have undergone the procedure in the forehead and periocular area while the area is immobilized with neurotoxin return for repeat neurotoxin treatment and show reduced or, occasionally, imperceptible wrinkles at rest relative to their appearance before the procedure.

SKIN TIGHTENING AND VOLUME CONTRACTION WITH OR WITHOUT VOLUME REPLACEMENT

The Pelleve procedure is also a valuable adjunct therapy to facial volume restoration. The midfacial skin envelope becomes lax as panfacial volume loss occurs. Contraction of the connective tissue bands that tether the skin to the deep fascia contracts and firms the soft tissue compartment. With decreased compliance, the volume delivered has a greater volumizing effect. I have used the Pelleve procedure as an adjunct to facial volume restoration for more than 3 years and seen a synergistic effect of triggering new collagen formation. With poly-L-lactic acid (PLLA), "seeds of new collagen growth" via a controlled foreign body reaction are laid down in the same anatomic plane that the Pelleve is triggering new collagen growth via a response to thermal injury. The PLLA injection

procedure can be administered immediately after the Pelleve procedure to bolster the lift and contraction achieved with a properly performed midface tightening (**Fig. 9**). This routine example shows how the skin envelope can be contracted to the residual volume even with an acute weight loss in a woman in her late 50s.

METHOD

It should be noted that this method is consistently referred to as a procedure, not a treatment, a semantic distinction important to obtaining consistent results. Most light-based technology and other RF energy devices have set dosing protocols that define a treatment session, usually developed to be within established safe dosing parameters. The use of the continuous RF energy delivery, with the end point being an obvious clinically evident smoothing and tightening of the skin, has to be approached as a procedure, not unlike a surgery in which certain steps are taken and customized to the patient's needs to reach an optimal end point. As with surgery, that end point should satisfy the provider and the patient.

In evaluating each patient before starting the procedure, standard 5 position photos, vertically oriented hairline to clavicle in height and pinna-to-pinna in width, should be taken. The subject's face should then be assessed for asymmetry side to side in cheek height and fullness and in the flair of the jaw line. See Video 1 online [www.facialplastic.theclinics.com]. With few exceptions, all patients have 3 to 10 mm of asymmetry in the vertical height and length of one side of the face compared with the other when measuring from the lateral canthus to a point on the jawline directly below it. The higher side is also most often fuller with greater overall midface volume, whereas the lower side is shorter with greater volume loss. It is important that this difference be demonstrated to the patient for 2 reasons. First, the patient

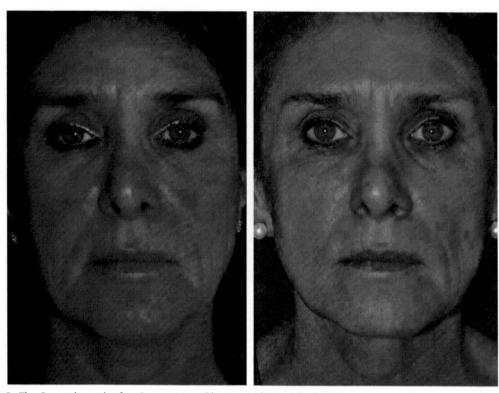

Fig. 9. The 6-month result after 2 treatments (despite 10-kg weight loss).

should not notice this difference for the first time in the postprocedure period and think that the procedure created the asymmetry. Second, it is vital to treat the high side first and exaggerate the asymmetry so that at the half-treated point, the patient will be impressed with the degree of change achieved. If the low side is treated first, the patients who may have never seen themselves as anything but symmetric in the past will be unimpressed if the low side is brought up even with the untreated high side. The flair of the body of the jaw is less often an issue, but, in many patients, one side tapers posteriorly at 45°, whereas the other side tapers back at 60°. If the providers fail to notice this asymmetry, they may grow frustrated trying to get the midface to taper symmetrically when the bony skeletal support is the cause, and not soft tissue fullness. Discussing these findings builds patient confidence in the providers' understanding of the anatomy and also opens the door to discuss volume replacement filler therapy to achieve more youthful height on the low side or balance the face overall after the skin sleeve has been tightened (**Fig. 10**).

All makeup should be removed from treatment areas; jewelry and hearing aids should be removed. Men should be clean shaven. Bearded skin cannot be treated because of the spark gap created by the hair density and thickness, but no

effect on underlying hair follicle growth has been observed clinically. The Pelleve procedure is performed on the facial skin surface where wrinkles and underlying laxity predisposing to wrinkles are present. A 7.5, 10.0, 15.0, or 20.0 mm monopolar electrode handpiece transfers the energy to the patient from the ellman S5 Surgitron RF generator and adhesive disposable return pad that is placed on the upper back skin between the shoulder blades. Pelleve gel is used on all treated skin and adjacent skin areas to avoid burn injury from applying the RF energy to unprotected skin. Only a thin layer is needed to provide smooth gliding of the electrode on the skin. The treatment electrode must always be in contact with the patient's skin and gel before activation to avoid generating a spark gap that can cause pain and a superficial burn similar in size to a razor nick. The treatment electrode should be deactivated before breaking contact with the skin. Any treatment of the periocular skin within the orbital rim requires plastic eye shields inserted after a topical anesthetic drop is applied to the cornea.

Using settings comfortable for the patient which can range from 15-80 depending on the area undergoing treatment, and no anesthetic of any kind that might impair heat perception, the area of skin is gradually heated to a surface temperature of 40°C to 45°C monitored by a handheld

Asymmetry of jaw flair

"High side" vs. "Low side"

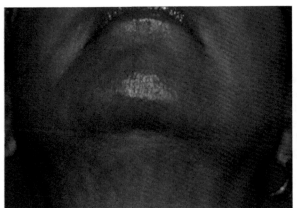
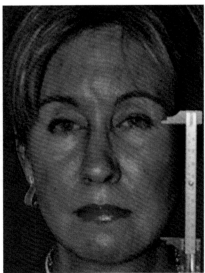

Fig. 10. Common congenital facial asymmetry.

infrared heat gun or the patient's response to the level of heat as "that's getting hot." After hundreds of treatments, the patient's level of pain perception has been observed to reliably predict skin surface temperature. The patient is advised that the sensation goes from warm to warmer but does not have to hurt to work and hotter does not mean a better result. The patients are encouraged to signal if they feel that the heat is about to get too hot to avoid allowing the heat to get to the point of the patient reflexively pulling away. Although the handheld infrared temperature gun is helpful in monitoring treatment temperatures, experience allows the treating personnel to move to adjacent areas or stop treating at the appropriate temperature. Close observation of skin color and texture as well as subtle body language projected by the patient prevents getting to uncomfortable treatment levels.

The ability to rely on patient feedback to guide the treatment comes from the fact that the tolerable target therapeutic temperature of 40°C to 44°C at the surface reflects a 20° differential at the dermal-subdermal junction, and the response to the gradual heating is consistent within a few degrees from patient to patient. Within that temperature range, based on thousands of observations by the author, patients report "that's getting hot" or a 7 to 8 out of 10 on a 10-point pain scale. There should be no pain if the provider remains aware of the tissue and patient response. At 45°C to 46°C, most patients spontaneously pull away. Surface temperatures of 48°C to 50°C, which can cause a necrotic thermal injury, cannot

be reached in an awake subject with no anesthesia. Temperatures less than 40°C does not denature type I collagen and does not give effective lasting results and can be tolerated indefinitely. The infrared temperature gun is useful in preventing undertreatment in patient's whose skin turns red easily at subthreshold temperatures, such as those with rosacea.

Passes of the energy are repeated after cooling the area with cold application to force solid tissue and collagen contractions. The cooling is transient, 10 to 15 seconds per area, and typically takes the tissue down to temperatures in the mid-20s. This heating and cooling is repeated until no additional visible or palpable tightening and smoothing is evident. Objectively this procedure translates to approximately 1 pass per decade of age plus or minus 1 pass (ie, 4 passes for a 42-year-old individual and 6 passes for a 65-year-old individual). Foreheads take fewer passes than the lower face and heavier skin takes more passes than thin skin. The cooling can be achieved with any reusable frozen cold pack or a stainless steel roller soaked in ice water. Typically, the face is treated half at a time, forehead to below the jawline, to allow comparison with the untreated side. Again, as a rule of thumb, 1 pass per decade of age is needed for optimum contraction, and 1 to 3 treatment sessions are needed 4 to 6 weeks apart for maximal long-term results. Single treatment sessions can last for 1 year or more in patients younger than 45 years, 2 treatments are needed for most patients, and 3 or more treatments may be required in extremely heavy or wrinkled skin. No special skin care before or after the treatment is needed, and patients can return to normal activities immediately.

RESULTS

In 4 years of observing hundreds of treated areas, all patients treated had good to excellent results. Although the number of treatment sessions needed may vary with age and skin condition, all skins smoothen and tighten when heated repeatedly in each session to a visible clinical end point. Additional sessions have always yielded greater smoothing and contraction, and no adverse effect has been seen with as many as 5 sessions in 6 months. Performed properly, the procedure should be painless and should present little risk of inadvertent superficial burn injury. Results can last for more than 1.5 years in many patients depending on age and indications, with some wrinkle results showing persistent improvement beyond 1.5 years (**Fig. 11**).

SUMMARY

The Pelleve procedure, done properly and to a truly significant clinical end point with each treatment, can reliably smooth and contract facial and neck skin without pain or downtime. The Pelleve represents a vital adjunct to filler procedures and any antiaging treatment plan, be it surgical or nonsurgical. The key to success in tightening and smoothing skin seems to be the ability to customize the dose, number of passes without concern for safety, discomfort, or cost. Additional safety in performing the Pelleve procedure comes in the form of GlideSafe treatment tips that will be pressure activated, greatly reducing the possibility of a spark gap if patient contact is lost.

TREATMENT PEARLS

- Always start the procedure on the side of the face where the midface appears higher and more full, so at the half-treated point, the result is obvious.
- Always assure you are in contact with the gel and skin before activating the electrode, and deactivate the electrode before breaking contact.
- Use a gloved hand and 4 × 4 sponges to stretch the skin in the lateral brow and lower lateral face while heating, and maintain the tension until cooling is complete.
- In areas, such as the midforehead, upper lip, lateral orbit, and neck, where wrinkle reduction is the first priority, do not apply cold for forced contraction after the last 1 to 2 passes so that the denatured collagen

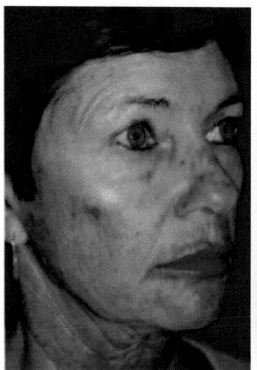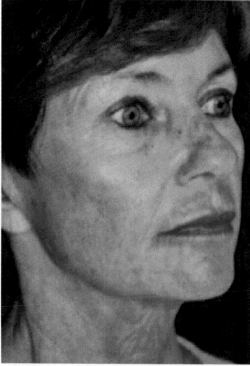

Fig. 11. Full face treated twice 6 weeks apart in January 2008 (January 23, 2008, to September 9, 2009).

can remain hot and amorphous. Physically smoothing over these areas firmly with 4 × 4 sponges may give even better long-term results.

- Encourage these patients to be pretreated with neurotoxin 2 weeks before their Pelleve procedure to avoid "wrinkling your work," and essentially allow the wrinkles to heal immobilized as if they were in a cast.

VIDEO ON PATIENT EVALUATION FOR PELLEVE PROCEDURE

A video showing patient evaluation prior to the performing the Pelleve Procedure is available online at www.facialplastic.theclinics.com. This video focuses on the assessment for asymmetry and other considerations to demonstrate for and discuss with the patient.

REFERENCES

1. Rusciani A, Curinga G, Menichini G, et al. Nonsurgical tightening of skin laxity: a new radiofrequency approach. J Drugs Dermatol 2007;6:377.
2. Fitzpatrick RE. Laser resurfacing. Adv Dermatol 1998; 13:463–501, 1998.
3. Zelickson BD, Kist D, Bernstein E, et al. Histologic and ultra structural evaluation of the effects of a radiofrequency-based non-ablative dermal remodeling device: a pilot study. Arch Dermatol 2004;140:204–9.
4. Javate R, Cruz R, Khan J, et al. Nonablative 4-MHz dual radiofrequency wand rejuvenation treatment for periorbital rhytides and midface laxity. Ophthal Plast Reconstr Surg 2011;27(3):180–5.
5. Fitzpatrick RE, Geronemus R, Goldberg D, et al. Multicenter study of noninvasive radiofrequency for periorbital tissue tightening. Lasers Surg Med 2003;33:232–42.
6. Fritz M, Counters JT, Zelickson BD. Radiofrequency treatment for middle and lower face laxity. Arch Facial Plast Surg 2004;6:370–3.
7. Arnoczky SP, Aksan A. Thermal modification of connective tissues: basic science considerations and clinical implications. J Am Acad Orthop Surg 2000;8(5):305–13.
8. Alster TS, Lupton JR. Nonablative cutaneous remodeling using radiofrequency devices. Clin Dermatol 2007;25:487–91.
9. Biesman BS, Baker SS, Carruthers J, et al. Monopolar radiofrequency treatment of human eyelids: a prospective, multicenter, efficacy trial. Lasers Surg Med 2006;38:890–8.
10. Kist D, Burns AJ, Sanner R, et al. Ultrastructural evaluation of multiple pass low energy versus single pass high energy radiofrequency treatment. Lasers Surg Med 2006;38(2):150–4.
11. Finzi E, Spangler A. Multipass vector (mpave) technique with nonablative radiofrequency to treat facial and neck laxity. Dermatol Surg 2005;31: 916–22.
12. Brown SA, Farkas JP, Arnold C, et al. Heat shock proteins 47 and 70 expression in rodent skin model as a function of contact cooling temperature: are we overcooling our target? Lasers Surg Med 2007; 39(6):504–12.

Radiofrequency: Thermage

Kristel D. Polder, MD[a,b,*], Suzanne Bruce, MD[b]

KEYWORDS

- Radiofrequency • Thermage • Nonablative procedures
- Aesthetic medicine

The demand for safe and effective modalities to improve laxity and appearance of wrinkles has steadily risen over the last several decades. Although ablative laser technology and surgical treatment, such as rhytidectomy and blepharoplasty, provide a proven, evidence-based method of rejuvenation of aging skin, patients often opt for procedures with less downtime and risk for complications, such as pigmentary changes, scarring, and infection. The development of minimally invasive procedures, such as nonablative laser and radiofrequency (RF) treatments, has boomed since the 1990s, leading to a paradigm shift in the field of aesthetic medicine. Patients are willing to accept less dramatic results if there is minimal recovery and risk.

One such nonablative system, the Thermage CPT (Solta Medical, Hayward, CA, USA) uses monopolar capacitively coupled radiofrequency (MRF) to tighten the skin and reduce laxity. This device garnered US Food and Drug Administration (FDA) approval for the treatment of periorbital wrinkles in 2002, facial rhytids in 2004, and all rhytids in 2005. Although there are other radiofrequency devices on the market, Thermage has the most literature and clinical trials published to date that support monopolar radiofrequency as

an effective modality for rejuvenation. Facial contouring and mild to moderate tightening is achieved through volumetric heating and dermal collagen remodeling, and epidermal cooling and the maintenance of an intact epidermis protects the skin from complications, such as infection, scarring, and pigmentary changes.

MECHANISM OF ACTION

The Thermage CPT system consists of 3 components: a generator, a cryogen unit, and a hand piece connected to a disposable treatment tip (**Figs. 1** and **2**).[1–6] The generator provides an alternating electrical current that creates an electric field through the skin that shifts polarity 6 million times per second. The charged particles change their orientation within the electric field. Heat is generated by the tissue resistance to particle movement. Precooling, parallel cooling, and postcooling is delivered via a digitally pulsed cryogen spray on the inside of the treatment tip, thereby protecting the epidermis. For this reason, MRF can safely be performed with all Fitzpatrick skin types (FST).[1] Pressure, current flow, and skin temperature (measured with thermistors inside the treatment tip surface) are monitored using

Author contributions: Drs Polder and Bruce had full access to all the data in the study and take responsibility for the integrity of the data and the accuracy of the data analysis; Study concept and design: Polder, Bruce; Acquisition of data: Polder, Bruce; Analysis and interpretation of data: Polder, Bruce; Drafting of the manuscript: Polder, Bruce; Critical revision of the manuscript for important intellectual content: Polder, Bruce; Study supervision: Polder, Bruce.
Financial disclosure: none reported.
Conflicts of interest: Dr Polder is a principal investigator and has received research support from Solta Medical and Dr Bruce is a consultant for Solta Medical.
[a] Department of Dermatology, University of Texas, 6655 Travis Street, Suite 650, Houston, TX 77030, USA
[b] Suzanne Bruce and Associates, The Center for Cosmetic Dermatology, 1900 Street James Place, Suite 650, Houston, TX 77056, USA
* Corresponding author. The Center for Cosmetic Dermatology, 1900 Street James Place, Suite 650, Houston, TX 77056.
E-mail address: kristelpolder@hotmail.com

Facial Plast Surg Clin N Am 19 (2011) 347–359
doi:10.1016/j.fsc.2011.04.006

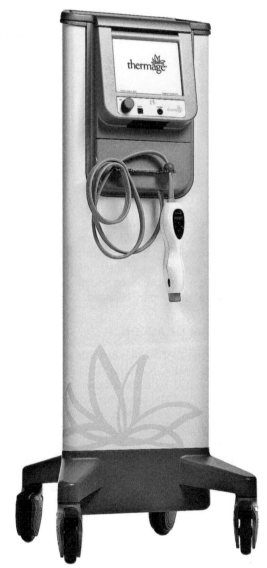

Fig. 1. The Thermage CPT system consists of a generator, a cryogen unit, and a hand piece connected to a disposable treatment tip.

a microprocessor in the treatment tip. Constant feedback from the treatment tip to the computer regulates whether a pulse is fired and the amount of energy fired from the tip. If the treatment tip is not in full contact with the skin surface, or if the skin temperature is too high, a pulse will not be discharged. Heating the dermis to the appropriate temperature while sparing the epidermis is essential for MRF to work and provide the optimal aesthetic result. The MRF system uses the reverse thermal gradient principle in which the epidermis is cooled and preserved while the deeper tissue (including dermal collagen) is heated (**Fig. 3**). The epidermis is kept at 40°C as the cryogen coolant

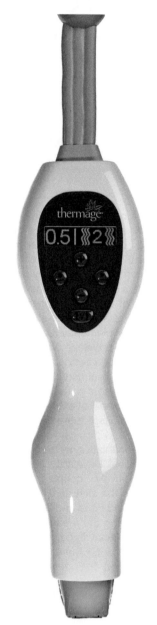

Fig. 2. The Thermage CPT hand piece display demonstrates the fluence setting on the left and the vibration setting on the right. Vibration may be delivered throughout the pulse and decreases pain as perceived by patients.

is delivered. Collagen denaturation occurs at approximately 65°C. Exposure to heating for 10 minutes results in 10% shrinkage of collagen fibers, whereas 60% shrinkage occurs after only 1.5 minutes at 80°C.[7] Thus, the higher the maximum temperature reached during heating, the greater the shrinkage. The MRF system heats the dermis to 65°C to 75°C, which has been confirmed in histologic studies.[8] If suboptimal

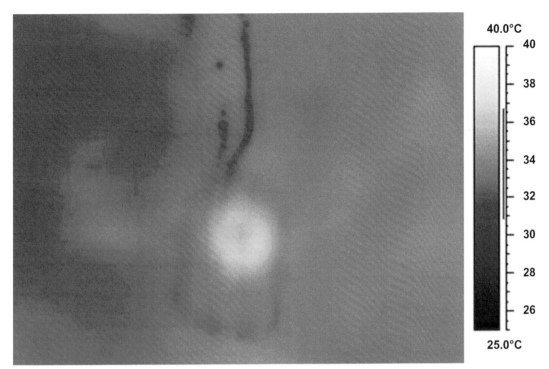

40.0°C

- 40
- 38
- 36
- 34
- 32
- 30
- 28
- 26

25.0°C

Fig. 3. The thermogram illustrates the heat generated by the radiofrequency energy delivered to the skin and subcutaneous tissue during a given pulse. The different colors demonstrate the heat gradient. Thirty seconds after one pulse of the Thermage CPT, 92% of the surface tissue is more than 34°C.

heat is generated, there will be no significant clinical improvement in laxity or rhytids. If excessive heat is generated, erosions, atrophy, scarring, or pigmentary changes may ensue.[9–11]

To ensure a controlled path of travel for the RF energy, a return pad is placed on patients' back and electrically connected to the generator module. Coupling fluid is applied before treatment to ensure full contact with the skin's surface. Cryogen spray is delivered throughout the treatment cycle, and the pressure and delivery of this cryogen coolant is electronically controlled. When the coolant canister is low, a message is displayed on the computer screen for notification.

The MRF device has undergone several name changes since its inception. Multiple names will be mentioned throughout this article, depending on when the clinical study was published. The first MRF device was the Thermacool TC (Thermage, Inc, Hayward, CA, USA) (2002), which was followed by the TC-3 (Thermage, Inc, Hayward, CA, USA) (2005), and then the NXT (Thermage, Inc, Hayward, CA, USA) in 2007. The Thermage CPT (Comfort Pulse Technology, Solta Medical, Hayward, CA, USA), the most recent device at the time of this publication, was released in August of 2009.

CLINICAL EFFICACY AND STUDIES

The ThermaCool TC system represented the first nonsurgical treatment for periorbital skin laxity and rhytids approved by the FDA. FDA clearance of the device took place in November of 2002 for periorbital rhytids, 2004 for facial laxity, and subsequently for the rest of the body in 2005. The initial device had been developed with a 1.0-cm^2 tip, which possessed a slow discharge time. The highest energy tolerated was used and a single pass was performed.[1–6] Because of significant pain, anesthetic blocks and oral pain medication was needed. Further, the results were modest. In 2004, the 1.0-cm^2 tip was then improved upon by a faster discharge time, and later, a larger tip was introduced. However, the treatment was still painful and the results remained modest. In 2006, Kist and colleagues[12] noted that twice the amount of collagen denaturation occurred when 3 passes were performed at lower energy settings rather than 1 pass at higher energy settings.[12,13] Even the highest energy settings did not produce as much collagen denaturation as 3 passes at the lowest settings. Histology was confirmed on facial preauricular skin treated before facelift surgery. This discovery represented a major shift in the treatment algorithm for MRF. Subsequent clinical studies confirmed the previous histologic findings.[9,14,15]

In 2003, Fitzpatrick and colleagues[1] treated 86 patients with a single treatment of the ThermaCool TC system with a follow-up of 6 months to assess periorbital tissue tightening. In this multicenter trial, wrinkle score improvements of at least 1 point on the Fitzpatrick scale were noted in 83.2%, whereas 61.5% of eyebrows were lifted by at least 0.5 mm. Abraham and colleagues[16] found a statistically significant increase in mean vertical brow height of 1.6 to 2.4 mm at 12 weeks when 35 patients with moderate facial aging were treated with a single session of MRF. Hsu and Kaminer[2] treated 16 patients between May 2002 and December 2002 with the ThermaCool TC on the lower face. Eleven of the patients had 3 areas treated, including the cheeks, jawline, and upper neck. Ten patients graded the treatment as mild to no improvement. Five patients graded the response moderate to excellent. Despite the disappointing results, this study brought forth a few points. First, 3-dimensional improvement was difficult to demonstrate via standard photography, and it was determined that more accurate methods were needed to measure skin tightening changes. Younger patients fared better than older patients in this trial, although because of the small numbers in this study, the results were not statistically significant. Third, patients that had all 3 areas treated had a higher percentage of moderate to excellent scores at follow-up.

Several smaller clinical trials indicated mild to moderate improvement in facial and eyelid laxity, with minimal down time and complications using the early ThermaCool TC system. Fritz and colleagues[17] treated 11 patients with a single MRF treatment and 9 patients with 2 MRF treatments. In this study, 2 treatments yielded higher scores in all categories of photographic analysis with the difference in improvement being statistically significant for the nasolabial folds ($P = .04$). Significant improvement in laxity after treatment was seen between the 1- and 4-month follow-up visits in both groups (single and 2-treatment groups). On self-assessment, patients who received 2 treatments reported more improvement than those in the single-treatment group 4 months after treatment ($P = .05$). Results were modest in both groups as noted by both physicians and patients, however. Despite the modest results, 75% (n = 15) reported that they would consider paying for additional treatment, and more than 50% (11/20) reported they would strongly consider doing so.

Tanzi and Alster[18] found significant improvement in cheek and neck laxity observed in the majority of a cohort of 50 patients treated with 1 session of MRF. Consistent with prior data, they found the nasolabial and melolabial folds more responsive to treatment than the jowls and mandibular ridge. A decreased response was found in the neck region. They found a 35% to 40% subjective improvement of nasolabial and melolabial folds and a 30% to 35% improvement in neck laxity. Jacobson and colleagues[4] treated 24 patients with laxity of the neck, nasolabial folds, marionette lines, and jawline with 2 passes performed on the forehead, 3 on the cheeks, and 1 on the neck. Each patient received 1 to 3 treatments spaced 4 weeks apart. Seventeen of the 24 patients demonstrated visible improvement at the 1-month follow-up evaluation. Bogle and colleagues[15] evaluated the multiple-pass, low-fluence algorithm for lower facial laxity in 66 patients at 3 treatment centers. At the 6-month follow-up, independent photographic review revealed improvement in 84% of patients. Patients were treated with 2 passes to the cheeks, upper neck, perioral area, chin, and submentum with the 1.5-cm tip, and 3 additional passes were performed at investigator discretion to areas needing the most skin tightening. The average number of pulses per treatment was 480. At the 6-month follow-up, 92% of patients had a measurable improvement in overall appearance.

MRF has also been shown to improve acne and acne scarring. Ruiz-Esparza and Gomez[19] evaluated the effects of one MRF session in 20 patients and 2 sessions in 2 patients at 72 J/cm², with a follow-up of 1 to 8 months. Patients had moderate to severe scarring, cystic, and active acne vulgaris. An excellent response (75% or better diminution in active acne lesion counts) was seen in 92% (n = 18). Acne was not made worse in any of these patients.

Meshkinpour and colleagues[20] treated 6 patients with hypertrophic scars and 4 patients with keloid scars with MRF. They found no significant differences between control and treatment sites clinically or with hematoxylin and eosin evaluation. There were differences in collagen morphology with increased collagen production (type III > type I) observed. This increase peaked between 6 and 10 weeks after treatment and did not return to baseline even after 12 weeks.

MRF AND FILLERS: COMBINATION THERAPY

As MRF is one part of a larger aesthetic armamentarium, many physicians began to combine MRF with botulinum toxin injections, filler injections, and light- and laser-based technology. Goldman and colleagues[21] conducted a randomized, evaluator-blind study of 36 patients to confirm or refute any possible subtractive effects on augmentation of the nasolabial folds when followed by 1320-nm Nd:YAG laser, 1450-nm diode laser, MRF, or intense pulsed light (IPL) treatment. Thirty-six patients were treated with hyaluronic acid (HA) gel (Restylane, Medicis Pharmaceutical Corp, Scottsdale, AZ, USA) on one side of the face and HA gel followed by one of the nonablative laser/MRF/IPL therapies on the contralateral side. An unblinded treating investigator administered HA gel to each nasolabial fold and bilateral postauricular regions, followed immediately by administration of one of the following treatments: 1320-nm Nd:YAG laser (CoolTouch, CoolTouch Corp, Solta Medical, Hayward, CA, USA), 1450-nm diode laser (Smoothbeam, Candela Corp, Wayland, MA, USA), MRF, or IPL therapy (Lumenis One, Lumenis Inc, Yokneam, Israel). The postauricular area was chosen as the site for retrieval of cutaneous biopsies without cosmetic detriment. Skin biopsies were obtained on the bilateral postauricular regions on postoperative days 0, 14, and 28 in every patient to assess the histologic effect of each laser, RF, or IPL therapy. Blinded investigator evaluations did not identify statistically significant differences in wrinkle severity scores between the nasolabial fold that were injected with HA alone compared with those treated with HA gel and the nonablative laser/IPL/RF modalities. Histologic studies from the small number of acceptable samples showed that HA gel was indistinguishable among patients and between laser/IPL/RF-treated and untreated sites. There was no evidence in this study that concomitant nonablative dermal treatment modified the implanted HA gel. The investigators concluded that clinical and extrapolated histologic data supported the use of laser/MRF/IPL directly over HA gel dermal implants without affecting patient safety or implant efficacy. Alam and colleagues[22] found similar results when RF treatment occurred at 2 weeks after implantation of hyaluronic acid and calcium hydroxylapatite in 5 patients. Each filler product was placed in the deep dermis, 3 cm apart on the forearm in each patient. Light microscopy did not reveal any differences in the filler material between the control arm and the experimental arm on punch biopsy 3 days after RF treatment. Further, Shumaker and colleagues[23] demonstrated the aforementioned findings in an animal model.

However, an earlier study (2005) by Sukal and Geronemus[24] reported one patient with postoperative biopsy-proven granulomas in the nasolabial folds that had previously undergone silicone injections. The granulomas resolved over a 1-year period with steroid injections.

CONTRAINDICATIONS

The Thermage CPT system is contraindicated in patients with a pacemaker, defibrillator, implantable cardioverter-defibrillator (ICD), or other implanted electronic device. An inquiry into the presence of metal implants, hardware, and braces is also important, and treatment should be avoided over these areas. The presence of active skin infection or pathology at the treatment site is a contraindication to treatment. Smoking, autoimmune conditions, prior radiation therapy, and other conditions that impair wound healing are also relative contraindications. Patients who are or might be pregnant are not treated with this device in the authors' practice. Regarding the Thermage Eyes procedure, patients should not have intraocular eye shields inserted if they have had recent corneal surgery, and therefore should not have the eye treatment. Further, after Lasik, patients should wait several months to heal before eye shields can be safely placed.[25]

PATIENT SELECTION

Patient selection is a critical aspect to achieving the desired outcome with MRF. MRF can be safely used in all Fitzpatrick skin types. Ideal candidates for MRF are between 35 and 60 years of age with mild to moderate facial and neck laxity and rhytids, crepey or wrinkled skin, after pregnancy, after weight loss, and with appropriate expectations (**Figs. 4A–6**).[25,26] Patients with severe laxity and deep rhytids are poor candidates for this procedure and would better benefit from surgical rhytidectomy. Patients who are not candidates for surgical intervention or who are unwilling to undergo surgical intervention for rhytids and laxity are also candidates for this minimally invasive procedure. Obese patients or those with extreme skin redundancy are poor candidates for Thermage.[26] Patients who are not ideal for the procedure are those with poor skin quality (excessive photodamage, severe elastosis), poor general or mental health, severely obese, or patients with fluctuating weight.[25] Patients on chronic corticosteroids or nonsteroidal antiinflammatory medication are also poor candidates for the MRF. This procedure is safe to perform on patients who have had prior rhytidectomy or blepharoplasty, laser surgery, botulinum toxin, or fillers.[21–23] Male patients can be treated with MRF without fear of facial hair loss from treatment. For MRF augmentation of the eyelids, optimal candidates are those with mild to moderate dermatochalasis, good skin tone,

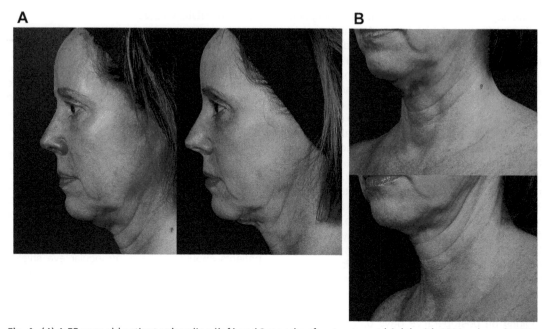

Fig. 4. (*A*) A 55-year-old patient at baseline (*left*) and 3 months after treatment (*right*) with 1200 pulses of MRF to the full face and neck. (*B*) A 55-year-old patient's lower jawline and upper neck at baseline (*above*) and 3 months after treatment (*below*) with 1200 pulses of MRF to the full face and neck.

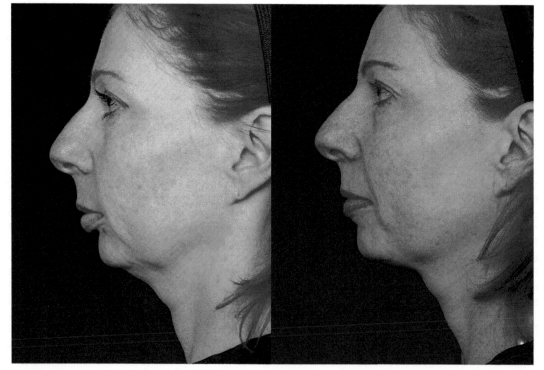

Fig. 5. A 43-year-old patient at baseline (*left*) and 3 months after treatment (*right*) with 900 pulses to the lower face and upper neck.

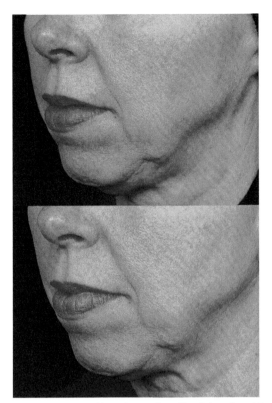

Fig. 6. A 57-year-old patient at baseline (*above*) and 3 months after treatment (*below*) with 900 pulses to the lower face and neck.

with no significant eyelid ptosis, eyebrow ptosis, or herniated orbital fat.[8] Ideal candidates either do not want or do not need blepharoplasty surgery. Those patients who have previously undergone blepharoplasty and who experience a gradual development of laxity are also good candidates for this procedure. Patients must be educated that results are less dramatic as compared with surgical alternatives.

PHOTOGRAPHY

Preoperative and postoperative photography is a necessity for patients undergoing the MRF procedure.[25,26] The authors' practice employs identical lighting, position of the patient, removal of jewelry and makeup, black headband, and a black cape to produce standardized photos (see **Figs. 4A–6**; **Figs. 7–9**). Patients are photographed via a frontal view, left and right side views, and a left and right three-quarter turn angle. Photographs are taken at baseline (pretreatment), at 3 months posttreatment, and at 6 months posttreatment.[25]

TECHNIQUE

Prior to treatment, patients should be educated about expected and potential side effects, complications, and informed consent should be obtained. Patients should be told that the treatment should feel hot, but not painfully hot. A 0 to 4 feedback system is often employed: (0) nothing; (1) warm (this does not hurt at all); (2) hot (just starting to hurt, but easily tolerable); (3) very hot (I can take it but not for long); (4) intolerable (do not do that to me again).[25] Patient feedback is important and is a safety mechanism that prevents epidermal overheating and resultant complications.[9–11]

Patients are positioned on the treatment table, with a grounding pad attached to them. All metal jewelry, makeup, and lotions should be removed before treatment. The treatment area should be gently cleansed. The cable connected to the device is clipped onto the grounding pad and secured, usually on the patients' back. A temporary grid system, supplied by the company, is placed on the treatment area, which guides the provider on pulse placement with the treatment tip. This grid uses a temporary ink transfer that guides the technician on where to place the tip. The grid size will correspond to the area being treated (a grid with larger squares for treatment on the buttocks and thighs is available). The skin should be cleaned with isopropyl alcohol. While the skin is still damp, the paper is placed ink side down over the treatment surface. The paper is dabbed lightly with isopropyl alcohol-moistened gauze until the grid shows through the paper. Prior to and during treatment, the membrane on the treatment tip should be checked to ensure integrity. If there is a breach in the membrane, the energy will not be applied properly and epidermal or dermal injury may result.

Pressure is evenly applied to the skin after coupling fluid is placed on the treatment area. A generous amount of coupling fluid should be used. If pressure is applied unevenly, an error message is displayed on the monitor, which prevents excessive energy from being delivered at one end of the treatment membrane. Pulses are laid down in an adjacent, but not overlapping, fashion. There are 3 main pass techniques: 2 single passes, 1 staggered pass, or 1 super pass. The super-pass technique is the one recommended for use with the most recent upgraded device, the Thermage CPT.[25] This technique corresponds to completing 1 row of squares followed by 1 row of circles on the grid, alternating rows. Staggered, partially overlapping pulses are no longer recommended with the Thermage CPT because this technique is thought to be too

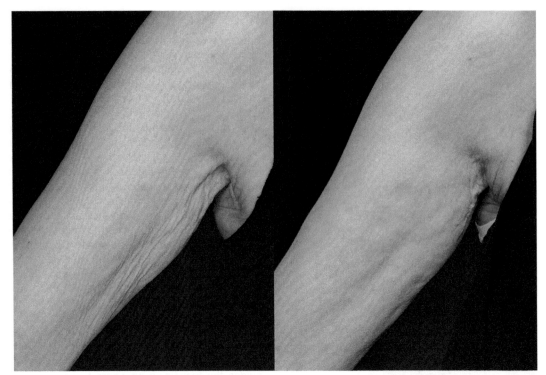

Fig. 7. A 62-year-old patient at baseline (*left*) and 3 months after treatment (*right*) with 400 pulses to the bilateral upper arms (200 pulses per arm, Body Tip 16.0 [Solta Medical, Hayward, CA, USA] used).

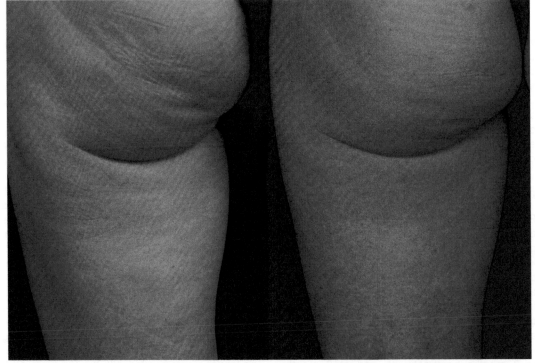

Fig. 8. A 48-year-old patient at baseline (*left*) and 3 months after (*right*) 400 pulses to the bilateral posterior inferior buttocks and upper thighs (200 pulses per side, Body Tip 16.0 [Solta Medical, Hayward, CA, USA] used).

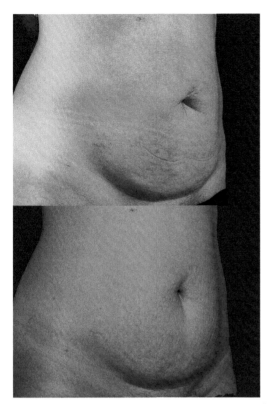

Fig. 9. A 46-year-old patient at baseline (*above*) and 15 months after (*below*) 800 pulses to the lower abdominal area.

aggressive with the upgraded device. Two passes are performed over the entire treatment area. Then, additional vector passes are performed in the direction in which the skin tightening/lift is desired (**Table 1**).[27,28] Three to 5 vector passes are performed in the direction of the desired lifting. If the upper lip is treated, wet gauze can be placed between the teeth and upper lip for comfort. When treating over bony prominences, many providers move the tissue such that more skin and subcutaneous fat is centered over the bony area, which decreases pain and sensitivity over the site during treatment. Similarly, treatment on the forehead can be more painful, therefore, fluence may need to be decreased at this site. Typically, fluence is also decreased when transitioning from the facial skin to the neck. Proper technique is essential on the neck so excess energy is not concentrated under the mandible, where superficial erosions may occur. Full contact with the treatment tip membrane is important to ensure the energy is dispersed appropriately.

Erythema, edema, and mild skin tightening are expected outcomes, and are indicators of clinical efficacy. The provider should observe the skin at all times during treatment, and patient feedback is important to determine if adverse events are occurring, such as epidermal injury. The clinical endpoint is visible or palpable tightening, which has been found to maximize long-term efficacy with the device.[1–6,15,18,25,26,28] The grid is removed after treatment with isopropyl alcohol and the skin is gently cleansed.

If patients are undergoing treatment of the upper and lower eyelids, sterile plastic eye shields must be placed to prevent ocular injury. We place 2 to 3 drops of proparacaine or tetracaine in each eye before ocular shield placement. A small amount of eye lubricant is applied to the sterile shield and secured in place. A small 0.25-cm^2 tip is used when treating the eyelids. A smaller grid is also applied to the treatment area when the eyelids are being treated. A nonoverlapping, nonstaggered method of applying pulses is performed over both upper and lower eyelids after coupling fluid is applied.[25]

Patients are given written instructions on postprocedure care, including expected side effects, timeline for follow-up photography, potential complications, and the clinic number to call if any questions or complications arise.

POSTPROCEDURE CARE

Erythema and edema are expected after MRF treatment. If erosions occur, patients are instructed to call the clinic, and are typically evaluated for concurrent infection or other complications. Biafine topical emulsion (OrthoNeutrogena, Titusville, NJ, USA) or Aquaphor healing ointment (Eucerin, Beiersdorf, Inc, Hamburg, Germany) can be applied to the erosions until they heal. Patients should be followed closely to ensure these lesions do not become infected and are treated appropriately. Cultures are indicated if the erosions develop honey crusting indicative of potential impetigo, or if there is persistent pain, erythema, pus, or drainage.

COMPLICATIONS

The incidence of complications with MRF is low.[9,10] Weiss and colleagues[9] performed a retrospective chart review of more than 600 consecutive patient treatments between 2002 and 2006 using the MRF device and found that the most common immediate and expected side effect was erythema and edema lasting less than 24 hours. Six patients reported edema lasting up to 1 week. Other reported side effects included acneiform eruptions and linear superficial crusts, both of which resolve by 1 week. Tenderness of the neck lasting 2 to 3 weeks was also rarely

Table 1
Tip selection

Area Treated	Lower Face	Lower Face and Neck	Full Face	Eyes Only	Eyes and Periorbital	Eyes and Full Face	Small Torso, Under Bra Areas, Just Above Knees	Average Torso, Thighs, Arms	Large Torso, Love Handles, Buttocks, Larger Thighs
Tip Suggested	Face tip 600 REPs	Face tip 900 REPs	Face tip 900 REPs	Eye tip 450 REPs	Eye tip 450 REPs plus face tip 100–200 REPs	Eye tip 450 REPs plus face tip 600–900 REPs	1 Body 16.0 tip 175–250 REPs	1–2 Body 16.0 tips 250–325 REPs	2–3 Body 16.0 tips 325 or more REPs
Full Passes	2 passes 4–5 vector passes	2–3 passes 4–5 vector passes	2–3 passes 4–5 vector passes	4–5 passes with eye tip	4–5 passes with eye tip 2–5 passes with face tip	4–5 passes with eye tip 2–5 passes with face tip	2 passes 1–2 vector passes	2 passes 2–3 vector passes	2–3 passes multiple vector passes
Procedure Time (min)	45–60	60–90	60–90	20–30	30–45	60–120	30–40	40–50	50–60 +

Abbreviation: REPs, repetitions, or pulses.

reported. This group found the overall rate of temporary unexpected adverse effects to be 2.7%. Fritz and colleagues[17] reported that most patients experienced mild to moderate erythema and mild edema after treatment in their small study of 20 patients; however, 1 patient experienced an exacerbation of her temporomandibular joint symptoms after her first treatment. These symptoms resolved fully after 2 months. Abraham and Ross[26] reported transient skin numbness in 5 patients (14%) after treatment; however, this was in the early studies using MRF with a high-fluence, single-pass algorithm that is no longer employed with MRF. As physicians adopted the low-fluence, multiple-pass technique, complication rates fell.

In 2007, De Felipe and colleagues[10] performed a retrospective review of 290 patients treated with 757 MRF treatments. This group found second-degree burns in 2.7% of their treatment sessions, with persistent erythema (1.22%), headaches, scarring, fat atrophy, burn in the return pad site, neuralgia, and facial palsy occurring less frequently. The group acknowledged that the facial palsy was possibly coincidental. The overall percentage of edema lasting 24 hours was 0.68%; edema lasting 48 hours was 0.53%; and third-degree burn with scar was 0.26% of 757 sessions of MRF performed.

De Felipe and Redondo studied an animal model to determine the etiology of fat atrophy post MRF treatment.[29] In contrast to the dermis, fatty tissue may more readily heat because of high inherent electrical resistance. The temperature in the fat is estimated to rise 7 times that of the dermis when treated with a radiofrequency device. Three age-matched pigs were tattooed with 3 16-cm^2 surface area (4 × 4) treatment squares per pig. Treatment was then performed using a 1-cm^2 tip. Area A was treated with 150 J/cm^2 (precooling was performed and skin contact occurred over 2.0 seconds); area C received a total of 4 seconds of cooling (precooled for 2 seconds, plus an additional frozen gel pack for 2 seconds) and the same amount of MRF at 150 J/cm^2; area B served as the control with no treatment. Treated and untreated areas were biopsied with a 6-mm punch biopsy at 4, 8, and 20 weeks after initial treatment. Area A was treated much the same way the earlier high-fluence, single-pass algorithm was performed (2 seconds of cooling followed by 2.3 seconds of 150 J/cm^2 MRF followed by 2 seconds of postcooling), and in all 3 pigs, a clinical scar developed, which was confirmed histologically. Area C was treated with the same energy density; however, precooling time was increased to 4 seconds and a frozen gel pack was applied

before treatment. No scars developed in area C; however, several depressions were noted 1 month after treatment. It was therefore postulated that the increased precooling resulted in heating of the deeper layers of tissue, leading to disruption of the fat lobules, including dissolution of adipocyte cell membranes at 8 and 20 weeks after treatment and confirmed on punch biopsy. In contrast, 2 seconds of precooling with treatment at 150 J/cm^2 allowed for more energy to heat the dermis, precipitating a dermal scar (area A). Atrophy has been attributed to pulse stacking and accumulation of heat in the lower layers of skin. Newer treatment tips (since 2007) deliver MRF more readily, decreasing the cycle of the tip, and have reduced posttreatment atrophy to almost zero. Further, coolant is now delivered concurrently throughout the entire treatment cycle on the CPT device. Finally, there is a 10-fold lower risk of subcutaneous fat atrophy (estimated risk based on incidents reported to the manufacturer, 1/10,000 cases) when more passes are performed at lower fluences.

As more and more physicians adopted the multiple-pass, low-fluence treatment algorithm, the overall adverse event rate has declined. With the newest treatment algorithm, the overall adverse event percentage has fallen to less than 0.05%.[11]

NONFACIAL TREATMENTS

Anolik and colleagues[30] performed a blinded, multicenter study evaluating the safety and efficacy of the MRF to treat mild to moderate abdominal skin laxity in 12 patients using the Thermage Multiplex Tip. All patients were women with no previous procedures or surgeries on or near the targeted treatment area, including cesarean sections; having less than 5% variation in body weight during the past year; and being within 20% of her body weight. Seven patients returned for all follow-up evaluations at 1, 2, 4, and 6 months after treatment. At each of the follow-up visits, a decrease in skin laxity was observed when compared with baseline assessment, and a decrease in waist circumference was also reported. Twelve patients demonstrated an average 1.4-cm reduction in waist circumference at the 1-month follow-up. The 9 patients who returned for the 6-month follow-up evaluation demonstrated an average 0.9-cm reduction in waist circumference from baseline. All patients but one demonstrated global aesthetic improvement. Patient satisfaction scores paralleled global aesthetic improvement scores. The percentage of patients claiming satisfaction (scores of either very or somewhat satisfied) among those who followed up was 89%, 80%, and 78% at follow-up visits 2, 4, and 6 months after treatment, respectively. Transient erythema and edema of treated skin was observed immediately following treatment and subsided within hours of the procedure. There were no unexpected side effects or adverse events observed during the trial.

Suh and colleagues[31] treated 37 FST III to IV patients with abdominal striae with both the 585-nm pulsed dye laser and the Thermacool TC. Patients underwent both treatments at baseline, and then were treated with the pulsed dye laser at fluences of 3.0 J/cm^2 (10 mm spot size) at weeks 4 and 8. Skin punch biopsies were performed on 9 of 37 patients, demonstrating increased and thickened dermal collagen. Staining of elastic fibers revealed increased uptake in the upper dermis or mid-dermis. All 9 specimens showed increased collagen, but only 6 specimens were found to have increased elastic fibers. Thirty-three of 37 patients were assessed as "good or very good" with respect to overall improvement of striae. Also, 33 (89.2%) of 37 patients had a net decrease in the width of the widest striae at week 12.

SUMMARY

In summary, MRF represents a minimally invasive method of facial, eyelid, neck, and nonfacial rejuvenation. Many clinical studies have shown this device to improve mild to moderate rhytids and reduce skin laxity. Although there are other radiofrequency devices currently available, MRF has the most literature and clinical trials published to date, which support this method as an effective modality for rejuvenation. Facial contouring and mild to moderate tightening is achieved through volumetric heating and dermal collagen remodeling. The optimal candidate for this procedure is a patient in his or her 30s to 60s with mild to moderate facial laxity that lacks the need for a surgical procedure. MRF using the Thermage CPT system offers minimal downtime with a favorable side-effect profile. Future studies should focus on the nonfacial use of the device on the upper arms, anterior thighs, as well as combination treatments with laser resurfacing, injectables, and intense pulsed light to determine qualitatively and quantitatively if additive effects on dermal collagen can be obtained.

TIPS FOR BEGINNERS

1. Realistic expectations must be set before the procedure.

2. Standardized photography is essential pretreatment and at 3 and 6 months after treatment. Many physicians also obtain immediate posttreatment photographs. Photographs taken at several angles assist in detecting subtle differences and 3-dimensional effects.

3. Absolute contraindications include treatment on patients with a pacemaker, defibrillator, ICD, or other implanted electronic device.

4. Appropriate patient selection is paramount for treatment with MRF.

5. The low-fluence, multiple-pass technique has been shown to attain greater collagen denaturation and skin tightening than the earlier single-pass, high-fluence technique.

6. Vector passes should be performed in the direction the tissue is desired to move.

7. The clinical endpoint is visible or palpable tightening, which has been found to maximize long-term efficacy with the device.

REFERENCES

1. Fitzpatrick R, Geronemus R, Goldberg D, et al. Multicenter study of non-invasive radiofrequency for periorbital tissue tightening. Lasers Surg Med 2003;33: 232–42.

2. Hsu TS, Kaminer MS. The use of nonablative radiofrequency technology to tighten the lower face and neck. Semin Cutan Med Surg 2003;22:115–23.

3. Iyer S, Suthamjariya J, Fitzpatrick RE. Using a radiofrequency energy device to treat the lower face: a treatment paradigm for a nonsurgical facelift. J Cosmet Dermatol 2003;16:37–40.

4. Jacobson LG, Alexaides-Armenakas M, Bernstein L, et al. Treatment of nasolabial fold and jowls with a noninvasive radiofrequency device. Arch Dermatol 2003;139:1371–2.

5. Ruiz-Esparza J, Gomez JB. The medical facelift: a noninvasive, nonsurgical approach to tissue tightening in facial skin using nonablative radiofrequency. Dermatol Surg 2003;29:325–32.

6. Narins DJ, Narins RS. Non-surgical radiofrequency facelift. J Drugs Dermatol 2003;2:495–500.

7. Arnoczky SP, Aksan A. Thermal modification of connective tissues: basic science considerations and clinical implications. J Am Acad Orthop Surg 2000;8:305–13.

8. Biesman BS. Advances in technology-based eyelid skin rejuvenation. J Cosmet Dermatol 2007;20:751–6.

9. Weiss RA, Weiss MA, Munavalli G, et al. Monopolar radiofrequency facial tightening: a retrospective analysis of efficacy and safety in over 600 treatments. J Drugs Dermatol 2006;5:707–12.

10. De Felipe I, Del Cueto SR, Perez E, et al. Adverse reactions after non-ablative radiofrequency: follow-up of 290 patients. J Cosmet Dermatol 2007;6:163–6.

11. Narins RS, Tope WD, Pope K, et al. Overtreatment effects associated with a radiofrequency tissue-tightening device: rare, preventable, and correctable with subcision and autologous fat transfer. Dermatol Surg 2006;32:115–24.

12. Kist D, Burns AJ, Sanner R, et al. Ultrastructural evaluation of multiple pass low energy versus single pass high energy radiofrequency treatment. Lasers Surg Med 2006;38:150–4.

13. Zelickson BD, Kist D, Bernstein E, et al. Histological and ultrastructural evaluation of the effects of a radio-frequency-based non-ablative dermal remodeling device. Arch Dermatol 2004;140:204–9.

14. Sasaki G, Tucker B, Gaston M. Clinical parameters for predicting efficacy and safety with nonablative monopolar radiofrequency treatments to the forehead, face and neck. Aesthet Surg J 2007;5:376–87.

15. Bogle MA, Ubelhoer N, Weiss RA, et al. Evaluation of the multiple pass, low fluence algorithm for radiofrequency tightening of the lower face. Lasers Surg Med 2007;39:210–7.

16. Abraham M, Chiang S, Keller G, et al. Clinical evaluation of non-ablative radiofrequency facial rejuvenation. J Cosmet Laser Ther 2004;6:136–44.

17. Fritz M, Counters JT, Zelickson BD. Radiofrequency treatment for middle and lower face laxity. Arch Facial Plast Surg 2004;6:370–3.

18. Alster TS, Tanzi E. Improvement of neck and cheek laxity with a nonablative radiofrequency device: a lifting experience. Dermatol Surg 2004;30:503–7.

19. Ruiz-Esparza J, Gomez JB. Nonablative radiofrequency for active acne vulgaris: the use of deep dermal heat in the treatment of moderate to severe active acne vulgaris (Thermotherapy): a report of 22 patients. Dermatol Surg 2003;29:333–9.

20. Meshkinpour A, Ghasri P, Pope K, et al. Treatment of hypertrophic scars and keloids with a radiofrequency device: a study of collagen effects. Lasers Surg Med 2005;37:343–9.

21. Goldman MP, Alster TS, Weiss R. A randomized trial to determine the influence of laser therapy, monopolar radiofrequency treatment, and intense pulse light therapy administered immediately after hyaluronic acid gel implantation. Dermatol Surg 2007;33:535–42.

22. Alam M, Levy R, Pavjani U, et al. Safety of radiofrequency treatment over human skin previously injected with medium-term injectable soft-tissue augmentation materials: a controlled pilot trial. Lasers Surg Med 2006;38:205–10.

23. Shumaker PR, England LJ, Dover JS, et al. Effect of monopolar radiofrequency treatment over soft-tissue fillers in an animal model: part 2. Lasers Surg Med 2006;38:211–7.

24. Sukal SA, Geronemus RG. Thermage: the nonablative radiofrequency for rejuvenation. Clin Dermatol 2008;26:602–7.

25. Thermage Treatment Reference Guide. Hayward (CA): Solta Medical; 2010. p. 1–37.

26. Abraham MT, Ross EV. Current concepts in nonablative radiofrequency rejuvenation of the lower face and neck. Facial Plast Surg 2005;21:65–73.

27. Finzi E, Spangler A. Multipass vector (mpave) technique with nonablative radiofrequency to treat facial and neck laxity. Dermatol Surg 2005;31:916–22.

28. Dover JS, Zelickson B, 14-Physician Multispecialty Consensus Panel. Results of a survey of 5,700 patient monopolar radiofrequency facial skin tightening treatments: assessment of a low-energy multiple-pass technique leading to a clinical end point algorithm. Dermatol Surg 2007;33:900–7.

29. De Felipe I, Redondo P. Animal model to explain fat atrophy using nonablative radiofrequency. Dermatol Surg 2007;33:141–5.

30. Anolik R, Chapas AM, Brightman LA, et al. Radiofrequency devices for body shaping: a review and study of 12 patients. Semin Cutan Med Surg 2009;28:236–43.

31. Suh DH, Chang KY, Son HC, et al. Radiofrequency and 585-nm pulsed dye laser treatment of striae distensae: a report of 37 Asian patients. Dermatol Surg 2007;33:29–34.

Aging Facial Skin: Infrared Broad Band Light Technologies

Macrene Alexiades-Armenakas, MD, PhD

KEYWORDS

- Infrared broadband light • Skin laxity • Rhytids
- Laser and related technologies

Skin tightening is a term often used to describe the treatment of skin laxity by laser and light-energy–based procedures, most notably radiofrequency and infrared wavelengths.[1,2] Skin laxity on the face and neck is manifested by progressive loss of skin elasticity, loosening of connective tissue framework, deepening and redundancy of skin folds, and progressive prominence of submandibular and submental tissues. A classification scale of skin laxity has been validated that categorizes progressive appearance of hallmark clinical findings into clinical laxity grades.[3] Intrinsic genetic factors and extrinsic factors, such as photoaging, contribute to skin laxity, as evinced by genetic skin disorders with mutations in filaggrin and other elastin genes, and the histopathologic findings of solar elastosis of photoaged skin, respectively.[3–5]

Although no device has yet to receive approval from the Food and Drug Administration (FDA) for treatment of skin laxity, it has become evident in the laser and light field that devices inducing volumetric heating, such as radiofrequency or infrared wavelengths, treat this condition with a process conventionally referred to as skin tightening.[1–3] Since its inception with the approval of the monopolar radiofrequency device Thermage (Solta, Hayward, CA, USA) in 2002 for the treatment of rhytids, volumetric heating has progressed with the development of further generations of radiofrequency devices, and more recently, the application of infrared wavelengths.[1,3,6] Combination bipolar radiofrequency and infrared laser or intense pulsed light were FDA approved for wrinkle reduction in 2006.[7] Subsequently, a combination unipolar and bipolar radiofrequency device was developed, which was FDA approved for rhytid reduction on-face and off-face in 2007.[8] Infrared wavelengths were then used for volumetric heating with the introduction of the 1100-nm to 1800-nm infrared light device (Titan, Cutera, Brisbane, CA, USA), which was FDA approved for deep dermal heating in 2006.[9] A variable-depth targeting infrared laser (1310 nm, Candela, Wayland, MA, USA) was also studied for skin tightening.[10] Thus, radiofrequency and infrared wavelengths have been used for the treatment of skin laxity, although until now reserved by FDA approval to the treatment of rhytids and/or deep dermal heating.

Skin-tightening technologies evolved rapidly over the past decade toward augmented efficacy, faster treatment times, and minimization of pain and side effects. Given that these technologies are applied on the skin surface, a major limiting factor to the delivery of adequate thermal injury to dermal targets was the heating of the epidermis and dermo-epidermal junction (DEJ). Initially, the application of high fluences with skin surface radiofrequency technologies were associated with severe pain and a low incidence (0.36%) of thermal burns.[6] In addition, this early protocol yielded dramatic improvement in a small subset of patients, and a lack of appreciable efficacy in most.[11] The pain and safety concerns resulted in a modification of the protocol to low fluence and increased pass

Disclosures: Dr Alexiades-Armenakas received a research grant to develop the mobile technique for the Titan device by Cutera. She does not serve as a consultant to any laser company nor does she hold stock or stock options in any laser company.
Department of Dermatology, Dermatology and Laser Surgery Center, Yale University School of Medicine, 955 Park Avenue, New York, NY 10028, USA
E-mail address: dralexiades@nyderm.org

Facial Plast Surg Clin N Am 19 (2011) 361–370
doi:10.1016/j.fsc.2011.05.001
1064-7406/11/$ – see front matter © 2011 Published by Elsevier Inc.

Notes to early users: Infrared Broadband Light Tips and Techniques

The application of infrared broadband light to the treatment of facial and neck skin laxity has contributed greatly to the laser, light-based, and energy-based technologies designed to deliver volumetric heating in the treatment of skin laxity. When applied and used properly, infrared broadband (1100 to 1800 nm) light yields consistent and reproducible improvements in skin laxity to the face and neck without recovery time, side effects, or significant complications.

Patient Consult

Early users are advised to start with careful patient selection. Patients with a baseline skin laxity of 2 to 3 on the 4-point quantitative laxity grading scale (**Table 1**) are optimal candidates; patients with severe skin laxity of grade 4 should expect the necessity for more treatment sessions to obtain appreciable improvement. Patients older than 65 are less responsive because of age-related changes in connective tissue.

The consultation should entail the presentation of all treatment options, including the surgical facelift.

The rare risk of a burn and the ensuing rare potential for a scar should be discussed during the informed consent process. The device is approved by the Food and Drug Administration for deep dermal heating and the application for the treatment of rhytids and skin laxity are off-label.

It is imperative to take baseline digital photographs of all patients so as to track progress with each treatment. Patients should be advised that results will start to become evident 2 weeks following the first treatment and that 2 to 3 monthly treatment sessions are required for significant improvement for patients with baseline laxity grade of 2 to 3 and 5 to 6 treatments for baseline laxity grade 3.5 to 4.0.

Technique

Early users are advised to start with the mobile technique at conservative fluences of 44 to 46 J/cm² for the face and 42 to 44 J/cm² to the neck. Apply ample aqueous gel to the area to be treated. A series of 8 passes to each row along the face and neck should be administered, so that the total pulse count for the face and neck should number 800.

As one develops experience with the device, the fluence may be titrated up to as high as 50 J/cm² for the face and 47 J/cm² for the neck as tolerated by the patient. Special attention should be given to treating the mandibular or bony prominences so that the sapphire tip is in full contact with the gel and parallel with the skin surface. Continual rapid movement of the tip is necessary to prevent discomfort and virtually eliminate the risk of burns. Total pulse counts for a face and neck treatment vary, depending on the size of the face and neck, and typically run between 200 and 400 pulses.

Maintenance and Follow-up

Patients should be followed at a 1-month interval and repeat photography is advised at each visit. Patients should be told at the outset that the final clinical outcome will take up to 6 to 12 months to manifest following the final treatment, paralleling the time course of neocollagenesis and neoelastogenesis. Maintenance treatments are generally advised once every 6 months.

---

counts, which greatly improved tolerability but lengthened treatment time to approximately 1 hour.[12] In an effort to increase the speed and efficiency of radiofrequency energy delivery to dermal structures, while allowing for cooling of epidermal and DEJ structures, a mobile protocol was developed.[8] A unipolar and bipolar radiofrequency device was used by moving the handpiece on the skin in a continuous motion, which was shown to render the treatment painless and virtually eliminate the risk of burns or complications.[8] In that publication, the rationale for this approach was put forth, demonstrating that the thermal relaxation time of the cutaneous pain sensory nerve fibers was substantially shorter than that of the dermal collagen fibers.[8] Mobile delivery of radiofrequency energy therefore allowed for cooling of these superficial sensory afferents while continuing to deposit energy into the large dermal targets, thereby precluding the firing of pain afferents and rendering the process painless.[8]

In 2006, an infrared broadband (1100 to 1800 nm) light device was introduced and FDA approved for deep dermal heating. It was soon applied to the treatment of skin laxity on the face and neck in a pilot study of 25 patients treated with a single-treatment infrared 1100-nm to 1800-nm broadband light with the stationary technique at 20 to 40 J/cm² and using topical anesthesia.[13] These findings were reproduced on

Table 1
Quantitative comprehensive grading scale of rhytides, laxity, and photoaging

Grading Scale	Descriptive Parameter	Categories of Skin Aging and Photodamage						
		Rhytides	Laxity	Elastosis	Dyschromia	Erythema-Telangiectasia (E-T)	Keratoses	Texture
0	None	None	None	None	None	None	None	None
1	Mild	Wrinkles in motion, few, superficial	Localized to nasolabial (nl) folds	Early, minimal yellow hue	Few (1–3) discrete small (<5 mm) lentigines	Pink E or few T, localized to single site	Few	Subtle irregularity
1.5	Mild	Wrinkles in motion, multiple, superficial	Localized, nl and early melolabial (ml) folds	Yellow hue or early, localized periorbital (po) elastotic beads (eb)	Several (3–6), discrete small lentigines	Pink E or several T localized 2 sites	Several	Mild irregularity in few areas
2	Moderate	Wrinkles at rest, few, localized, superficial	Localized, nl/ml folds, early jowels, early submental/submandibular (sm)	Yellow hue, localized po eb	Multiple (7–10), small lentigines	Red E or multiple T localized to 2 sites	Multiple, small	Rough in few, localized sites
2.5	Moderate	Wrinkles at rest, multiple, localized, superficial	Localized, prominent nl/ml folds, jowels and sm	Yellow hue, po and malar eb	Multiple, small and few large lentigines	Red E or multiple T, localized to 3 sites	Multiple, large	Rough in several, localized areas
3	Advanced	Wrinkles at rest, multiple, forehead, periorbital and perioral sites, superficial	Prominent nl/ml folds, jowels and sm, early neck strands	Yellow hue, eb involving po, malar and other sites	Many (10–20) small and large lentigines	Violaceous E or many T, multiple sites	Many	Rough in multiple, localized sites
3.5	Advanced	Wrinkles at rest, multiple, generalized, superficial; few, deep	Deep nl/ml folds, prominent jowels and sm, prominent neck strands	Deep yellow hue, extensive eb with little uninvolved skin	Numerous (>20) or multiple large with little uninvolved skin	Violaceous E, numerous T little uninvolved skin	Little uninvolved skin	Mostly rough, little uninvolved skin
4	Severe	Wrinkles throughout, numerous, extensively distributed, deep	Marked nl/ml folds, jowels and sm, neck redundancy and strands	Deep yellow hue, eb throughout, comedones	Numerous, extensive, no uninvolved skin	Deep, violaceous E, numerous T throughout	No uninvolved skin	Rough throughout

This 4-point grading scale has been extensively tested and used for evaluating laser and energy-based cosmetic treatments.
From Alexiades-Armenakas M. Rhytides, laxity, and photoaging treated with a combination of radiofrequency, diode laser, and pulsed light and assessed with a comprehensive grading scale. J Drugs Dermatol 2006;5(8):731–8; with permission.

a subsequent study of 13 patients with facial and neck skin laxity treated with 2 monthly sessions at 30 to 36 J/cm^2 and 3 passes, with 6-month follow-up.[14] A study in Asian skin used 32 to 40 J/cm^2, 3 passes, and 3 successive monthly treatment sessions with descriptive improvements in facial skin laxity reported.[15] Of import, among 63 total treatment sessions using the stationary technique, 7 incidences of vesiculation and blistering were reported.[15] Another split-face study in Asian skin demonstrated descriptive improvement following 2 infrared broadband (1100–1800 nm) light treatments at 36 to 46 J/cm^2 on the treated side at 3-month follow-up.[16] One incidence of blistering occurred among the 23 patients treated.[16] In addition, topical anesthesia was required, as the stationary application of the device was associated with significant discomfort. Another study of 9 patients demonstrated that application of topical anesthesia followed by infrared broadband light treatment at 30 to 40 J/cm^2 in 1 to 2 sessions yielded descriptive improvements in skin laxity at 1-month follow-up.[17]

The mobile energy delivery approach was subsequently applied to infrared broadband light 1100 to 1800 nm (Titan, Cutera, Brisbane, CA, USA) in an effort to augment fluence delivery, patient tolerance of high fluences, and to increase safety.[18] As was the case for mobile radiofrequency delivery, the mobile delivery of infrared broadband light precluded the need for topical anesthesia, rendered the treatment painless, and safely allowed for a 30% increase in fluence dosage delivered per pulse as well as an increase in the pass count to 8 passes.[18] The clinical outcomes for the treatment of skin laxity with this procedure was assessed through quantitative grading using a tested laxity grading scale and demonstrated augmented clinical efficacy as compared with the stationary technique.[18] The mobile delivery of infrared broadband (1100 to 1800 nm) light yielded consistent clinical improvement in all subjects in the study and afforded a 0.2 laxity grade improvement per treatment on the 4-point grading scale while rendering the procedure painless and free of side effects or complications.[18]

CLINICAL EXAMINATION AND PATIENT HISTORY

The classification of neck laxity and photoaging into quantitative grades has been previously published and evaluated for clinical trial use by the author (see **Table 1**). Patients with a baseline laxity grade of 2.0 to 3.0 are ideal candidates; patients with a baseline grade of 3.5 to 4.0 are advised that more treatment sessions are necessary to

attain appreciable improvement. Patients older than 65 are less likely to respond to skin surface–applied nonablative treatments, and therefore are strongly discouraged from this approach. Patients with a history of thyroid or parathyroid disease or neoplasia are contraindicated. Baseline and follow-up photography amphas, three-quarter view, and from both side views are necessary. As aforementioned, patients should be offered all the treatment options for treating their skin laxity, including but not limited to injectables, laser and light-based treatments, surgical facelifting and no treatment. The rare but real risk of a thermal burn and scar should be discussed during informed consent, in addition to the usual and customary risks and complications of any medical procedure. Premedication and anesthesia are not necessary.

METHOD OF DEVICE OR TREATMENT APPLICATION
Protocol

Patient preparation
No topical anesthetic is needed for the procedure. A thin, 1-mm layer of aqueous ultrasound gel is applied. The typical treatment areas include the lower face and neck, excluding the thyroid region (see **Fig. 1**).

Treatment intervals
Patients with baseline laxity grades 2 to 3 should receive 2 to 3 treatments with infrared broadband (1100 to 1800 nm) light at 2-week to 4-week intervals.

Mobile pulse application
Each light pulse is administered in a mobile continuous fashion within a localized area measuring approximately 1 handpiece width laterally and vertically. The handpiece is moved with the initiation of each pulse, making oval/circular movements extending approximately 1 width laterally to the handpiece tip and 1 length of the handpiece tip vertically. The pulses are delivered in succession along each row of facial or neck skin. A series of 4 to 5 pulses are administered across small grid areas, followed by 6 to 8 passes to each grid area, totaling approximately 200 to 400 pulses per treatment. The pulses should be administered in a linear fashion along the jawline, along the upper neck, and in the submental area. The precise segments or grid areas include the lower cheek, mid-to-upper cheek, mandible, upper lateral neck, and submandibular and submental areas. The passes are administered in succession to each linear area before commencing in a new area. A minimum of 4, but preferably 7 to 8 passes along each segment each covering an area of

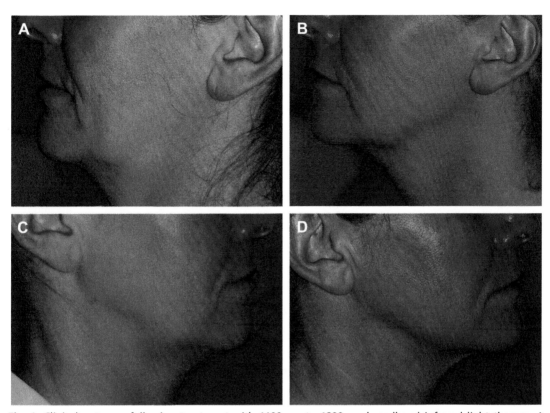

Fig. 1. Clinical outcome following treatment with 1100-nm to 1800-nm broadband infrared light therapy. A patient with skin laxity to the lower face and neck at baseline (*A* and *C*) and 1 month following 2 treatments (*B* and *D*). A significant reduction in skin laxity is noted.

approximately 1.5 cm² should be administered. See Video 1, Titan Mobile, online for demonstration of procedure.

Dose/fluence
Precooling, parallel cooling, and postcooling of the epidermis is applied through continuous contact with a sapphire tip. Each mobile pulse is delivered at a fluence of 46 J/cm² to the face, 45 J/cm² to the mandible, and 44 J/cm² to the neck. The fluence is commenced at 46 J/cm² for the mobile protocol to the face; 45 J/cm² to the mandible; and 44 J/cm² to the neck. If the patient senses momentary transient discomfort, the fluence should be titrated down by 1 J/cm² for a final target range on the face of 44 to 50 J/cm²; for the neck, 42 to 47 J/cm² mobile. For superior periorbital regions, the mobile technique is initiated at fluences ranging from 20 to 24 J/cm². One to 2 adjacent pulses may be administered to each brow extending to the lateral periorbital region. A total of 4 to 5 passes should be delivered and are comfortably tolerated by the patient. Good contact with ample aqueous gel is crucial.

Clinical evaluations
Clinical results should be evaluated using the comprehensive 4-point grading scale from photographs at baseline, and 1-month, 3-month, and 6-month follow-up visits after the final treatment.

Pain evaluations
Pain should be evaluated while administering each pulse and the fluence titrated up or down to the point of tolerability by the patient to maximize total energy delivery and safety.

Postoperative Care
Postoperative erythema resolves within minutes to hours and no postoperative care is needed.

RESULTS
Clinical Findings
Clinical results in skin laxity and rhytid reduction will begin to become evident starting 2 weeks following the first treatment session. Progressive improvements in skin laxity and rhytids will continue to be observed over several months, reaching a maximum benefit at 6 to 12 months.[15,18]

This correlates histologically with the completion of the time course of neocollagenesis.[1,18,19] In the clinical study assessing the mobile infrared delivery technique, 22 female patients aged 40 to 75, 19 white and 3 Asian, were treated and assessed by quantitative grading.[18] All subjects completed and responded to treatment. Photographic examples of laxity reduction in patients during the follow-up interval are shown in **Figs. 1** and **2**.

Quantitative Assessments

The mean treatment number was 2.1 ($\pm$ 0.9) and mean follow-up interval was 1.9 ($\pm$ 1.0) months. The mean baseline laxity grade was 2.9 $\pm$ 0.5 and mean posttreatment laxity grade was 2.5 $\pm$ 0.6, with a mean difference in prelaxity versus postlaxity grades of 0.4 $\pm$ 0.3 (95% confidence interval [CI] for mean difference: 0.2540, 0.5415;

and a mean percentage improvement in laxity grading scores of 14.1% $\pm$ 11.3%). Paired t test comparison demonstrated that the difference between the laxity grading scores before and after treatment were statistically significant with a P value less than .0001 (**Table 2**).[18]

Pain Evaluations

Use of the standard stationary technique results in discomfort and requires topical anesthesia at fluences exceeding roughly 30 to 35 J/cm^2. With the mobile technique, the procedure should be painless at fluences of 44 to 50 J/cm^2. In the clinical study assessing the mobile technique, the treatment discomfort was rated as a mean of 0.7 ($\pm$ 0.6) on a 0 to 10 Visual Analog Scale grading scale.[18] By patient questionnaire asking the patient to rate the procedure as painless, mildly painful,

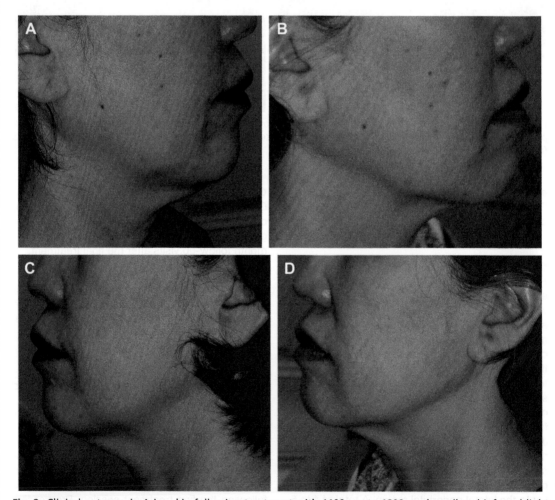

Fig. 2. Clinical outcome in Asian skin following treatment with 1100-nm to 1800-nm broadband infrared light therapy. An Asian-skinned patient with skin laxity to the lower face and neck at baseline (*A* and *C*) and 1 month following 2 treatments (*B* and *D*). A significant reduction in skin laxity is noted. No adverse events or side effects were observed.

Table 2
Comparison of laxity grading scores before and after treatment with infrared light using mobile delivery Paired *t* Test for Laxity Pre-Laxity Post Grading Scores[18]

	N	Mean	SD	SE
Laxity Pre	22	2.875	0.539	0.115
Laxity Post	22	2.477	0.597	0.127
Difference	22	0.3977	0.3242	0.0691

The mean pretreatment and posttreatment laxity scores and mean difference between pretreatment and post-treatment scores, standards of deviation (SD), standards of error of the means (SE), paired *t* test, and confidence intervals (CI) across the 22 patients in the study were calculated and are shown in the table. The posttreatment values represent the laxity grading scores at a mean follow-up interval of 1.9 (range 1–3) months following a mean of 2.1 (range 1–3) treatments.

95% confidence interval for mean difference: 0.2540, 0.5415.

t test of mean difference = 0 (vs not = 0): *t* value = 5.75; *P* value = .000.

The data show statistically significant difference between before and after measurements (*P*<.0001).

Data from Alexiades-Armenakas M. Assessment of the mobile delivery of infrared light (1100–1800 nm) for the treatment of facial and neck skin laxity. J Drugs Dermatol 2009;8(3):221–6.

moderately painful, or painful, sensation during the treatment was rated as painless by 100% (22 of 22) of patients.[18] In a separate question asking patients whether they sensed rare (<5) transient moments of heat pain versus frequent (more than 5) moments of heat pain versus persistent heat pain during the procedure, 18% (4 of 22) of patients reported only rare transient moments of heat pain during the course of the procedure. None (0%) of the patients reported the procedure as painful or as sensing frequent or persistent heat pain sensation during the treatment.[18]

Safety

Immediately following treatment, minimal erythema is noted, which resolves within 1 to 3 hours. No crusting, dyspigmentation, or scarring should be observed. It is imperative to use adequate gel and maintain full contact of the sapphire tip with the gel and skin surface to prevent any epidermal injury.

DISCUSSION

Skin laxity, manifested by progressive loss of skin elasticity, loosening of connective tissue framework, deepening and redundancy of skin folds, and progressive prominence of submandibular

and submental tissues, is caused by a combination of intrinsic genetic factors and extrinsic factors, such as photoaging.[3–5] Intrinsic genetic factors influence skin laxity, such as in cases of cutis laxa, a genetic disease caused by mutations in elastin and fibulin genes, and of progeria or premature aging syndromes caused by mutations affecting telomere shortening, laminins, and DNA repair.[20–23] It is possible that progressive skin laxity during aging is caused by polymorphisms or acquired mutations in these candidate genes or by external factors affecting the corresponding proteins they encode. Photoaging is an extrinsic cause of skin laxity, resulting in solar elastosis and the corresponding loss of skin elasticity. Molecular biologic findings support such an etiology: disorders of elastin degradation, such as floppy eyelid syndrome, are characterized by excessive elastin degradation resulting in extreme skin laxity of the eyelids.[23] Thus, a combination of genetic and external factors likely contributes to the progressive skin laxity observed with aging.

Although the targeting of skin laxity through skin surface–applied tightening technologies has yet to be acknowledged as a distinct application by the FDA, the laxity grading scale used here has been validated in prior and current studies of radiofrequency and infrared treatments, and most recently fractional resurfacing.[3,7,8,10,24] In the application of this laxity grading scale to the mobile infrared protocol, quantitative analysis of clinical results demonstrated statistically significant improvements in laxity grades following treatment with infrared (1100 to 1800 nm) light.[18] Using this protocol of infrared broadband light delivery, the mean pretreatment score was 2.9 ± 0.5, mean posttreatment score was 2.5 ± 0.6, and the mean improvement in prelaxity versus postlaxity grades was 0.4 ± 0.3 (95% CI: 0.2540, 0.5415).[18] These represented a statistically significant difference between before and after measurements (*P*<.0001) (see **Table 2**). The mean percentage improvement in laxity grading scores was 14.1% ± 11.3% following a mean of 1.9 serial treatments.[18]

Mobile delivery of infrared light compares favorably to prior skin surface–applied skin-tightening technologies in laxity grade improvements. A prior study of combination bipolar radiofrequency with intense pulsed light and diode (900 nm) laser assessed with the same quantitative grading scale demonstrated a mean percentage improvement in laxity grading scores of 9.9% (95% CI: 6.6, 13.2).[7] In a randomized, split-face study with blinded evaluations comparing serial unipolar versus bipolar radiofrequency treatments demonstrated mean percentage improvements in laxity scores of 4.6% ± 4.8% and 7.3% ± 3.5%, respectively, although the data were not statistically significant.[8] A variable-depth targeting infrared (1310 nm) laser treatment was also assessed for the treatment of skin laxity using the same quantitative grading scale, and demonstrated a mean percentage improvement in laxity scores of 7.9% (95% CI: 3.6, 12.3).[10] Thus, the quantitative laxity grading scale used here has been tested previously, and the current study has demonstrated efficacy of this infrared device in treating skin laxity following an average of roughly 2 treatments and a mean of 2 months of follow-up with statistically significant results. This translates from a practical standpoint into a treatment that yields clinically evident improvements in skin laxity within a short time period and after few treatments, which is desirable for patient satisfaction.

Earlier clinical studies using infrared broadband (1100 to 1800 nm) light device used the stationary technique at lower fluences, which was associated with peri-procedural pain, the requirement of topical anesthesia, and a reported higher incidence of clinical burns in those studies. In the first pilot study, infrared light was used at 20 to 30 J/cm^2 on the face and neck for the treatment of skin laxity in 25 patients.[13] Topical anesthetic was used in some of the cases and the clinical outcomes were variable, with some patients showing no improvement.[13] A subsequent study of 13 patients with facial and neck skin laxity treated with 2 monthly sessions at 30 to 36 J/cm^2 and 3 passes, with 6-month follow-up, demonstrated consistent improvement in the vast majority of subjects.[14] A study in Asian skin used fluences of 32 to 40 J/cm^2, 3 passes, and 3 successive monthly treatment sessions with descriptive improvements in facial skin laxity reported.[15] However, in that study of 63 total treatment sessions, 7 incidences of vesiculation and blistering were reported, suggesting that the stationary treatment technique may have a low risk of thermal burns particularly in darker skin types.[15] A subsequent split-face study in Asian skin demonstrated descriptive improvement following 2 infrared broadband (1100–1800 nm) light treatments at 36 to 46 J/cm^2 on the treated side at 3-month follow up.[16] Once again, an incidence of blistering occurred among the 23 patients treated with the stationary technique.[16] Although these studies clearly demonstrated reproducible efficacy for infrared broadband light in the treatment of skin laxity, the stationary technique required topical anesthesia, used lower fluences, and was associated with a higher complication rate in darker skin types.

Most recently, the implementation of the mobile technique in the application of infrared broadband light allowed for 30% higher fluences to be applied painlessly and without any observed complications, while maintaining quantifiable, consistent efficacy in laxity grade improvements on the face and neck.[18] Given that the continuous mobility allows for the cooling of pain sensory fibers at the DEJ (short thermal relaxation times) and the DEJ itself, while continuing to deposit energy into the large collagen fibrils and other dermal targets (long thermal relaxation times) as discussed in prior work, it is likely that this mobile protocol increases the safety of the procedure by minimizing the risk of epidermal and DEJ thermal burns.[10]

Histologic evaluations of the infrared 1100-nm to 1800-nm broadband light effects on skin have supported the induction of collagens and elastin synthesis. In a rat model, induction of collagen type I in excess of collagen type III was demonstrated by immunostaining in skin sections obtained up to 90 days and 45 days after irradiation, respectively.[25] Interestingly, in postabdominoplasty human skin, irradiation with 30, 45, and 60 J/cm^2, 4 passes, demonstrated a difference in the level of collagen fibril alteration among the different fluences. Lower (30 J/cm^2) fluences showed less collagen fibril alteration on electron microscopy at the 0-mm to 1-mm depth as compared with 1-mm to 2-mm depth, owing to the effects of contact cooling at lower fluences. For 45 and 65 J/cm^2, the entire field demonstrated contracted collagen fibrils.[26] These findings correlate with augmented clinical efficacy in treating rhytids and laxity observed with the mobile technique at high (>46 J/cm2) fluences.[18] Finally, infrared 1100-nm to 1800-nm broadband light is 1 of 2 skin-tightening technologies that have been shown to induce both neocollagenesis and neoelastogenesis.[19] Recently, human skin biopsies following irradiation at 36 J/cm^2 using the stationary technique were obtained at 1, 2, and 3 months after treatment.[19] In sun-protected skin, immunostains demonstrated significant increases in type I collagen until 1 month, and in type III collagen and elastin through month 3. In sun-exposed skin, these studies showed increases in type I collagen through month 2, and type III collagen and elastin through month 3.[19] The combined induction of both neocollagenesis and neoelastogenesis likely explain the clinical impact on both rhytids and skin laxity.

SUMMARY

The application of infrared broadband light is the more recent addition of nonsurgical laser and light-based treatment for skin laxity and rhytids. Infrared broadband light, when used with the mobile technique, offers a painless, safe, nonsurgical alternative treatment option for the treatment of skin laxity on the face and neck. The application of the mobile technique allows for 30% higher fluences to be used, does not require topical anesthesia, renders the treatment painless, and allows for increased pass counts as compared with the stationary approach. A clinical study using quantitative assessments of facial and neck skin laxity grading following mobile infrared broadband light treatment, showed a mean percentage improvement of 14.1% ± 11.3% following a mean of 1.9 treatments, a statistically significant difference between before and after measurements (P<.0001).[18] Prior studies using a stationary technique also demonstrated appreciable clinical improvements in skin laxity and correlated these findings with neocollagenesis and neoelastogenesis over a 6-month to 12-month time course.[13–17,25] The consistency of clinical improvement in skin laxity supports the use of this approach for moderate to advanced skin laxity of the face and neck.

SUPPLEMENTARY DATA

Supplementary video related to this article can be found at doi:10.1016/j.fsc.2011.05.001.

REFERENCES

1. Alexiades-Armenakas M. Laser skin tightening: non-surgical alternative to the face lift. J Drugs Dermatol 2006;5(3):295–6.

2. Gold MH. Tissue tightening: a hot topic utilizing deep dermal heating. J Drugs Dermatol 2007; 6(12):1238–42.

3. Alexiades-Armenakas MR, Dover JS, Arndt KA. The spectrum of laser skin resurfacing: non-ablative, fractional and ablative laser resurfacing. J Am Acad Dermatol 2008;58(5):719–37 [quiz: 738–40].

4. Milewicz DM, Urban Z, Boyd C. Genetic disorders of the elastic fiber system. Matrix Biol 2000;19(6):471–80.

5. Uitto J. The role of elastin and collagen in cutaneous aging: intrinsic aging versus photoexposure. J Drugs Dermatol 2008;7(2 Suppl):s12–6.

6. Fitzpatrick R, Geronemus R, Goldberg D, et al. Multicenter study of noninvasive radiofrequency for periorbital tissue tightening. Lasers Surg Med 2003; 33(4):232–42.

7. Alexiades-Armenakas M. Rhytides, laxity, and photoaging treated with a combination of radiofrequency, diode laser, and pulsed light and assessed with a comprehensive grading scale. J Drugs Dermatol 2006;5(8):731–8.

8. Alexiades-Armenakas MR, Dover JS, Arndt KA. Unipolar versus bipolar radiofrequency treatment of rhytides and laxity using a mobile painless delivery method. Lasers Surg Med 2008;40:446–53.

9. Taub AF, Battle EF Jr, Nikolaidis G. Multicenter clinical perspectives on a broadband infrared light device for skin tightening. J Drugs Dermatol 2006;5(8):771–8.

10. Alexiades-Armenakas MR. Non-ablative skin tightening with a variable-depth heating 1310 nm laser in combination with surface cooling. J Drugs Dermatol 2007;6(11):1098–103.

11. Hsu TS, Kaminer MS. The use of nonablative radiofrequency technology to tighten the lower face and neck. Semin Cutan Med Surg 2003;22(2):115–23.

12. Bogle MA, Ubelhoer N, Weiss RA, et al. Evaluation of the multiple pass, low fluence algorithm for radiofrequency tightening of the lower face. Lasers Surg Med 2007;39(3):210–7.

13. Ruiz-Esparza J. Near painless, nonablative, immediate skin contraction induced by low-fluence irradiation with new infrared device: a report of 25 patients. Dermatol Surg 2006;32(5):601–10.

14. Goldberg DJ, Hussain M, Fazeli A, et al. Treatment of skin laxity of the lower face and neck in older individuals with a broad-spectrum infrared light device. J Cosmet Laser Ther 2007;9:35–40.

15. Chua SH, Ang P, Khoo LS, et al. Nonablative infrared skin tightening in Type IV to V Asian skin: a prospective clinical study. Dermatol Surg 2007; 33(2):146–51.

16. Chan HH, Yu CS, Shek S, et al. A prospective, split face, single-blinded study looking at the use of an infrared device with contact cooling in the treatment of skin laxity in Asians. Lasers Surg Med 2008;40: 146–52.

17. Ahn JY, Han TY, Lee CK, et al. Effect of a new infrared light device (1100–1800 nm) on facial lifting photodermatology. Photodermatol Photoimmunol Photomed 2008;24:49–51.

18. Alexiades-Armenakas M. Assessment of the mobile delivery of infrared light (1100–1800 nm) for the treatment of facial and neck skin laxity. J Drugs Dermatol 2009;8(3):221–6.

19. Tanaka Y, Matsuo K, Yusuriha S. Long-term evaluation of collagen and elastin following infrared (1100–1800 nm) irradiation. J Drugs Dermatol 2009;8(8):708–12.

20. Rodriguez-Revenga L, Iranzo P, Badenas C, et al. A novel elastin gene mutation resulting in an autosomal dominant form of cutis laxa. Arch Dermatol 2004;140(9):1135–9.

21. Markova D, Zou Y, Ringpfeil F, et al. Genetic heterogeneity of cutis laxa: a heterozygous tandem duplication within the fibulin-5 (FBLN5) gene. Am J Hum Genet 2003;72(4):998–1004.

22. Ding SL, Shen CY. Model of human aging: recent findings on Werner's and Hutchinson-Gilford

SmartLifting Fiber Laser–assisted Facial Rejuvenation Techniques

Richard D. Gentile, MD, MBA

KEYWORDS

- Laser lipolysis • Laser facial sculpting
- Laser facial contouring

HISTORY OF LASER LIPOLYSIS AND INTERNAL AESTHETIC FIBER LASER–ASSISTED SURGERY

The history of laser lipolysis is brief and has been summarized well by DiBernardo,[1] who notes that Apfelberg[2] is credited for describing the laser-fat interaction in 1992, and that publications by Blugerman,[3] Schavelzon and colleagues,[4] and Goldman and colleagues[5] followed in which each showed their own experience with lasers on adipose tissue. Badin and colleagues[6] also highlighted the important tissue retraction that he noted with his technique of laser lipolysis. Ichikawa and colleagues[7] published on the histologic evaluation of tissue treated with laser lipolysis, showing the destructive changes of heat-coagulated collagen fibers and degenerated fat cell membranes with dispersion of lipid after laser irradiation of human specimens. These histologic changes correlate with clinical changes seen by both physician and patient. Further, the hemostatic properties of the 1064-nm wavelength have been well documented and are discussed later. The thermal effect produced by the neodymium-doped yttrium-aluminum-garnet (Nd:YAG) laser (1064 nm) in the adipose tissue promotes better hemostasis, resulting in less surgical trauma and wound healing with fewer adverse sequelae. In addition to the histologic evidence, the clinical evaluation shows improved postoperative recovery, resulting in a more rapid return to daily activities with an excellent aesthetic result. The application of laser lipolysis to facial and neck rejuvenation, in conjunction with the advanced facial rejuvenation techniques of SmartLifting,

were introduced by Gentile[8] in 2007. The initial procedures were performed with the SmartLipo 1064-nm laser but, on introduction of the SmartLipo MPX, the 1064/1320-nm multiplexed laser was used. Although these lasers were introduced for the purpose of lipolysis, it became evident that, for the facial plastic surgeon, the lasers had significant hemostatic and tissue-tightening effects. External laser treatment of human skin does produce a remodeling of dermal collagen and elastin fibers as well as the stimulation of neocollagen. In other aesthetic devices, the epidermis and dermis presented itself as an obstruction to getting optical or electrical energy into the deeper dermal and subcutaneous layers. Internal aesthetic lasers bypass this obstruction and hence are better positioned to perform thermodermoplasty or shrink-wrapping of the facial and neck skin envelope. The use of internal aesthetic lasers is a new modality and the benefits of these innovative or technology-enabled techniques can be assessed by examining the factors listed in **Table 1** regarding the potential benefits provided by introduction of a new technology-enabled technique. New technology should not only introduce another particular technique, it should be proved to offer the specific benefits that are detailed in **Table 1**.

THE INTRODUCTION OF INTERNAL LASER USE FOR AESTHETIC FACIAL AND NECK REJUVENATION

The Cynosure SmartLipo laser was the first laser to be approved by the US Food and Drug

Facial Plastic & Aesthetic Laser Center, 6505 Market Street A103 & Northeastern Ohio College of Medicine, Youngstown, OH, USA
E-mail address: dr-gentile@msn.com

Facial Plast Surg Clin N Am 19 (2011) 371–387
doi:10.1016/j.fsc.2011.05.011

Table 1
Technology innovations mediating transformational change in aesthetic surgery

Criteria for assessing improved outcomes in aesthetic surgery resulting from technology innovations	Reduces anesthetic requirements for procedure Reduces operating time for procedure Reduces complications or morbidity for procedure Reduces recovery time for procedure Facilitates new technical approaches lacking in conventional or existing techniques More than 1 novel application is possible with the new technology

Administration for laser lipolysis. In addition to the laser lipolysis indication, the laser is approved for the surgical incision, excision, vaporization, ablation, and coagulation of soft tissue. All soft tissue is included, such as skin, cutaneous tissue, subcutaneous tissue, striated and smooth tissue, muscle, cartilage meniscus, mucous membrane, lymph vessels and nodes, organs, and glands. Since the 2006 introduction of subcutaneous laser-based lipolysis techniques, other laser companies have introduced similar products and many have introduced different wavelengths for the specific indication of laser lipolysis. Other wavelengths for laser lipolysis include 980 nm, 1440 nm, and 1444 nm.

EARLY CLINICAL STUDIES AND OBSERVATIONS

The original SmartLipo laser (**Fig. 1**) delivered 1064-nm optical energy though a 300-μm fiber at 6 W (**Fig. 2**A). All subsequent Cynosure SmartLipo and SmartLipo MPX lasers use a 600-μm fiber (see **Fig. 2**B) and now the 1000-μm fiber (see **Fig. 2**C) for high-power laser lipolysis. The 600-μm optical fiber is introduced into a 1-mm diameter stainless steel microcannula of variable length and is used for facial laser-assisted procedures. The laser is fired through the distal end of the fiber, which protrudes 2 mm beyond the tip of the cannula. The distal end of the fiber interacts with the facial and neck soft tissue. For visualization purposes, an aiming laser source is provided in the beam path providing the precise location of the fiber tip, indicating where the laser is working. For most facial and neck anatomic regions, a 6-W to 12-W, 100-microsecond pulsed laser at 40 Hz and 150 mJ was used. The SmartLipo MPX laser, which is capable of blending both the 1064-nm and 1320-nm wavelengths, was used in more recent studies and is used today in completing these procedures. The Nd:YAG laser produced photomechanical and thermal effects that dissected

the tissue quickly and easily. In addition, the hemostatic properties of the Nd:YAG laser allowed for the coagulation of small blood vessels in the subcutaneous plane with preservation of the dermal plexus of vessels. Multiplexing the 1064-nm and 1320-nm wavelengths provides some unique advantages. SmartLipo with MultiPlex (known as SmartLipo MPX, **Fig. 3**) allows individual as well as sequential emission of 1064-nm and 1320-nm wavelengths. The sequential firing of these 2 wavelengths in combination maximizes the positive properties of both. The combination of these wavelengths increases the efficiency of laser lipolysis and offers a more evenly distributed laser energy profile that benefits superficial and deep treatment. These 2 wavelengths emitted

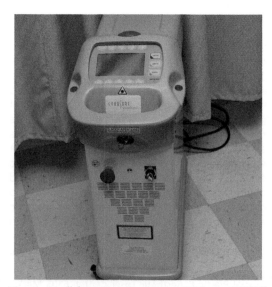

Fig. 1. Small-footprint SmartLipo 1064-nm Nd:YAG Laser. The SmartLipo laser was initially approved at 6 W and underwent power upgrades to 18 W before advancing to the MPX and now TriPlex versions.

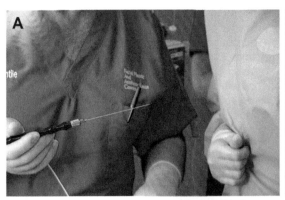
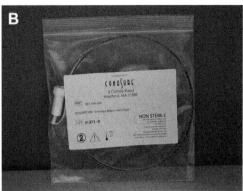
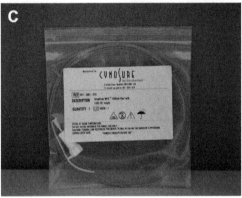

Fig. 2. (*A*) Original 300-μm fiber used for lipolysis and tissue coagulation, (*B*) 600-μm fiber, (*C*) 1000-μm fiber. The laser fibers have also progressed from a small, 300-μm fiber to now the larger 1000-μm fiber.

sequentially offer a more efficient vascular coagulation through the conversion of hemoglobin to methemoglobin.[7] The 1320-nm wavelength heats the blood, converting hemoglobin to methemoglobin. The 1064-nm wavelength has a 3 to 5 times greater affinity for methemoglobin than for hemoglobin, thereby increasing absorption and resulting in more efficient coagulation, leading to enhanced skin tightening. SmartLifting is noted to permit easier flap separation in typically difficult-to-reach areas such as the buccal labial folds (BLF) and the corner of the mouth and infracommissural BLF, also known as marionette lines, when completing full rhytidectomy. The wavelength characteristics and thermodynamic photospectrum of the 1064-nm and 1064-nm/1320 multiplexed lasers and comparative thermal volumes are shown in **Fig. 4**.

>   1064-nm wavelength characteristics (see **Fig. 4**A)
>   1320-nm wavelength characteristics (see **Fig. 4**B)
>   Multiplexing (see **Fig. 4**C)
>   Comparative thermal volumes (see **Fig. 4**D).

HEMOSTASIS AND FIBER LASER FLAP ELEVATION

After the observations of early 2008 and on my discussions with Cynosure regarding the clinical hemostatic properties observed, we began to investigate the intrinsic hemostatic properties of other laser for facial flap elevation. What we wanted to determine was how the SmartLipo and SmartLipo MPX lead to the profound and desirable hemostatic effects when used before facial flap elevation, as shown in **Fig. 5**. Do other fiber lasers show an equal or proportionate hemostatic effect? With proper patient consent, we compared the use of the pulsed 1064-nm and pulsed 1064/1320-nm laser with a 980-nm continuous-wave laser. In these clinical studies, the power was set to 10 W and the procedures were completed. The results of the studies indicated that, although the 980-nm laser glided through subcutaneous tissue more easily, the net hemostasis was poor and the procedure was about the same as performing a rhytidectomy without the benefits of laser-enhanced hemostasis. Photographs of the study are shown in (**Figs. 6 and 7**). The study was

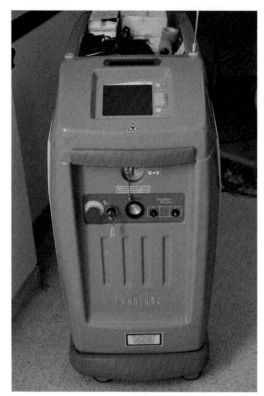

Fig. 3. SmartLipo MPX. The MPX or Multiplex permits laser use in either the 1064-nm or 1320-nm mode or Multiplex, which is sequential emission of 1064 nm and 1320 nm in 3 blends.

microdissection tunnels (**Fig. 8**). We initially performed this with a low-wattage Nd:YAG laser fiber introduced through a stainless steel cannula and operating at 6 W. With the advent of more powerful laser lipolysis units, higher optical energy is possible, but rarely should the power settings exceed 15 W. We generally use 9 to 12 W for most areas of the face, and the higher settings can be used with caution in the very thin midline neck in patients with heavy necks. The second new technology that was introduced in the past few years is the barbed suture used in open surgeries differing from the previous closed techniques. One of the problems with barbed sutures in closed procedures was the inability of tissue repositioned to stay where it was placed because of the considerable dermal attachments of the skin to the deeper soft tissues and the tendency of these dermal attachments to return the tissues to their original position. The dermal attachments eventually led to a gradual descent of the tissues, which made the subtle results of these techniques very short lived. The ability to laser undermine the tissue and to elevate the skin flap off the dermal attachments in most of the procedures releases the deeper tissue and permits a more durable repositioning of the deeper soft tissues. Concurrent skin excision also contributes to more durable results in a minimally invasive procedure. The ability to use internal barbed sutures in the open technique is a work in progress and, now that we can release the skin from the deeper tissues in an atraumatic and hemostatic fashion, different suturing patterns will develop in search of the ideal pattern of suture plication or imbrication, the ideal being a technique that produces the longest-lasting and most aesthetically pleasing results and maintains quick recovery classification.

quantified by sponge use when completing the procedure, and roughly 5 times as many sponges were used on the continuous-wave 980-nm side as on the pulsed 1064-nm and 1064/1320-nm lasers (see **Figs. 6**B and **7**C). Other clinical findings were that the patients had longer bruising, swelling, and induration after the subcutaneous treatment with the 980-nm continuous-wave laser, which is most likely caused by more blood extravasating into the superficial soft tissues. SmartLipo was also compared with the 1444-nm pulsed laser, which also did not show hemostatic properties as significant as the 1064-nm and 1064/1320-nm multiplexed laser.

SMARTLIFTING TECHNIQUES

SmartLifting evolved from the application of 2 new technologies in facial surgery. The first is the use of subcutaneous laser techniques for hemostasis and for developing the facial flap in the most ideal plane. The laser helps define the facial flap and creates a dissection plane by creating multiple

LaserFacialSculpting Surgical Techniques

Until late 2007, most in-office procedures that included SmartLipo techniques were completed by using the laser for laser lipolysis, liposculpting, and the concurrent tightening of the facial soft tissues through tissue coagulation that follows interstitial laser lipolyis. The first procedures usually did not have external temperature monitoring, so it is likely that the tissue tightening that was obtained was less than is possible now because thermal end points have been introduced that bring the skin temperature to the highest possible temperature without inducing skin necrosis. These studies were first completed by DiBernardo and Reyes,[9] who showed that epidermal necrosis was associated with external skin temperatures approaching 48° to 52°C.

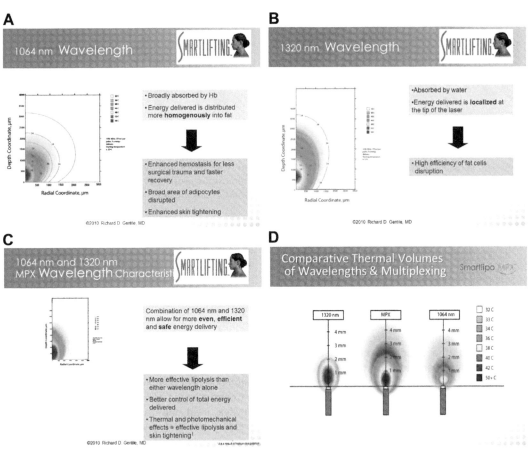

Fig. 4. (*A*) The 1064 wavelength characteristics and photothermal footprint, (*B*) 1320 wavelength characteristics and photothermal footprint, (*C*) 1064/1320 multiplexed wavelength characteristics and photothermal footprint; (*D*) relative thermal volume of laser pulse.

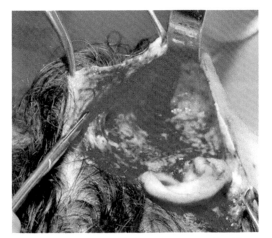

Fig. 5. Very dry surgical field with uncauterized laser-elevated facial skin flap. The surgical field beyond the incision is shown with little bleeding to 5.5 cm of dissection.

DiBernardo and Reyes[9] published their results showing the degree of skin tightening available with subcutaneous laser irradiation, with the thermal end points being not exceeding 42°C.[9] Because the techniques for SmartLifting procedures have evolved, we present the various techniques from the most fundamental to the more extensive. The subcutaneous technique without any concurrent rhytidectomy techniques is referred to as LaserFacialSculpting (LFS). LFS enables firming of the soft tissues and skin tightening, which also leads to contour improvements. Most of the procedures with concurrent rhytidectomy techniques (hybrid techniques) used the initial subcutaneous LFS techniques before elevating the skin flaps and performing various deep tissue lifting maneuvers. These techniques include the UltraMiniLift, UltraMiniNeckLift, and the LaserSmartLift. The UltraMiniLifts are minimal-incision techniques and use self-retaining sutures.

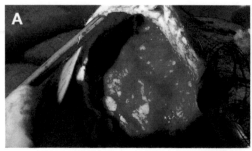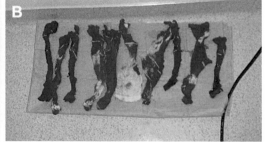

Fig. 6. (A) A 980-nm continuous-wave laser-elevated flap with poor hemostasis; (B) sponge count. The continuous-wave 980-nm diode laser does not have strong hemostatic properties because of its pulse configuration. The net result was no better hemostasis than a with traditionally elevated face-lift flap.

The protocol for LFS procedures includes marking the face and neck of the patient into grids depicting the subcutaneous laser treatment zones of the lateral and midface as well as the lateral and central neck. The grids for the lateral face and midface are shown in (Fig. 9). The treatment zones for the lateral and central neck are shown in (Fig. 10). After marking, the access ports for both the tumescent anesthesia and the laser access are marked (Fig. 11). As shown, these small incisions are located in the temple, anterior to the lobule and in the posterior hairline. A modified Klein tumescent solution is then infiltrated. The composition of the modified Klein solution infiltrated is shown in Table 2. Just before the tumescent infiltration, 20 mL of 0.5% Xylocaine with 1:200,000 parts epinephrine is infiltrated into the grids. The tumescent solution is infiltrated with the use of a compression sleeve on the liter bag of tumescent fluid dispensed through an infiltration cannula attached to a control cannula. After 8 to 10 minutes, the laser is inserted and treatment of each grid is accomplished. Because superheating a treatment area can lead to thermal necrosis, we always treat the more distal grid first before passing into the grids adjacent to the portals.

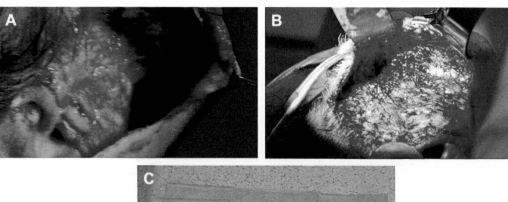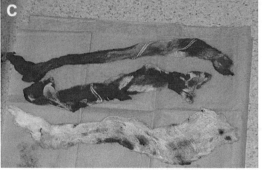

Fig. 7. (A) SmartLipo MPX 1320-nm laser-elevated flap. (B) 1064-nm/1320-nm multiplexed (C) sponge count 1320 nm. The MPX shows excellent hemostasis in either the 1064-nm, 1320-nm, or blended mode.

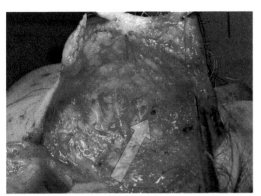

Fig. 8. Microdissection tunnels created by laser dissection. The major benefit of laser-assisted flap elevation is the development of microdissection tunnels, which makes the elevation similar to tearing paper with serrations.

This sequence reduces the laser exposure to the more proximal grids and prevents the overtreatment of the sites closest to the insertion points. The treatment end points for LFS procedures is 40 to 42° for skin flaps that are not elevated. In skin flaps that will be elevated and skin placed under tension, we use 36° as the end point as well as easy pass ability of the cannula, recognizing that there is less need to try to achieve maximal skin contraction because skin excisional techniques are also being used. The typical patient undergoing LFS techniques has early laxity of the face and neck with fatty deposition and associated

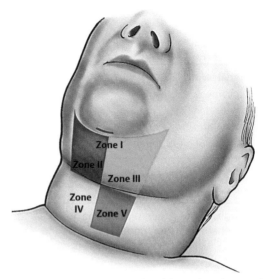

Fig. 10. LFS treatment grids of lateral and central neck. Central and lateral treatment zones for the middle neck.

jowling. As jowling and facial and neck laxity increase, different rhytidectomy techniques may be necessary to achieve a satisfactory aesthetic result. Patients who desire facial firming and do not want incisions or a rhytidectomy are also good candidates for the procedure. Several LFS patients undergoing firming and sculpting procedures are shown in (**Figs. 12 and 13**).

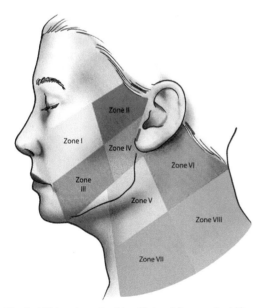

Fig. 9. LFS treatment grids of lateral face and midface. The treatment grids used for delineating the treatment areas in facial treatment zones.

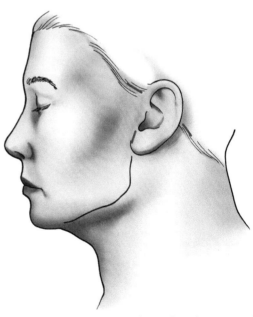

Fig. 11. Access incisions are located in the temporal hair tuft, anterior to lobule and posterior pariental hair line. The incisions are utilized for tumescent infiltration and fiberlaser surgery.

Table 2
Modified Klein solution

Component	Amount
Normal saline	1000 mL
Xylocaine	500–1000 mg
Epinephrine	0.5–0.65 mg
Sodium bicarbonate	10 mEq
Tramcinolone (optional)	10 mg

LFS Focused Applications

Although most of our procedures involve more comprehensive laser undermining of the facial and neck skin, there are applications where more limited approaches can be useful. LFS and Ultra-MiniLift procedures both cover most of the mid-face and lower face and neck (see **Figs. 9** and **10**). In isolated jowl fat excess, subplatysmal fat, isolated herniated orbital fat, or prominent nasal labial folds, the laser can be used to selectively sculpt the subcutaneous fat and soft tissue. The sculpting technique may require deep laser energy application or an open approach, especially for subplatysmal and orbital fat. Thermal monitoring is important to prevent overtreatment of the dermal-epidermal component creating thermal necrosis. If treating herniated orbital fat, laser corneal shields are essential to prevent inadvertent injury. Deeper treatment with the laser must also consider that larger-bore blood vessels are not as easily coagulated as the smaller vessels

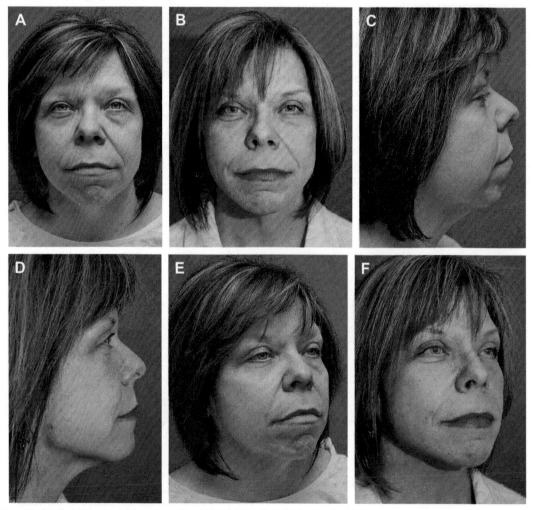

Fig. 12. (A–F) A 50 year old undergoing LFS. This patient is shown before and 9 months after LFS with chin augmentation and microablative skin rejuvenation. The noticeable thinning of her face is evident, with contour enhancements of the mandibular border.

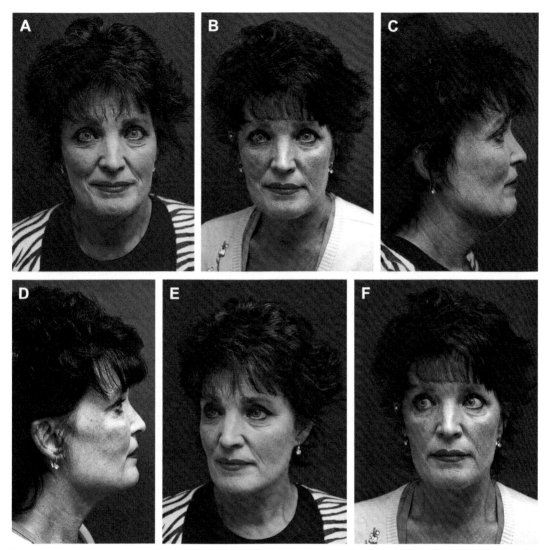

Fig. 13. (*A–F*) A 50 year old undergoing LFS. This patient is shown before and 6 months after LFS with microablative skin rejuvenation. She shows an almost complete correction of her midline fullness with no skin excision.

and the technique should be practiced with extreme care when using deeper laser energies in the lower face and neck. LFS relies on laser lipolysis, tissue coagulation, and dermal tightening to achieve the desired aesthetic end points.

UltraMiniLift Surgical Technique

A significant benefit of subcutaneous laser dissection is that it readily separates the skin from the deeper subcutaneous tissues with significant hemostasis. This benefit permits the surgeon to consider lifting procedures and suture techniques for the superficial muscular aponeurotic system performed through a limited incision. Because the dissection is controlled, with little bleeding,

the surgeon can be less concerned about having access to bleeding sites that would require the passage of cautery devices. The ability to obtain hemostasis frequently requires wide access and a larger skin incision. The UltraMiniLift was developed to permit a vertical elevation of the jowl via a small temporal-tragal incision (**Fig. 14**). The procedure involves performing LFS as described via the 3 portals, making the larger incision and elevating a facial skin flap of 5 to 5.5 cm through the limited incision. Liposculpture of the jowl is frequently performed after LFS, especially in the heavier jowl or face. Buccal fat may be contributing to large jowls and must be considered when completing the surgery; in those patients, buccal fat reduction may be completed. Next the

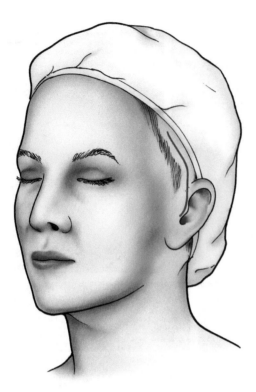

Fig. 14. Temporal-Tragal incision used for UltraMini-Lift. The UltraMiniLift is performed through a limited superior-based temporal-tragal incision. The incision may occasionally extend just past the lobule if necessary for contouring the skin.

midface and jowl are elevated with the Quill suture technique termed the mixed-plane rhytidectomy (**Fig. 15**). This technique does not include any lower face or neck sutures. After the plication is completed, redundant skin is excised from the temporal-tragal incision (**Fig. 16**). In some patients, repositioning of the temporal hair tuft is necessary

to avoid an elevated hairline of the temporal hair tuft. The UltraMiniLift can be combined with limited-access platysmaplasty or neck lifting (discussed later) because of the ability of the surgeon to widely undermine the midline and lateral neck skin through a small incision. Results of UltraMini-Lift procedures can be enhanced with the use of ablative fractional skin rejuvenation. A patient undergoing UltraMiniLift is shown in **Fig. 17**.

UltraMiniNeckLift Surgical Technique

The process of consultation with patients about their interest in facial rejuvenation involves a complete understanding of what the patient expects and also what they believe is possible with advances in facial rejuvenation procedures. In developing quick recovery methods, there are several discussions that must be completed during this process. Smaller incisions or less invasive methods can be used in the patient's treatment plan, but these do not always result in the best overall aesthetic result for the patient. In some minimal-incisions techniques, the bruising and swelling may be on a par with what may be seen in some minilift procedures. Patients must be counseled in such a way that gives them a complete understanding of what the final result can or will be and what the recovery time should be. In some of the LFS procedures and UltraMiniLifts, the maturation phase of the result can take as long as 6 months to finalize, and the patient may understand that quick recovery is not equated with the quick achievement of postoperative results in some of these procedures. In attempting to bridge the results obtainable with LFS techniques and minilifts, we started to implement some platysmaplasty techniques through very limited incisions with no skin excision. After following these patients for up to 6 months, it became evident that platysmaplasty techniques

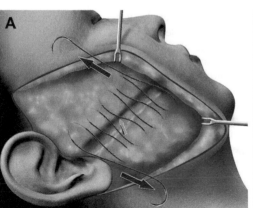
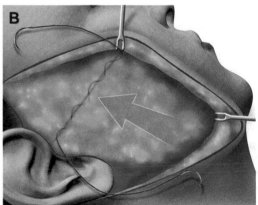

Fig. 15. (A, B) Jowl lift in UltraMiniLift. This mixed-plane rhytidectomy technique using a Quill self-retaining suture is used to elevate the jowl in patients who may need extra elevation to contour the mandibular border.

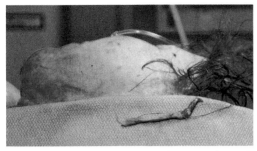

Fig. 16. Limited skin excision in UltraMiniLift. In the UltraMiniLift, a limited amount of skin is removed. The technique relies on skin contraction via tissue tightening to achieve its end points.

via minimal incisional approaches did contribute to enhanced neck results in certain patients. This conclusion has been especially evident in male patients with significant midline laxity, who would be expected to benefit only from face-lift and neck-lift combined procedures. The technique for these patients includes performing LFS before focusing on the neck via the midline and posterior neck incision. We use a hammock platysmaplasty or midline platysmal overlap approach that was first described by Fuente del Campo.[10] In our modification of the overlap technique, we use Quill self-retaining sutures and then purse string the lateral component to the mastoid periosteum. The technique is shown in **Fig. 18**. Patients undergoing Ultra-MiniNeckLift procedures are shown in **Figs. 19–21**.

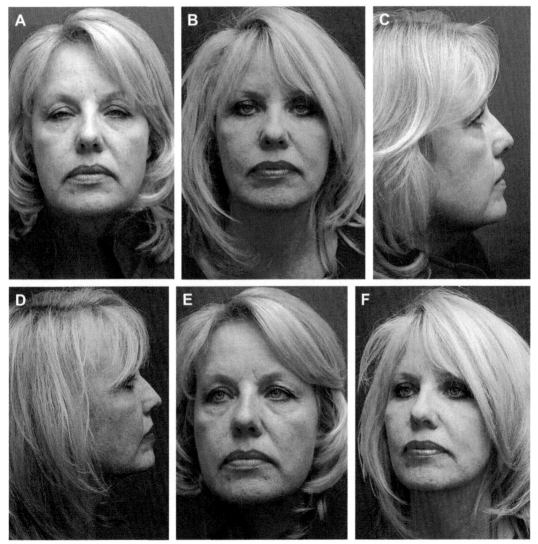

Fig. 17. (A–F) 53 year old undergoing UltraMiniLift. This patient is shown 1 year after undergoing UltraMiniLift with upper and lower blepharoplasty. The reduction in vertical height of the face is shown with a more youthful contour.

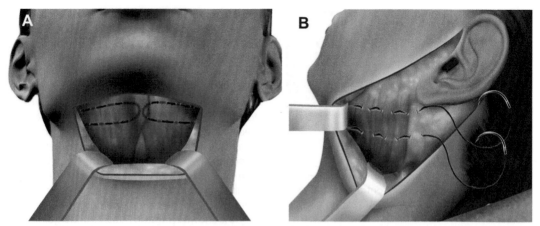

Fig. 18. (*A, B*) Quill Hammock Platysmplasty or UltraMiniNeckLift. The LFS procedure may be enhanced by minor platysmal surgery. In patients undergoing LFS, the surgical field in the central neck is hemostatic and permits platysmal modification to be accomplished with minimal bleeding. The graphic shows an open approach but the procedure uses minimal access incisions.

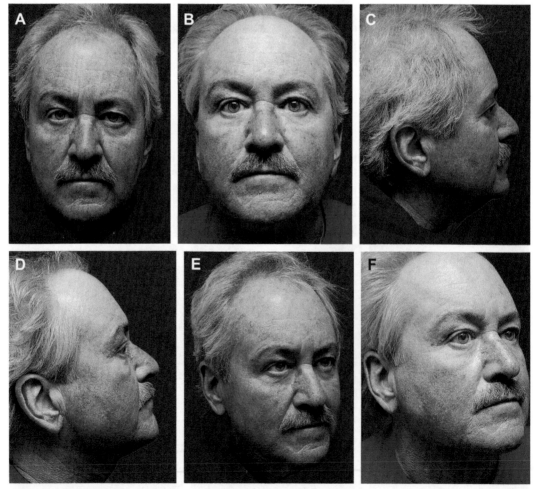

Fig. 19. (*A–F*) Male patient undergoing UltraMiniNeckLift. Midline neck fullness in men may require additional support with the Quill Hammock Purse String Platysmaplasty shown. This can be accomplished via small incisions and provides strong support to the neck.

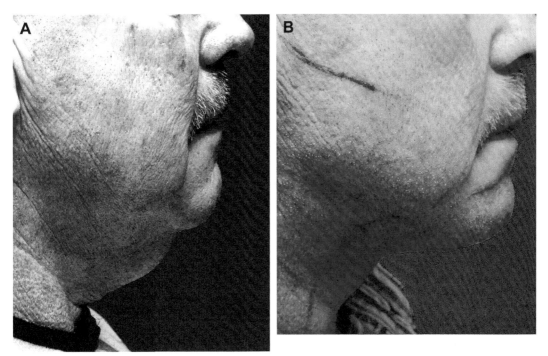

Fig. 20. (*A, B*) Male patient show 48 hours after LFS with UltraMiniNeckLift. Quick recovery characteristics of the UltraMiniNeckLift are seen in this patient, shown 3 days after surgery with minimal bruising and swelling.

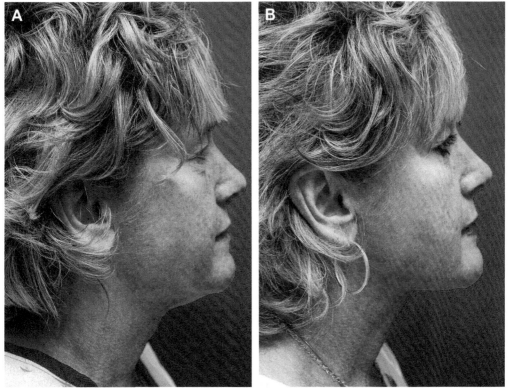

Fig. 21. (*A, B*) A 52 year old female patient shown 6 weeks after LFS with UltraMiniNeckLift. Early neck aging is corrected with the combination of neck tightening and self-retaining platysmal sutures.

LaserSmartLift Surgical Technique

The LaserSmartLift is the most frequently performed SmartLifting procedure and represents the combination of an LFS procedure with a mixed-plane rhytidectomy. LFS is first performed before marking and elevating a 5-cm to 6-cm intermediate facial flap. The incision is depicted in **Fig. 22** and is variable in the posterior neck, reflecting the skin redundancy or lack thereof. In some patients, a limited posterior incision is made. Some patients require a slight extension into the hairline and, for severe neck skin redundancy, the incision extends well into the hairline. After elevating the skin flap, the upper and lower Quill sutures are placed consistent with the mixed-plane rhytidectomy technique and the skin is redraped and trimmed of excess. In most patients, we reposition the temporal hair tuft by excising a Burrow triangle and moving the hairline downward, as is done with a classic Hamra deep-plane rhytidectomy. Patients with low temporal hair tufts may not require repositioning. It is rare for us to perform midline medial platysmaplasty procedures unless there is extensive subplatysmal fat that needs to be addressed or very heavy medial platysmal bands. A patient undergoing the LaserSmartLift procedure is shown in **Fig. 23**.

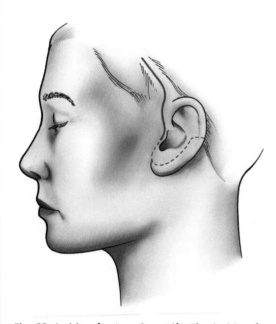

Fig. 22. Incision for LaserSmartLift. The incision for the LaserSmartLift is similar to other rhytidectomies but the posterior limb is adjusted to account for the amount of neck skin expected to be removed.

LaserSmartLift Extended Surgical Technique

In some circumstances, the flap elevation is longer than 6 cm to permit certain adjunctive procedures. In patients with extremely deep nasal labial folds, we perform an upper face dissection along the zygomatic major muscle extending past the nasal labial fold and crease. In some circumstances, the mouth has pronounced melolabial folds and, in these patients, we dissect past the depressor anguli oris and release the mandibular cutaneous ligaments. We frequently section the depressor anguli oris in these patients. Some patients have prominent buccal fat and, when the mixed-plane plication is performed, excessive fullness in the midface may result. In these patients, a subtotal excision of the buccal fat pad is accomplished. Patients undergoing extended LaserSmartLifts are shown in **Fig. 24**.

COMPLICATIONS

Since 2007, we have used SmartLifting techniques in more than 500 procedures and have seen few complications. The complications encountered can be those that would have occurred with or without the use of the laser to undermine the facial skin flaps, such as hematomas or seroma, or other complications typically associated with facial and cervical rhytidectomy. Although the specific data do not exist to prove or disprove a lower hematoma rate or bruising or swelling reduction, our observations are that these are all generally lower in patients treated with the subcutaneous laser before rhytidectomy. One benefit of laser flap elevation is that the laser tends to elevate the flap with a flap thickness that is ideal for flap viability. With laser flap undermining, there is little variability in flap thickness, which is especially useful in revision rhytidectomy with the lasers ability to easily penetrate scar tissue during the flap separation.

Epidermal and Dermal Necrosis

Although laser flap elevation may be suspected of increasing the incidence of flap necrosis, this has not been a finding in many cases. Unlike trunk and extremity laser lipolysis, the energy settings for the SmartLifting are low, rarely exceeding 9 to 12 W. With these lower energies and a selective slow heating of the flap, we have not seen dermal and epidermal necrosis in these patients that would exceed the expected incidence of 3%. Like non–laser-assisted flap elevation, it can and does occur, but it is extremely rare. We have had 2 episodes of minor blistering and necrosis near the lateral canthal area that occurred most likely

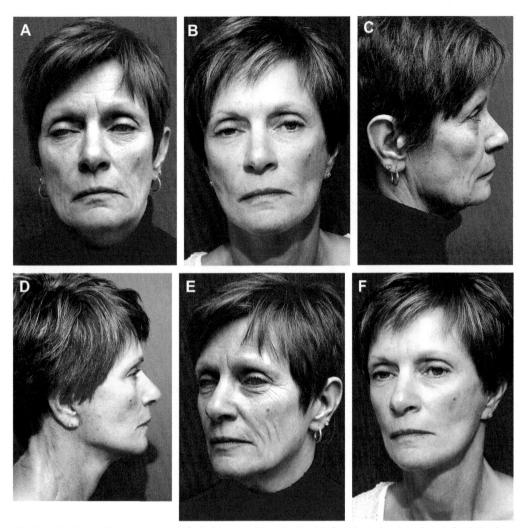

Fig. 23. (*A–F*) Patient after LaserSmartLift. A 54 year old patient with facial, perioral, and neck laxity is shown 6 months after undergoing LaserSmartLift.

because of the laser being used without the benefit of enough tumescent fluid; these also occurred before using extensive thermal monitoring of the region. One of the patients with thermal injury is shown in **Fig. 25** and most likely had dermal involvement caused by electrocautery use, but this occurred during a LaserSmartLift. We find it unnecessary and inadvisable to do extensive laser undermining inside the limits of the orbital rim. We have had 1 episode of full-thickness cervical blistering and skin necrosis despite thermal monitoring and this was most likely due in part to using more than 15 W to perform the neck elevation (**Fig. 26A**). When using the higher energies, the rate of temperature increase is more unpredictable and overshooting the upper limit for skin

safety can occur. With the advent of thermal guides and better appreciation of the thermodynamics of the skin heating process, fewer of these complications will occur. All complications occurring as a result of thermal injury and skin necrosis have responded well to conservative treatment. The patient in **Fig. 26** has undergone a limited scar revision with good aesthetic results. With thermal monitoring, we have not seen any thermal-related complications.

Neural Injury

It is recognized that the greatest fear of using lasers subcutaneously in the face is that the energy will be uncontrolled and facial motor nerve

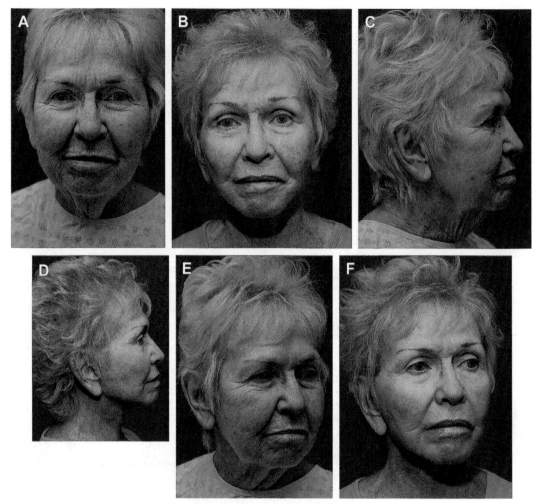

Fig. 24. (*A–F*) Patient after LaserSmartLift (extended neck and midface). LaserSmartLift extended to encompass extensive laxity of face and neck. Patient is shown 9 months after extended LaserSmartLift, upper blepharoplasty, and fractional laser skin rejuvenation of lower eyelids and upper lip.

injury will occur. With hundreds of successful SmartLifting procedures, this is not a complication that occurs provided the laser and surgical guidelines are followed. It is important to always see the aiming beam of the laser when elevating the skin flap and, if the laser is passed too deeply, it is possible to cause neural injury. We have seen several short-term, marginal mandibular neuropraxias in several patients, all of which resolved within weeks. We occasionally see these

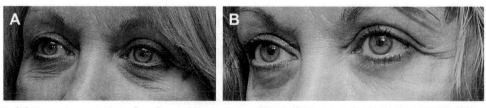

Fig. 25. (*A*) Hyperpigmentation after thermal dermal interaction adjacent to left epicanthus. (*B*) After treatment with intense pulsed light and filler with complete resolution. This patient had minor thermal injury caused by either laser energy or, most likely, electrosurgical collateral injury. (*A*) Hyperpigmentation of the skin occurred. (*B*) Successful treatment with pulsed light treatment and filler to dermis.

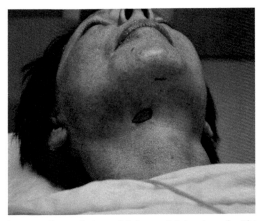

Fig. 26. Thermal dermal injury of lateral neck. This type of injury is usually evident with skin blistering at the end of the procedure. Patient also with full-thickness injury caused by either laser energy or electrosurgical collateral damage. This injury was treated with Kenalog injection followed by scar revision with a satisfactory aesthetic outcome.

neuropraxias in our patients having non–laser-elevated rhytidectomy, and attribute these temporary neuropraxias to liposuction trauma more than thermal trauma. There have been no permanent nerve injuries in any patient undergoing SmartLifting procedures. As with traditional rhytidectomy, there is temporary interruption of cutaneous sensory nerves during the flap elevation and repositioning phases of the rhytidectomy, and the resolution of the temporary sensory deficits is identical to the resolution of non–laser-elevated rhytidectomies.

REFERENCES

1. DiBernardo BE. Laser lipolysis with sequential emission of 1064 and 1320 nm wavelengths. Available at: http://www.cynosure.com/products/...mpx/DiBernado-Lipolysis-White-Paper.pdf. Accessed June 7, 2011.
2. Apfelberg D. Laser-assisted liposuction may benefit surgeons and subjects. Clin Laser Mon 1992;10:259.
3. Blugerman G. Laserlipolysis for the treatment of localized adiposity and "cellulite." In: Abstracts of the World Congress on liposuction surgery. Dearborn (MI): 2000.
4. Schavelzon D, Blugerman G, Goldman A, et al. Laser lipolysis. In: Abstracts of the 10th International Symposium on cosmetic laser surgery. Las Vegas (NV): 2001.
5. Goldman A, Schavelzon D, Blugerman G. Laser lipolysis: liposuction using Nd:YAG laser. Rev Soc Bras Cir Plast 2002;17:17–26.
6. Badin AZ, Gondek LB, Garcia MJ, et al. Analysis of laser lipolysis effects on human tissue samples obtained from liposuction. Aesthetic Plast Surg 2005; 29(4):281–6.
7. Ichikawa K, Miyasaka M, Tanaka R, et al. Histologic evaluation of the pulsed Nd:YAG laser for laser lipolysis. Lasers Surg Med 2005;36(1):43–6.
8. Gentile RD. SmartLifting: a technological innovation for facial rejuvenation. Lasers Surg Med 2006;38(1):26–32.
9. DiBernardo BE, Reyes J. Evaluation of skin tightening after laser-assisted liposuction. Aesthet Surg J 2009;29(5):400–7.
10. Fuente del Campo A. Midline platysma muscular overlap for neck restoration. Plast Reconstr Surg 1998;102(5):1710–4 [discussion: 1715].

Laser Therapy in Latino Skin

Anthony M. Rossi, MD, Maritza I. Perez, MD*

KEYWORDS

• Laser therapy • Latino • Hispanic • Phototypes

DEFINING SKIN OF COLOR AND THE LATINO POPULATION

Defining skin of color can be a challenge; a universal definition is not known. The terminology skin of color encompasses not only cultural aspects, but historical ones as well. There are also religious and geographic considerations to consider. The term skin of color can refer to individuals of certain racial and ethnic groups who share similar defining characteristics. Certain skin type populations are not only defined by the hues of their skin but also by the cutaneous diseases and reaction patterns that they share. Races are groups of people defined by the continent from which they originated. Although it is a matter of perspective for who is defining skin of color it is generally believed that skin of color identifies racial groups with darker skin hues other than that of white skin. This definition includes groups such as Africans, Asians, Native Americans, and Pacific Islanders. The United States is unique with its larger heterogeneous population. The US Census Bureau recognizes 5 racial categories: American Indian or Alaska Native; Asian; Black; Native Hawaiian or Pacific Islander; and White. There is a genetic basis as well for skin of color. Lamason and colleagues[1] identified the SLC24A5 gene, which is localized to the melanosome, as the determinant of the skin pigmentation gradient between blacks and whites. West Africans possess the normal form of the SLC24A5 gene, which produces brown skin, whereas whites of European descent possess a modified SLC24A5 gene. This gene produces fewer and smaller melanosomes, which results in a white skin type.

Individuals who possess skin of color can also be defined by ethnicity. An ethnic group, or ethnicity, is a group of people whose members identify with each other through a common heritage, common language, and culture, which often includes religion and a tradition of common ancestry. Members of an ethnic group are conscious of belonging to the group and recognize the group's distinctiveness from other ethnicities. In the United States the fastest increasing ethnic group is the Hispanic or Latino population. The term Latino was officially adopted by the United States government in 1997 to define the ethnicity as Hispanic for anyone who is of Spanish descent, speech, or ancestry. According to US Census population projections for 2050 it is estimated that the nonwhite skin of color population will equal that of the non-Hispanic white population and 29% of those will be Latinos. The US Census encompasses the Mexican, Cuban, Puerto Rican, Central American, South American, and other populations of Spanish descent as being part of the overarching Hispanic/Latino ethnic group. This ethnic group is composed of diverse populations and their skin hues can range from white to black.[2] Correspondingly the Hispanic/Latino population is composed of various ancestries, which include white, Native Indian, African, and European descents. As a result of the eclectic makeup of this ethnic group it can be challenging to put forth strict guidelines regarding diagnosis and treatment of skin conditions that occur. Skin of color has distinct reaction patterns to cutaneous disease and this must be taken into consideration when approaching treatment options. With the rapid increase in patients with skin of color in the

Disclosure: This author has nothing to disclose (A. M. R.). Dr Mariza Perez is a consultant for Cutera.
There was no outside funding for this project.
Department of Dermatology, St Luke's Roosevelt Hospital, 1090 Amsterdam Avenue, Floor 11, New York, NY 10025, USA
* Corresponding author. 25 Tamarack Avenue, Danbury, CT 06811-4829.
E-mail address: miptulla@aol.com

Facial Plast Surg Clin N Am 19 (2011) 389–403
doi:10.1016/j.fsc.2011.05.002
1064-7406/11/$ – see front matter © 2011 Elsevier Inc. All rights reserved.

facialplastic.theclinics.com

patient population it is imperative that the physician takes into account the cultural, genetic, and physiologic aspects of each population.

There is a paucity of research and epidemiologic information regarding the Latino/Hispanic ethnic group. Sanchez[3] identified the top common skin disorders affecting this group. In the private and hospital-based dermatology setting acne vulgaris, eczema/contact dermatitis, photoaging, facial melasma, and hyperpigmentation ranked among the more commonly encountered problems. In contrast, a comparative practice survey carried out at the St Luke's Roosevelt Hospital Skin of Color Center in New York City, between 2003 and 2004, revealed that the top most common skin disorders in the black population are: acne vulgaris, dyschromia, contact dermatitis, and alopecia and seborrhea dermatitis. These contrasting epidemiologic results show that within the realm of skin of color, all are not the same[4] and a "1 treatment fits all" policy cannot be applied.

Although there is a paucity of medical knowledge on the differences between skin structure and function between racial and ethnically distinct skin, differences do exist. Reed and colleagues[5] showed that skin phototypes V and VI, when compared with skin phototypes II and III, required more tape strippings to disrupt the epidermal barrier. This finding implies that the more compact cornified skin layers in the darker skin types displayed increased epidermal barrier function and a quicker recovery time. This finding was not true of white skin compared with Asian skin, showing that this inherent property was related to skin phototype and not race. In a study by Sugino and colleagues[6] the ceramide content variability of different skin phototypes was measured. Ceramides are the major lipid constituent of lamellar sheets present in the intercellular spaces of the stratum corneum. These lamellar sheets are believed to provide the barrier property of the epidermis. Therefore externally supplied ceramides function by incorporating into the intercellular lipid of stratum corneum to replace the depletion that occurs with aging and environmental damage such as from surfactant exposure. Topical ceramide has been shown to improve barrier function of damaged skin both acutely and chronically, as assessed by reduced transepidermal water-loss assays. This improved barrier can reduce skin sensitivity and responsiveness to environmental insult, leading to reduction in skin appearance problems such as redness and potentially the manifestations of aging. The lowest ceramide levels were in black skin, followed by whites, Hispanics, and Asians. Ceramide levels are directly proportional to water content and inversely proportional to transepidermal water loss. Whether these structural differences lead to functional differences for patients of Latino/Hispanic skin type is still under investigation, with more rigorous studies needed to assess irritability and erythema induction in skin of color.

Melanocytes within the epidermis are an important structure when assessing differences in skin of color. Melanocytes are derived from neural crest cells and migrate into the basal layer of the epidermis. These cells transfer melanosomes containing melanin into neighboring keratinocytes. One of the main functions of melanin is to provide ultraviolet (UV) radiation protection. It is known that melanocyte number is constant among all races.[7] The differences in clinically perceived skin color depend on the amount, density, and distribution of melanin within the melanosome and inherent melanocyte activity. Therefore the differences in melanosome density, size, and aggregation correlate with the differences in skin pigmentation. Fair-skinned individuals have more stage I and II melanosomes, which are small, more aggregated, and degraded quicker in the stratum corneum compared with darker-skinned individuals who have stage IV melanosomes, which are larger, nonaggregated, and degraded at a slower rate.[8] In skin of color, the higher number of larger, nonaggregated melanosomes correlates with a higher absorption of UV light. Darkly pigmented skin has average minimal erythema doses 15 to 33 times greater than that of white skin, with variation depending on skin tone. The melanin pigment in black skin is a neutral density filter, which reduces all wavelengths of light equally.[9] This is important to consider when treating skin of color, especially Latino skin, which can run the gamut of phototypes.

The dermis is a highly vascular structure, which is compromised of multiple components and houses appocrine and eccrine glands. Darker skin types compared with lighter phenotypes have a thicker and more compact dermis with smaller collagen fiber bundles, more numerous, larger, and multinucleated fibroblasts, and numerous and larger melanophages. There is greater eccrine gland activity when comparing black patients with white patients, with Hispanic patients possessing gland activity between that of black and white eccrine gland activity.[10] All these structural differences lead to important implications in assessing and treating skin of color, especially the Latino population. In the epidermis the increased melanin content implies a lower rate of skin cancer overall; however, the risk and rate of skin cancer is still real. The increased melanosome dispersion implies less pronounced photoaging. However, also because of this situation the pigmentary disorders that do arise in skin of color are a result of both biologic inheritances and cultural practices. The higher rate of pigment alteration after adulteration of skin of color is also concerning and therefore must be addressed beforehand. In the dermis the more multinucleated and larger fibroblasts correlate with the greater incidence of keloids experienced in darker phototypes.[11]

With the Hispanic population being the fastest increasing population in the United States, treating people of this ethnic/racial grouping is a growing priority. Although the census may group certain ethnic backgrounds into an encompassing category of Hispanic, biology does not. Therefore when treating a patient who identifies themselves as Hispanic, the keen physician must accurately assess and tease out the phototype and phenotype of that patient's skin. The Hispanic population encompasses the range of phototypes and therefore 1 rule cannot apply to all Latinos/Hispanics. Dr Leal, dermatologist in an academic center in Monterrey, Mexico, has tried to decipher the best way to predict the propensity of white phototype Latinos to postinflammatory hyperpigmentation. His studies have revealed that pigmentation of palmar and digital creases is the best predictable factor for postinflammatory hyperpigmentation in Latinos. Dr Leal and colleagues (personal communication pending manuscript publication, 2010) has divided the color diversity of the palmar and digital creases into 0 to 3, with the higher number indicating a darker skin tissue response despite skin phototype (**Fig. 1**). With a solid understanding of laser physics and properties and tissue interactions dermatologic lasers can be used in all patients regardless of skin color. Safe use of these lasers strongly depends on proper selections of laser wavelengths and suitable laser parameters. Some overarching principles can be applied to all patients undergoing a dermatologic laser procedure. Test spots are strongly encouraged in all patients with darker and even lighter phenotypes with dark palmar and digital creases, allowing the physician and patient to assess the efficacy and safety of the specific laser before undergoing a complete procedure. This strategy also inadvertently strengthens the physician-patient bond and establishes a trusting relationship. Also, preoperative expectations and goals need to be communicated and the inherent risks and complications need to be addressed beforehand. When treating patients with darker phenotypes less aggressive parameters are recommended to minimize unwanted adverse effects, with the realization that multiple treatments are usually necessary in patients with darker phototypes.

PROPERTIES OF LASERS

When treating skin phototypes IV to VI with laser therapy the challenge is to deliver efficacious and reproducible results and minimize unwanted adverse reactions. Careful patient selection and choice of laser are of the utmost importance. Laser is an acronym for light amplification by the stimulated emission of radiation. Lasers were introduced around 1960 and have steadily gained acclaim and usage. Lasers are made up of multiple

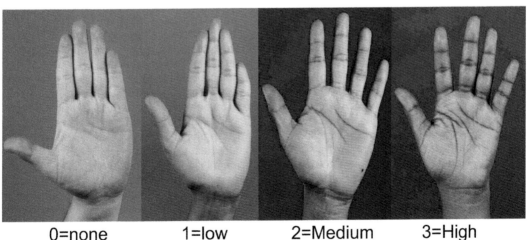

0=none   1=low   2=Medium   3=High

Fig. 1. Pigmentation of palmar and digital creases as a predictive factor for postinflammatory hyperpigmentation, with 0 having the least amount of postinflammatory pigmentation and 3 having the highest possibility of postinflammatory hyperpigmentation.

components, including the pumping system, or energy source, and the lasing medium, which supplies the electors needed for the stimulated emission of radiation and which also determines the wavelength of the laser. The lasing medium can be gaseous, liquid, or solid. Inherent properties of lasers include the fact that the light emitted from the laser beam is monochromatic, coherent (in phase), collimated (parallel), and of high intensity or energy. Laser light can then be delivered, depending on the machine, in a continuous, quasi-continuous, or pulsed fashion, either in millisecond or nanosecond durations. For a laser to exert an effect on the skin, the laser light must be absorbed, as put forth by the Grothus-Draper law.[12] Reflected and transmitted light therefore does not cause an appreciable clinical effect. Reflection primarily occurs at the epidermal level, whereas scattering occurs predominately in the dermal layers. Forward and sideways scattering decreases the power of the light delivered, whereas backscattering increases the power within the tissue. Longer wavelengths of laser light and larger spot sizes correlate with less scattering.

One of the main principles underscoring the use of laser therapy is the concept of the target chromophore. The 3 main endogenous chromophores of the skin include hemoglobin and oxyhemoglobin, melanin, and water. Each chromophore has a unique absorption spectrum and a peak absorption wavelength within. Melanin absorbs broadly across the action spectrum, whereas oxyhemoglobin and reduced hemoglobin absorb strongly in the UV, blue, green, and yellow regions of the spectrum. Tattoo ink is an example of a clinically significant exogenous chromophore. Therefore for the appropriate clinical effect to be achieved one must choose the correct wavelength of light that corresponds to the intended target chromophore. The thermal relaxation time, or the time necessary for the target tissue to cool down to half the temperature to which it is heated, needs to be taken into account when laser therapy is used because it is important to minimize any unwanted surrounding tissue destruction. Smaller objects cool faster than larger ones. If the target is heated for longer than its thermal relaxation time, there is ensuing diffusion of the thermal energy to the surrounding structures, causing unwanted nontargeted tissue damage. By choosing a pulse duration equal to or less than the thermal relaxation time of the target chromophore, one ensures that the heat delivered is confined to the target chromophore; this is known as the theory of selective photothermolysis.[13] The thermal relaxation times of the intended chromophores therefore are important when choosing the pulse duration of the laser.

The thermal relaxation time for the melanosome is approximately 250 nanoseconds and the corresponding typical pulse duration is 10 to 100 nanoseconds. For vessels in port wine stains with diameters ranging from 30 to 100 μm the corresponding thermal relaxation time is 1 to 10 milliseconds and therefore the appropriate pulse duration is 0.4 to 20 milliseconds. Terminal hair follicles have a thermal relaxation time of about 100 milliseconds and a suitable pulse duration is from 3 to 100 milliseconds. When treating darker skin phototypes it is crucial to choose longer pulse duration within the appropriate range. This strategy ensures that the energy is delivered over a longer period, which allows for less surrounding tissue injury outside the targeted chromophore. Energy fluence relates to pulsed lasers and is the amount of energy absorbed by the target. Fluence is measured in the unit of Joules per square centimeter. Irradiance is used for continuous laser systems because there is no fixed pulse duration and it is measured in the unit of Watts per square centimeter (cross-sectional area).

Although there is no difference in the melanocyte density between Latino skin and lighter skin types, in darker-skinned individuals there is an increase in the number of melanin granules within the basal layer. This large amount of melanin within the epidermis of Latino skin and darker skin types competitively absorbs laser light targeted for other chromophores. With the absorption spectrum of melanin ranging from 250 to 1200 nm, great care and diligence must be taken when using laser light on Latino skin. The laser light, targeted for dermal chromophores, is absorbed by epidermal melanin, with subsequent conversion to heat causing nonselective thermal injury to the epidermis. This situation can lead to blistering, burns, pigment alteration, and possible scarring.

Laser parameters that suit skin of color in regards to safety include longer wavelengths, a long pulse duration, and efficient cooling. The use of longer wavelengths is essential when treating Latino and equivalent skin types. Because melanin has a broad absorption spectrum, the use of a longer wavelength minimizes absorption by melanin. The longer wavelengths target deeper dermal structures and reduce heat transfer to the melanocytes within the epidermis. Longer pulse duration also helps minimize unwanted effects. The longer pulse duration delivers the laser light more slowly, which results in a slower heating of the epidermis. Accordingly the epidermis is allowed to cool more efficiently, reducing rapid heating and destruction of melanosomes. Because the thermal relaxation time of melanosomes is less than 1 microsecond, equivalent to 250 to 1000 nanoseconds, the melanosome is avoided when using pulse durations in the millisecond range. The third parameter essential to treating Latino skin is the use of an efficient cooling system. Epidermal damage can also be minimized by effective use of skin cooling directed at the superficial epidermis. The 3 basic types of skin cooling are precooling, parallel cooling, and postcooling. When pulse duration is less than 5 milliseconds, the time needed for the epidermis to cool is minimal and therefore precooling is suitable. For longer pulse durations in the 5-millisecond to 10-millisecond range, parallel cooling is efficient. Postcooling is also used to minimize bruising, erythema, and pain. In darker skin types excessive cooling can also cause melanocyte destruction, leading to postinflammatory pigment alteration. The use of test spots is encouraged when treating Latino or any skin of color. Immediate tissue responses can be evaluated 10 to 15 minutes after firing a test pulse and the clinical outcome can be assessed around 1 month later.

APPLICATIONS OF LASERS IN THE TREATMENT OF LATINOS

Using the principle of selective photothermolysis allows the use of vascular laser systems for a multitude of dermatologic conditions in skin of color. The vascular lasers when used at appropriate settings can be used for the light and dark skin tones in the Latino population. The main vascular chromophore is oxyhemoglobin. Vessels within lesions such as port wine stains are around 30 to 100 μm in diameter and have a thermal relaxation time ranging from 1 to 10 milliseconds. For larger leg veins that have diameters of 1 mm the thermal relaxation time is around 1 second. The lasers that are able to target vascular structures include the pulsed dye laser (585, 590, 595, 600 nm); variable-pulsed potassium titanyl phosphate (KTP) (532 nm); frequency doubled neodymium:yttrium aluminum garnet (Nd:YAG) (532 nm); long-pulsed alexandrite (755 nm); long-pulsed diode laser (800 nm); and long-pulsed Nd:YAG (1064 nm) laser. Intense pulsed light (IPL) with a wavelength range of 400 to 1200 nm can also be used for vascular targets in lighter- skinned individuals. The use of pulsed lasers allows the appropriate amount of energy to be delivered to the vascular target, minimizing heat dissipation to surrounding structures. The thermal relaxation time for cutaneous vasculature is 1 to 10 milliseconds for vessel diameter of 30 to 100 μm and the pulse duration of the traditional pulse dye laser is 450 microseconds, which is shorter than the target relaxation time, ensuring sufficient energy absorption by oxyhemoglobin and resultant red blood cell

coagulation. The pulsed dye laser is the treatment of choice for vascular lesions such as port wine stains, facial telangiectasias, and some superficial hemangiomas. Extended applications include verrucae, hypertrophic scars, and striae distensae. Newer pulsed dye lasers are ones with deeper penetrating wavelengths in the 590-nm to 600-nm range and a slightly longer pulse duration of 1.5 milliseconds, which is closer to the 1-millisecond to 10-millisecond thermal relaxation time of cutaneous vasculature. Ultralong or variable-pulsed dye lasers allow pulse duration of up to 40 milliseconds, which can treat larger-caliber vessels. Pulsed dye lasers have fluences up to 40 J/cm^2 and pulse durations from 0.45 to 40 milliseconds.

Phototypes IV to VI have epidermal melanin that acts as a competitive chromophore against hemoglobin and oxyhemoglobin. Epidermal melanin has a higher absorption coefficient than hemoglobin in the range of pulsed dye lasers. Therefore there is a risk of epidermal injury such as blistering, crusting, and resultant dyspigmentation. Also because of this competition less fluence is able to reach the target vasculature. Higher fluences are therefore necessary to achieve the desired clinical response but using fluences that are too high potentially damages the highly melanized epidermis. By decreasing the fluence to protect the epidermis, the physician must compensate by performing multiple treatments to achieve the desired clinical outcome. The 585-nm wavelength pulsed dye laser penetrates to a depth of 1.2 mm. The longer 595-nm wavelength allows for a slightly deeper penetration; however, the absorption coefficient of oxyhemoglobin is 3 times higher at 585 nm than 590 nm, which makes the 585-nm pulsed dye laser superior in treating the vascular lesions such as port wine stains. The 585-nm and 595-nm lasers are both suitable for fair-complexioned phototype IV skin. For darker phototypes V and VI, longer wavelengths should be used. In addition, longer pulse durations are safer in darker-skinned Latinos. With the pulsed dye laser treatment a resultant violaceous to purpuric discoloration of the treated area is expected. The duration of the resultant discoloration depends on the pulse duration selected, the skin phototype, and the amount of chromophore. With pulse durations less than 1.5 milliseconds the discoloration may last from a few days to weeks. If a longer pulse duration is used the discoloration is more transitory. Test spots should be used to determine the correct fluence for the particular skin type. As lesions like port wine stains lighten subsequent treatments likely require higher fluences to achieve clinical resolution. Transient hyperpigmentation has been reported in 44% to 46% of patients.[14] Longer pulse durations around 6 milliseconds allow clearance of vascular targets at relatively higher fluences such as 6 to 8 J/cm^2, while still remaining below the purpura threshold (around 12 J/cm^2). The use of a larger spot of 10 mm and speeds of 1 Hz allows for rapid treatment. The use of concomitant cooling devices is essential to minimize discomfort and increase the safety in darker skin types. For vascular lesions that require fluences above the purpuric threshold the physician can use multiple long pulses on top of one another during the same session. This technique is called pulse stacking and it improves efficacy without producing purpura. The pulsed dye laser can also be used at subpurpuric fluences to treat hypertrophic scars and keloids in the skin of color population. This laser shows histologic improvement of collagen remodeling.

The 800-nm diode laser has a fluence range of 10 to 100 J/cm^2 and a pulse duration range of 5 to 400 milliseconds. The diode laser can be used to target vascular structures such as leg veins or can be used for hair removal. Because hemoglobin has a small absorption peak in the 700-nm to 900-nm range the long-pulsed diode laser can be used to treat larger-caliber veins. The longer wavelength of the long-pulsed diode is in the near-infrared spectra (720–1200 nm). These longer wavelengths are absorbed less by melanin and penetrate deeper into the skin but their absorption by hemoglobin is less.

The long-pulsed 1064-nm Nd:YAG laser has a multitude of uses in the Latino population with skin of color. The longer wavelength Q switched laser systems in general work best for pigmented skin. The 1064-nm Nd:YAG laser produces less interference with epidermal melanin because the longer wavelength penetrates deeper into the skin; however, the absorption by hemoglobin is less than that of other lasers. The longer wavelength and pulse duration up to 100 milliseconds can treat vessels with diameters greater than 1 mm. The long-pulsed 1064-nm Nd:YAG can effectively photocoagulate superficial and deep vessels up to a diameter of 3 mm. This laser can be used to target venulectasias, such as spider veins and blue reticular veins, in the deep reticular dermis. However, when treating vasculature high fluences are needed so caution is advised when trying to treat large vessels in skin of color with this system. When used at fluences of 80 to 130 J/cm^2 at a pulse duration of 10 to 16 milliseconds approximately 75% of veins with diameters of 0.5 to 3 mm cleared within 3 months after a single treatment. The long-pulsed 1064-nm Nd:YAG laser when used with a pulse duration range from 1 to 100 milliseconds is useful for clearing deeper and larger facial vessels in darker-skinned phototypes.[15] See **Box 1** for laser treatment protocol for traumatic scars, postsurgical scars, and keloids.

Laser-assisted hair removal is able to achieve a permanent reduction of hair and this is a frequently sought after procedure in the Latino population. Previously hair laser removal in darker phototypes, such as phototype IV and above, was more of a challenge because of the risk of resultant pigment alteration with the earlier laser systems.

Box 1
1064-nm Nd:YAG (Genesis) laser treatment protocol for traumatic scars, postsurgical scars, and keloids

1. Traumatic Scars:

   a. Fluence starts at 12 J/cm^2 and increases because patient can tolerate up to 18 J/cm^2
   b. Use 500 pulses for small scars and 2000 pulses maximum for larger scars (>3 cm)
   c. One treatment per week for 3 weeks
   d. After 3 treatments wait 3 months; if needed start another set of 3 treatments with 1 treatment per week for 3 weeks
   e. Usually maximum is 2 sets of treatments; most patients take only 1 treatment

2. Postsurgical Scars:

   a. Wait 6 weeks to 3 months after surgery depending on the patient's healing process
   b. Start at 14 J/cm^2 and escalate to 18 J/cm^2 depending on patient's tolerance
   c. Use 500 pulses for small scars and a maximum of 2000 pulses for larger scars (>3 cm)
   d. 1 treatment per week for 3 weeks
   e. Repeat another session of 3 treatments 1 week apart after 3 months if necessary

3. Keloids:

   a. Week 1: inject intralesional triamcinolone 10 mg/mL for a total of 3 mL maximum
   b. Weeks 2, 3, 4, 5, 6, and 7: commence 1064-nm Nd:YAG (Genesis, Cutera, CA, USA) laser treatments; start at a fluence of 13 J/cm^2 and escalate up to 18 J/cm^2 as per patient's tolerance
   c. Give 2000 pulses per keloid
   d. One treatment weekly for 6 total treatments
   e. At week 8 reevaluate: if necessary give another intralesional triamcinolone 10 mg/mL injection at week 8 and then another round of 1064-nm Nd:YAG laser treatments at weeks 9, 10, 11, 12, 13, and 14
   f. Reevaluate in week 15
   g. Intralesional triamcinolone 5 mg/mL for 1 mL total volume in the periphery of lesions when active; no recurrences seen in 5 years

With the advent of lasers with longer wavelengths, longer pulse durations, and efficient cooling devices, all skin types can be treated with lasers for hair removal without side effects. The use of longer wavelengths penetrates to a deeper depth, lessening the degree of absorption by the epidermal melanin and ensuing less pigment destruction by the laser intended for the targeted melanin in the hair follicle. Melanin absorption decreases as wavelength increases. The longer wavelengths penetrate deeper into the dermis where the hair follicle resides. The terminal hair has a diameter of about 300 μm and a thermal relaxation time of 100 milliseconds. Therefore the pulse durations used for laser hair removal are in the range of 3 to 100 milliseconds. In the darker subsets of Latinos it is important to use longer pulse duration (around 30–100 ms) to aid in slowly heating the intended melanin chromophore in the hair follicle and to protect the epidermis. The longer pulse duration ensures a slower heating of the chromophore and resultant slower heating of the epidermis, which decreases epidermal thermal damage. The use of concomitant cooling devices further protects the epidermis from collateral thermal damage. In darker skin excessive cooling should be avoided as well because of possible pigment alteration. Two lasers that are appropriate for use in Latino skin up to phototypes IV are the diode laser, 810 nM, and the Nd:YAG laser at 1064 nM for Latinos up to phototypes VI. Both lasers require multiple treatments (usually more than would be required in the lighter skin phototypes) because of the need to increase pulse duration and decrease fluence to protect epidermal melanin. During each treatment an appropriate tissue response includes perifollicular edema lasting from minutes to hours. Excessive pain, frank erythema, graying of the skin, and blistering should not be encountered and indicate that the fluence may be inappropriately high.

The diode laser can be used to target the follicular melanin chromophore for use in hair removal. High fluences can be achieved when using long pulse durations. Permanent hair loss of around 20% to 35% per treatment has been reported with the diode laser.[16] In darker phenotypes 75% to 90% hair reduction was reported after 8 to 10 treatments at 10 J/cm^2 and 30 milliseconds pulse duration. Longer pulse durations of 100 to 400 milliseconds allow for higher fluences of 20 to 30 J/cm^2.[17] Longer pulse durations of 100 milliseconds or greater should be used when treating skin phototypes V and VI.

The 1064-nm Nd:YAG is considered to be the safest for hair removal in the darker pigmented population. It is suitable for use in all skin types I to VI. Mean hair reductions of 44% for the face and 50% for body areas were reported at fluences of 30 to 60 J/cm^2 and a 10-millisecond to 30-millisecond pulse duration. For phototypes V and VI the pulse duration is safest at 30 milliseconds or greater. Alster and colleagues[18] reported successful use of the long-pulsed 1064-nm Nd:YAG with a pulse duration of 30 milliseconds or longer for facial hirsutism. A greater than 50% reduction in facial hair was achieved in 6 months in patients with phototypes V and VI.

A rare but notable adverse effect called paradoxic hypertrichosis can occur, especially when subtherapeutic fluences are used for laser hair removal. This phenomenon has a low incidence, ranging from 0.6% to 10% and it most commonly occurs on the face and neck, but can occur in other places such as the back, especially in men. It also tends to occur in an adjacent area of untreated skin. Paradoxic hypertrichosis was first reported with the use of the IPL system, but has also been reported with the long-pulsed 755-nm alexandrite, the 810-nm diode laser, and 694-nm ruby laser. So far no case reports have cited this effect with the 1064-nm Nd:YAG laser. It is hypothesized that subtherapeutic thermal injury to the follicular vasculature, from suboptimal laser fluences, can affect follicular cycling in a way that induces terminal hair growth rather than inducing miniaturization. The heat-induced inflammatory reaction from a suboptimal fluence may increase blood flow to the follicular papilla and therefore supply growth factors to the follicle. Bouzari and colleagues[19] also theorized that the suboptimal thermal injury that does not destroy the follicle may induce follicular stem cell differentiation and growth by increasing the level of heat shock proteins such as heat shock protein 27 in the tissue. Goldberg and colleagues[20] reported that paradoxic hypertrichosis occurs more frequently in patients with skin types III or greater as well as those with undiagnosed hormonal conditions. Most reports have come from Mediterranean countries where most of the population is of a darker skin type. This situation may occur because patients of darker skin type have a greater tendency to shift from vellus to terminal hairs. Willey and colleagues[21] reported several factors that they believe contribute to the failure to destroy the follicle and therefore cause paradoxic hypertrichosis. These factors include hair thickness, with thinner hairs being harder to destroy; hair color, because darker hairs are more efficiently heated; depth of hairs, with deeper anagen hairs being harder to heat; underlying hormonal conditions; use of hormone supplements; presence of posttreatment side effects, suboptimal treatment fluences; anatomic site (face and neck); sex, because of a female preponderance but this finding may be from a sampling error; and darker skin types (III–VI). Treatment of paradoxic hypertrichosis includes continuing the laser hair removal but using a higher-energy fluence or changing to the 1064-nm Nd:YAG laser.

The Nd:YAG laser has also been reported to treat pseudofollicilitis barbae in the population with skin of color. For this application, especially in the beard area, the physician must be aware of the bridging effect. The terminal beard hairs are thick and therefore retain more heat, which can lead to scarring. Therefore when using the Nd:YAG laser in this area or any hair with a high density of thick terminal hair it is essential to decrease the fluence and increase the pulse duration. The Nd:YAG can also be used as an adjuvant therapy for acne keloidalis nuchae.

ABLATIVE LASERS

Ablative skin resurfacing is a useful treatment of photoaging, rhytides, hyperpigmentation, scars, and lesions such as epidermal nevi and seborrheic keratoses. Resurfacing removes the old epidermis via the process of ablation and stimulates contraction and remodeling of the dermis after treatment through the process of coagulation. The heat generated under the ablative layer of tissue denatures and shrinks collagen, causing a visible tightening of the skin. Ablative resurfacing produces a controlled partial-thickness burn of the epidermis and partially of the dermis, so its use in phototypes V and VI is not indicated because of the risk of scarring and hyperpigmentation, as well as delayed-onset hypopigmentation. Continuous-wave CO_2 lasers were used in the 1980s and 1990s to resurface photodamaged skin. The chromophore in ablative resurfacing is water. The CO_2 laser (10,600 nm), erbium:YAG (Er:YAG) laser (2940 nm), and the 2790-nm erbium:yttrium-scandium-gallium-garnet (Er:YSGG) laser (Pearl Laser, Cutera, CA, USA) are effective ablative lasers. The water absorption coefficients for the 3 wavelengths mentioned earlier differ by an order of magnitude (103 cm-1 for CO_2 laser at 10,600 nm, 104 cm-1 for Er:YAG laser at 2940 nm, and 102 cm-1 for Er:YSGG laser at 2790 nm). The 10,600-nm CO_2 laser is strongly absorbed by tissue water and the penetration is dependent on the water content of the tissue. With pulse duration of less than 1 milliseconds, the CO_2 laser penetrates 20 to 30 μm into the skin and residual thermal damage can be confined to 100 to 150 μm in depth. The fluence required to achieve vaporization of water is 5 J/cm^2. Also the diameter of the beam factors in, with

smaller beams reaching higher fluences and quicker tissue vaporization. Beam diameters of greater than 2 mm induce no vaporization heating and increase the risk of deep thermal damage. There are 2 types of CO_2 lasers: a pulsed system that delivers energy in individual pulses of about 1 milliseconds or less, and a continuous-wave CO_2 laser that delivers a continuous wave over a focally scanned area. The Er:YAG laser emits infrared light with a wavelength of 2940 nm, which is close to the absorption peak of water and produces an absorption coefficient 16 times that of the CO_2 laser. The penetration depth of the Er:YAG laser is limited to about 1 to 3 μm of tissue. This depth allows for more precise ablation of the skin, with minimal thermal damage to the surrounding tissues. However, because there is less thermal damage, there is less coagulation and less collagen production, creating the need for multiple passes for better efficacy. Newer ablative lasers such as the variable-pulsed Er:YAG, the 1540-nm and 1420-nm fractional Er:YAG and the fractional 10,600-nm CO_2 laser allow for resurfacing treatments with less downtime, edema, erythema, and scarring. There is a faster healing time than seen with conventional ablative lasers; however, multiple treatments are necessary. Again side effects include scarring, hyperpigmentation, hypopigmentation, and infection.

The newer 2790-nm Er:YSGG laser (Pearl Laser; Cutera) is at a wavelength that is slightly less than the 2940-nm Er:YAG. The 2940-nm Er:YAG laser emits a wavelength of 2940 nm, which is close to the absorption peak of water and yields an absorption coefficient 16 times that of the CO_2 laser. The 2790-nm Er:YSGG laser has a slightly shorter wavelength and is believed to ablate the top 10 to 30 μm of the epidermis and at less than that the epidermis is coagulated. Also the residual thermal damage is believed to stimulate new dermal collagen synthesis.

FRACTIONAL ABLATION

Ablative fractional resurfacing with laser uses fractionated technology to produce microscopic columns of controlled dermal tissue ablation and vaporization, which are surrounded by thermally induced annular coagulation zones of denatured collagen. Interspersed between these ablated regions are areas of untreated tissue, which are believed to allow a nidus of recovery tissue, leading to less downtime. By delivering the energy fractionally, greater depth of penetration, ranging from 300 mm to more than 1 mm, can be achieved. The resultant dermal remodeling is reflected by the greater degree of tissue contraction and collagen production compared with nonablative fractional treatment. Immunohistochemical studies have shown the induction of epidermal heat shock protein and persistent collagen remodeling with wound-healing response lasting up to 3 months after fractional ablative CO_2 laser treatment.[22] Fractional ablative CO_2 lasers seem to have a better safety profile compared with traditional ablative lasers. This situation is because of the interspersed untreated cutaneous tissues, allowing for complete reepithelialization in about 3 to 6 days, compared with 2 to 3 weeks with traditional ablative lasers. Most published articles have been in type I phototypes and there are some reports of its use in Asian patients; however, postinflammatory hyperpigmentation is of greater concern in darker phototypes.[23]

These ablative devices are not suitable for use in skin types V to VI because of the higher incidence of scarring and resultant dyspigmentation. There is a paucity of literature regarding use of fractionated ablative lasers in skin type IV, and these lasers in lighter Latino skin should be used with caution and extensive preoperative counseling. The use of perioperative measures such as hydroquinone,

tretinoin, and sunscreens is important, as well as postoperative avoidance of the sun, trauma, and infection to produce the best results and least permanent dyspigmentation. Also prophylaxis with antiviral medication should be used for herpes simplex virus suppression.

NONABLATIVE LASERS

To circumvent the challenges of ablative laser resurfacing, nonablative resurfacing laser technology emerged. This technology provides a treatment modality to improve pigment disorders and skin texture, as well as subtle rhytides, without removing the epidermis. Therefore there is less risk of scarring and dyspigmentation with less downtime. However, there are less impressive results clinically compared with the ablative laser technologies. The 1320-nm Nd:YAG laser is commonly used for skin rejuvenation. This laser heats dermal water at 50 to 300 μm. It produces collagen enhancement and remodeling by distributing the energy throughout the dermis because the target chromophore is the water within the papillary and midreticular dermis. There is also

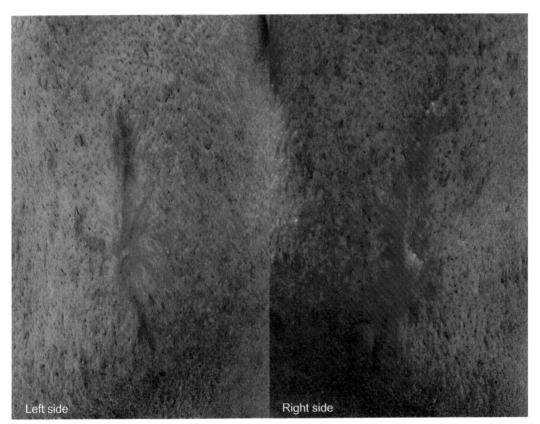

Left side

Right side

Fig. 2. Bilateral facial keloids left side treated with intralesional triamcinolone 10 mg/mL 1.5 mL total volume and 1064-nm Nd:YAG (Genesis, Cutera, CA, USA) laser: 2000 pulses (6 treatments total). Right side: treated with intralesional triamcinolone 10 mg/mL alone 1.5 mL total volume.

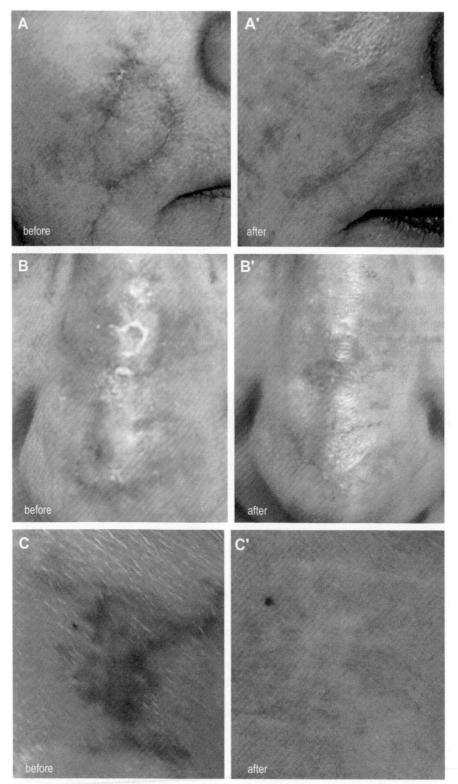

Fig. 3. (*A*, *B*, *C*) Postsurgical scars treated with the 1064-nm Nd:YAG (Genesis, Cutera, CA, USA) laser with 2000 pulses for collagen remodeling. Three treatments 1 week apart. (*A'*, *B'*, *C'*) After treatment.

epidermal spongiosis and swelling of the epidermal basal layer, which implies that there is epidermal injury taking place. This subclinical epidermal injury helps to improve skin texture.[24]

FRACTIONAL NONABLATIVE THERAPY

Fractional resurfacing or fractional photothermolysis is another nonablative approach used in skin resurfacing. This technology fractionally ablates areas of skin and leaves intervening areas of normal skin that allow a more rapid healing of the ablated columns. Unlike other nonablative lasers that do not have a direct effect on the epidermis, fractional photothermolysis improves skin texture.

The laser is a 1550-nm midinfrared erbium doped laser (Fraxel SR, Mosaic, SoltaMedical, CA, USA), which causes cylindrical areas of thermal damage to the epidermis and upper dermis, spaced at 1000 to 3000 microscopic treatment zones of photothermolysis per square centimeter in density. These are called microthermal zones and each is about 70 to 150 μm wide and with a vertical dimension of 400 to 700 μm into the dermis. About 15% to 25% of the skin surface is ablated per treatment.[25] The stratum corneum stays intact, which allows for a more rapid healing time and less risk of infection. There is also dermal remodeling, and histologically there is epidermal and dermal necrosis, which is confined to the microthermal treatment zones. There is no confluence of these injury zones. This fractional therapy is indicated for all skin types but most studies have been performed in skin phototypes I to IV. This therapy is used in phototypes IV and above but caution should be exercised because the creation of these microthermal zones of destruction can lead to postinflammatory hyperpigmentation and scarring in the darker skin types. Once again a test spot is warranted before commencing treatments. The posterior auricular location is a suitable test spot. The test spot can be initiated at a low-density and low-energy setting and gradually increased with multiple passes. In darker phototypes regional treatment can be appropriate for selective disorders such as acne scarring or melasma. Prophylaxis with hydroquinone for 1 month before therapy is advised, and the use of antiviral agents to suppress herpes simplex virus infection is warranted. Contraindication to fractional therapy

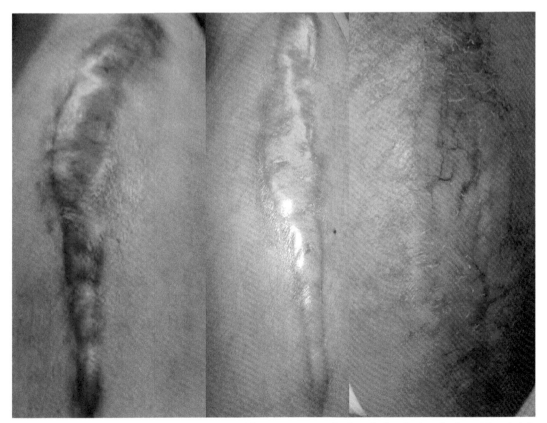

Fig. 4. 1064-nm Nd:YAG (Genesis, Cutera, CA, USA) laser treatment plus intralesional triamcinolone 10 mg/mL for the treatment of a keloid.

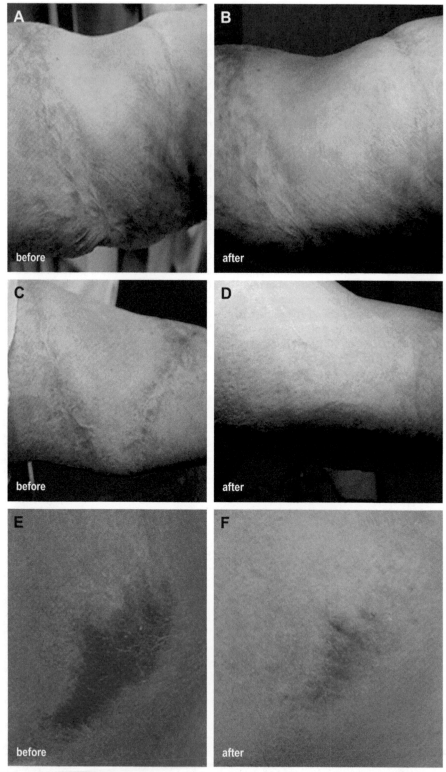

Fig. 5. 1064-nm Nd:YAG (Genesis, Cutera, CA, USA) treatment of posttraumatic scars: (*A*) before, (*B*) after, (*C*) before, (*D*) after, (*E*) before, and (*F*) after.

included oral retinoid use, a history of keloids, and tanned skin.

The long-pulsed 1064-nm laser has also been used in a nonablative fashion. Goldberg and colleagues reported neocollanogenesis in electron micrographic evaluation of skin treated with the long-pulsed 1064-nm laser. Furthermore, Lipper and Perez[26] studied the use of the nonablative 1064-nm Nd:YAG laser for treatment of facial acne scarring. Nine of 10 enrolled patients with moderate to severe facial acne scarring received 8 sequential 1064-nm Nd:YAG treatments (laser

Table 1
Select lasers and their uses in the Latino/Hispanic population

Laser	Target Chromophore	Skin Phototypes and Applications	Settings: Fluence (J/cm^2) Pulse Duration (ms)
Vascular			
Variable-pulsed KTP laser (532 nm)	Oxyhemoglobin (long-pulsed) Melanin/pigment (Q switched)	All phototypes: Facial telangiectasias; venous malformations; cherry angiomas	Fluence: Up to 240 Pulse: 1–100
Pulsed dye laser (585, 590, 595, 600 nm)	Oxyhemoglobin	All phototypes: port wine stains; telangiectasias; scars; verruca	Fluence: Up to 40 Pulse: 0.45–40
Long-pulsed Nd:YAG (1064 nm)	Oxyhemoglobin	All phototypes: venulectasias, telangiectasia, blue reticular veins	Fluence: 5–900 Pulse: 2–200
Diode (800 nm)	Oxyhemoglobin	All phototypes: spider leg venulectasias	Fluence: 10–100 Pulse: 5–400
Hair Removal			
Diode (800, 810 nm)	Melanin	Hair removal: skin types I–VI	Fluence: 10–100 Pulse: 100 ms (darker phototypes)
Nd:YAG (1064 nm)	Melanin	Hair removal: skin types I–VI	Fluence 0–600 Pulse: >30 ms
Fractional			
Fractionated 1550-nm erbium doped fiber laser (Fraxel)	Water	Resurfacing; scars; rhytides; dyspigmentation: use with caution in phototypes IV and above	Melasma phototypes III–VI: Energy: 6 mJ Density: 250 MTZ/ cm^2 Passes: 8 Total density: 2000 MTZ/cm^2
Nonablative			
Nd:YAG 1064 nm	Dermal collagen; water	Resurfacing; scars; keloids: all phototypes	Fluence: 14 J/cm^2, Pulse: 0.3 ms 5-mm spot size, 7-Hz pulse rate, 2000 pulses per side of face
Ablative			
CO$_2$ 10,600 nm	Water	Total ablative resurfacing: use with caution in skin types IV	Fluence 5–7 J/cm^2 Pulse: <950 µs
Er:YAG laser (2940 nm)	Water	Total ablative resurfacing: use with caution in skin types IV	Fluence: 1–50 mJ/cm^2 Pulse: 250 µs– 50 ms
Er:YSGG laser (2790 nm) (Pearl, Cutera)	Water	Total ablative resurfacing: use with caution in skin types IV	Fluence: 3.5 J/cm^2 Pulse 0.4 ms Overlap: 0%–20%

parameters 14 J/cm^2, 0.3 ms, 5-mm spot size, 7-Hz pulse rate, 2000 pulses per side of face). Patients were graded for the presence and severity of 3 scar morphologies, which included superficial or rolling, medium-depth or boxcar, and deep or ice pick scars. Scar improvement was noted in all treated patients with minimal discomfort and no downtime. Chan and colleagues[27] also reported the use the 1320-nm Nd:YAG laser for rhytid reduction. Twenty-seven women received 3 passes every 4 to 6 weeks for 5 to 6 treatments, and patients reported a 4.9 out of 9.8 improvement in wrinkle reduction. An unexpected result was the increase in epidermal thickness, which suggests that the epidermis may be more affected than previously believed.

Perez and colleagues treated keloids and hypertrophic scars with the 1064-nm Nd:YAG laser at a pulse duration of 300 microseconds (Rossi A, Perez MI. The Use of the 300 microsecond 1064nm Nd:YAG Laser in the Treatment of Keloids. Submitted for publication.). The fluence used was 13 to 18 J/cm^2, spot size of 5 mm, and 2000 pulses. The wavelength allows penetration into and selective photothermolysis of the dermis, with resultant reduction in the deranged collagen of the keloids and neocollagenesis. Although the exact mechanism is unclear, this neocollagenesis may improve the bulk of these lesions through collagen remodeling, and it is also possible that the thermal injury may affect keloidal collagen through cytokine release and stimulation of fibroblast proliferation (**Figs. 2–5**).

SUMMARY

Table 1 reviews the lasers discussed and their applications in the Latino/Hispanic ethnic group. Although there are many laser treatment options that included both ablative and nonablative technologies in the population with skin of color and in the Latino population a combination approach is best used. Reports of using fractional ablative and nonablative lasers in skin types IV have shown promising results. These lasers are most often also used with medical treatments such as chemical peels for dyschromias as well as hydroquinones and topical retinoid therapy. When approaching a patient of Latino descent one must individualize the patient into a specific skin phototype, because this population has highly variable skin pigmentation. One treatment does not fit all and nor do certain parameters. There are more and more studies regarding using these laser technologies in skin of color and more specifically skin phototypes IV to VI. Not every laser is intended for use in darker skin phototypes. The efficacy and use of laser therapy in the Latino population are limited by possible adverse effects caused by competing melanin in the skin. When dealing with skin types V and VI one must be aware that ablative and fractionally ablative procedures are not appropriate because the risks of scarring and dyspigmentation outweigh any potential gain. Safe use of lasers includes using test spots before commencing all treatment plans. The use of longer wavelengths and longer pulse durations to protect epidermal melanin as well as using concomitant cooling devices help to ensure safe lasing in darker phototypes. Although an individual patient may be represented by a specific ethnic group, there can be extreme variation within the group and therefore each treatment should be individually tailored.

Notes to Early Users:

- The Latino/Hispanic ethnic group is a rapidly increasing population and their specific dermatologic problems should be addressed
- The learning curves are different for each specific laser and one should familiarize oneself with each system before starting treatment
- Laser treatments should be patient tailored, because there is no "1 parameter fits all" approach
- The use of test spots is encouraged before commencing treatment
- In darker skin types (phototypes IV–VI), the use of longer-wavelength lasers, longer pulse durations, and effective epidermal cooling are parameters to help ensure epidermal protection and less collateral thermal damage
- Ablative and fractional laser procedures should be used by experienced physicians only and with caution in any pigmented skin and should not be used on skin types V or above

---

REFERENCES

1. Lamason RL, Manzoor-Ali PK, Mohideen, et al. SLC24A5, a putative cation exchanger, affects pigmentation in zebrafish and humans. Science 2005;310:1782–6.
2. US Census Bureau. Population growth. Available at: http://www.census.gov/. Accessed May 3, 2011.
3. Sanchez MR. Cutaneous diseases in Latinos. Dermatol Clin 2003;21:689–97.
4. Taylor SC. Epidemiology of skin diseases in ethnic populations. Dermatol Clin 2003;21(4):601–7.

5. Reed JT, Ghadailly R, Elias PM. Effect of race, gender, and skin type on epidermal permeability barrier function. J Invest Dermatol 1994;102:537.

6. Sugino K, Imakawo G, Maibach H. Ethnic difference of stratum corneum lipid in relation to stratum corneum function. J Invest Dermatol 1993;100:597.

7. Starkco RS, Pinkus H. Quantitative and qualitative data on the pigment cell of adult human epidermis. J Invest Dermatol 1957;28:33.

8. Masson P. Pigment cells in man. In: Miner RW, et al, editors, The biology of melanosomes, vol. IV. New York: New York Academy of Sciences; 1948. p. 10–7.

9. Kaidbey KH, Agin PP, Sayre RM, et al. Photoprotection by melanin: a comparison of black and Caucasian skin. J Am Acad Dermatol 1979;1:249–60.

10. Homma H. On appocrine sweat glands in white and Negro men and women. Bull Johns Hopkins Hosp 1956;38:365.

11. Taylor SC. Skin of color: biology, structure, function, and implications for dermatologic disease. J Am Acad Dermatol 2002;46:S41–62.

12. Anderson RR, Parrish JA. Selective thermolysis; precise microsurgery by selective absorption of pulsed radiation. Science 1983;220:524–7.

13. Anderson RR, Parrish JA. The optics of human skin. J Invest Dermatol 1981;77:13–9.

14. Sommer S, Sheehan-Dare RA. Pulsed dye laser treatment of port wine stains in pigmented skin. J Am Acad Dermatol 2000;42:667–71.

15. Anderson RR. Lasers in cutaneous and aesthetic surgery. Philadelphia: Lippincott-Raven; 1997. p. 25–51.

16. Baugh WP, Trafeli JP, Barnette DJ Jr, et al. Hair reduction using a scanning 800nm diode laser. Dermatol Surg 2001;27:358–64.

17. Greppi I. Diode laser hair removal of the black patient. Lasers Surg Med 2001;28:150–5.

18. Alster TS, Bryan H, Williams CM. Long pulsed Nd:YAG laser assisted hair removal in pigmented skin. A clinical and histological evaluation. Arch Dermatol 2001;137:885–9.

19. Bouzari N, Firooz AR. Lasers may induce terminal hair growth. Dermatol Surg 2006;32:460.

20. Schmults CD, Phelps R, Goldberg DJ. Nonablative facial remodeling: erythema reduction and histologic evidence of new collagen formation using a 300-micro- second 1064-nm Nd:YAG laser. Arch Dermatol 2004;140:1373–6.

21. Willey A, Torrontegui RN, Azpiazu J, et al. Hair stimulation following laser and intense pulsed light photo-epilation: review of 543 cases and ways to manage it. Lasers Surg Med 2007;l39:297–301.

22. Rahman Z, MacFalls H, Jiang K, et al. Fractional deep dermal ablation induces tissue tightening. Lasers Surg Med 2009;41(2):78–86.

23. Hunzeker CM, Weiss ET, Geronemus RG. Fractionated CO2 laser resurfacing: our experience with more than 2000 treatments. Aesthet Surg J 2009; 29(4):317–22.

24. Fatemi A, Weiss MA, Weiss RS. Short-term histologic effects of nonablative resurfacing: results with a dynamically cooled millisecond domain 1,320 nm Nd:YAG laser. Dermatol Surg 2002;28:172–6.

25. Manstein D, Herron GS, Sink RK, et al. Fractional photothermolysis: a new concept for cutaneous remodeling using microscopic patterns of thermal injury. Lasers Surg Med 2004;34:426–38.

26. Lipper GM, Perez M. Nonablative acne scar reduction after a series of treatments with a short-pulsed 1,064-nm neodymium:YAG laser. Dermatol Surg 2006;32(8):998–1006.

27. Chan HH, Urn LK, Wong DS, et al. Use of 1,320nm Nd:YAG laser for wrinkle reduction and the treatment of atrophic acne scarring in Asians. Lasers Surg Med 2004;34:98–103.

Laser Therapy in Black Skin

Heather Woolery-Lloyd, MD[a],*, Martha H. Viera, MD[b],
Whitney Valins, MD[a]

KEYWORDS

- Laser therapy • Melanin • Laser complications in black skin
- Hyperpigmentation

Patients of African descent often require special consideration when it comes to receiving cosmetic procedures, specifically with laser, light, and energy-based procedures. They are particularly vulnerable because any kind of significant trauma, be it from a laser or other device, can cause permanent pigmentary changes and scarring. For the clinician, cosmetic procedures in patients with skin of color can therefore be challenging. Because of enhanced technology and scientific advances, the demand to seek procedures to address these patients' cosmetic concerns has reached new heights. Patients with skin of color have various motivations and goals including attaining an even skin tone, removing unwanted hair, and/or reducing the signs of aging. The American Society of Plastic and Reconstructive Surgery revealed that cosmetic procedures among minority patients increased from 12% of all cosmetically treated patients in 1992 to 20% in 1998. Of the 11,000,000 esthetic procedures performed in the United States in 2005, 6% were African American (up from 4%), 8% were Hispanic (up from 5%), and 4% were Asian (up from 3%).[1,2]

This article provides a systematic overview of laser, light, and other energy devices for patients of African descent. It also reviews complications in skin of color and some treatment options for these adverse events.

MELANIN, UV REACTIVITY, AND PHOTOPROTECTION

Dermal melanin is produced by melanocytes in the basal layer of the epidermis; however, there is no difference in melanocyte number among races. Instead, skin color is determined by the size and distribution of melanosomes.[3] Melanin absorbs and scatters energy from UV light and visible light to protect epidermal cells from UV damage. The photoprotection offered by melanin in darkly pigmented skin greatly influences the UV-induced differences seen in black and white skin. After long-term exposure to sunlight, the epidermis of black skin displays only minor changes, in contrast to the enlarged, cellular stratum lucidum layer that is observed in sun-exposed white skin.[4] Photoprotection is a definite advantage for those with skin of color.

ADVANTAGES AND DISADVANTAGES

Along with the advantage of photoprotection, dark-skinned individuals also present with a delay in photoaging. In a survey of age-matched white and black women, with a mean age of 43, 65% of black women reported that their skin was not wrinkled compared with only 20% of white women,[5] revealing a marked distinction in perceived photoaging.

Disclosures: Heather Woolery-Lloyd, MD, is a speaker for Cutera. Martha Viera, MD: none. Whitney Valins: none.
[a] Department of Dermatology and Cutaneous Surgery, University of Miami Miller School of Medicine, 1600 NW 10th Avenue, Miami, FL 33136, USA
[b] Department of General Surgery, University of Miami, 1120 NW 14th Street, 4th Floor, Miami, FL 33136, USA
* Corresponding author.
E-mail address: woolerylloyd@yahoo.com

At the same time, there are other unique cosmetic concerns for those with skin of color. Inflammation or injury to the skin is almost immediately accompanied by alteration in pigmentation, namely hyperpigmentation or hypopigmentation. As follows, patients are most concerned with post-inflammatory pigment changes. In a survey of the cosmetic concerns in women of color (81 African, 16 Hispanic, 3 Asian), with a mean age of 41, 86% reported hyperpigmentation or dark spots, and 80% reported blotchy or uneven skin as their greatest concern.[5]

ACNE SCARS
Ablative Devices

CO_2 lasers have been used for the treatment of acne scars in ethnic skin; however, the laser's usefulness has been limited by the risk of hyper-pigmentation and scarring. For this reason, other modalities have been investigated for optimum acne scar treatment in ethnic skin.[6]

Fractional Devices

Nonablative fractional resurfacing is used for photorejuvenation in all skin types and is especially useful for the treatment of acneiform scarring in ethnic skin.[7] Nonablative fractional resurfacing is performed using a midinfrared laser, which creates microscopic zones of thermal injury, called micro-thermal zones (MTZs), with an energy-dependent diameter ranging from 100 to 160 μm. At the energies commonly used for facial rejuvenation (8–12 mJ/MTZ), the depth of penetration ranges from 300 to 700 μm.[8] Relative epidermal and follicular structure sparing account for rapid recovery without prolonged downtime. Melanin is not at risk of selective, targeted destruction; therefore, fractional resurfacing has been used successfully in patients with skin of color.

There are several fractional devices available, with the most extensively studied being 1550-nm erbium-doped fiber laser (Fraxel, Reliant Technologies Inc, San Diego, CA, USA). In a study of the efficacy of this laser in Japanese patients with acne scars, one treatment consisted of 4 passes of the device to attain a final microscopic treatment zone of thermal injury with a density of 1000 to 1500/cm². The fluence was 6 mJ per microscopic treatment zone. The treatment was repeated up to 3 times at 2-week to 3-week intervals and clinical improvement was achieved in all the patients. Rare adverse events included mild transient erythema, whereas no patients showed scarring or hyperpigmentation as a result of treatment.[9]

Another study evaluated the Fraxel for the treatment of acne scars in 27 Korean patients with skin types IV and V. Patient self-assessments demonstrated excellent improvement in 30%, significant improvement in 59%, and moderate improvement in 11% of patients. No patients developed hyperpigmentation.[10]

Although the safe and effective use of nonablative fractional resurfacing in Asian patients is well documented, there are few published studies in skin types VI or in African American patients. In one retrospective review of 961 treatments in patients of all skin types, the rate of hyperpigmentation was 11.6% in skin type IV (n = 8) and 33% in skin type V (n = 3). The ethnicities of these patients were not specified.[11]

Nonablative fractional resurfacing represents a relatively safe and effective option for Asian patients with skin of color for the treatment of acne scars and photoaging. Patients of African descent have been less extensively studied; however, in these patients conservative settings (low densities) are necessary to minimize the risk of hyperpigmentation.[12]

Nonablative Devices

In a study comparing the 1320-nm Nd:YAG and the 1450-nm diode laser in the treatment of atrophic scars of patients with skin types I to V, both devices led to clinical improvement without significant side effects.[13]

A short-pulsed nonablative Nd:YAG (Laser Genesis, Cutera, Inc, Brisbane, CA, USA) has been studied in skin types I to V for the treatment of acne scars. Settings were 14 J/cm², 0.3 milliseconds, 7 Hz, with a 5-mm spot size. The study included 9 patients who were treated every 2 weeks for a series of 8 treatments. Each side of the face was treated with a total of 2000 pulses. Three blinded physician observers used a grid on pictures of the patients to count scars at baseline and after the final treatment. They found a 29% improvement in the scar severity score. Eight of 9 patients reported improvement in their acne scars ranging from 10% to 50% improvement. This non-ablative Nd:YAG laser offers another safe and well-tolerated option to treat acne scars in patients of African descent.[14] It is important to note that a series of 8 or more treatments are required to achieve improvement. This device has an excellent safety profile in all patients, including skin type VI, and is most effective in shallow acne scars. Deep ice-pick acne scars remain a challenge with all laser modalities in skin of color.

PHOTOREJUVENATION

As mentioned previously, in patients with skin types IV to VI, photoaging is delayed and less severe. In African American individuals, photoaging is more prominent in lighter-complexioned individuals. In addition, it may not be apparent until the late fifth or sixth decade of life and clinically can appear as fine wrinkling, mottled pigmentation, and dermatosis papulosa nigra. In Asian and Hispanic patients, photoaging is also manifested by solar lentigos and prominent pigmentary changes.[15]

Light-Emitting Diode

Light-emitting diodes (LEDs) offer another advancement in visible spectrum, monochromatic light therapy for photoaged skin. Typically, LEDs in devices are arrayed in panels with each LED emitting visible light in a ± 10-nm to 20-nm band around the dominant emitted wavelength. Energy output is less than 25 W, representing a fluence of about 0.1 J/cm^2.[16] The mechanism of this device is thought to act by targeting stimulation of fibroblast mitochondrial metabolic activity. In addition, concomitant upregulation of procollagen and downregulation of matrix metalloproteinase I has been demonstrated.[17] Although there are no studies on LEDs in ethnic skin, based on the mechanism of action, these devices should be and are generally considered safe in darker racial ethnic groups.

LASER HAIR REMOVAL
Alexandrite

The alexandrite laser has been studied in skin types IV to VI. In one study, a long-pulsed 755-nm laser with a 40-millisecond pulse width was used to treat 150 patients with skin types IV to VI. A test site with a fluence of 16 J/cm^2 was first performed and energy fluence was selected according to response. A small complication rate (2.7%) was reported; however, only 2 patients with skin type VI were included in the study and both developed blistering.[18] A smaller study of the alexandrite (755-nm, 3-millisecond pulse width) included 4 African American women with Fitzpatrick skin type VI. In this study, lower fluences were used (8–14 J/cm^2) and no side effects were noted.[19] Although treatment of skin types IV to VI is possible with the alexandrite, the associated risk is still great in these patients.

Diode

The Diode laser has been studied with greater success in the treatment of darker-skinned patients. The 800-nm diode laser was studied with pulse widths of 30 milliseconds and 100 milliseconds. Adrian and Shay[20] reported that

although both settings could be used safely, longer pulse widths (100 ms) allowed higher fluences to be used with fewer complications. Another study used the 810-nm Diode laser to treat 8 African American patients with skin types V and VI. These patients were treated with a lower fluence of 10 mJ/cm^2 and a pulse width of 30 milliseconds. Despite the lower fluence, transient blistering and pigment alterations were noted in some patients.[21] Overall, although the diode laser offers increased safety over the alexandrite laser in African American patients, complications remain an issue.

Nd:YAG

The long-pulsed Nd:YAG is the safest laser for hair removal in darker skin types, owing to 2 factors. First, the wavelength of this laser (1064 nm) is at the end of the absorption spectrum of melanin, and is sufficient to achieve significant thermal injury in dark coarse hairs while sparing epidermal pigment. Second, the adjustable pulse width of long-pulsed Nd:YAG lasers allows the laser energy to be delivered over a longer period of time allowing for the heat to dissipate with sufficient epidermal cooling.

The long-pulsed Nd:YAG is the treatment of choice for hirsutism and pseudofolliculitis barbae in African American patients with skin types V to VI, because of their typically coarse, dark hair. It is both safe and highly effective at achieving permanent hair reduction after a series of treatments.[22,23]

Challenges with the long-pulsed Nd:YAG in darker skin types arise in patients with dark skin but fine hair. In these patients, permanent hair reduction is more challenging because the fluence and pulse width that are necessary to achieve permanent reduction of fine hair are risky in darker skin types. In these cases, it is important to educate the patient on the limitations of laser-assisted hair reduction. Patients must have realistic expectations and understand that lasers can offer an excellent hair-management program but may not offer permanent long-term removal of fine hairs. Many patients who fall into this category still prefer laser because of the elimination of irritation and dyschromia frequently seen with shaving, waxing, or threading.

SKIN TIGHTENING

In contrast to photoaging, increasing skin laxity with advanced age is equally common in all skin types. Older patients commonly seek treatment for the jowls and nasolabial folds, which are prominent signs of aging, whereas younger patients seek treatment of the abdomen after pregnancy. Many African American patients seek nonsurgical interventions because of the significant risk of scarring in this patient population.

The concept behind noninvasive skin tightening devices is to spare epidermal injury while directing injury only to the site of maximal energy absorption in the dermis. This injury is speculated to create new collagen and elastic fibers and may contribute to immediate tightening owing to denaturation and contraction of existing collagen fibers.[24,25] A number of devices were created for this purpose; however, appropriate patient selection is crucial to achieve significant success. The ideal patient is one with mild to moderate skin laxity and lack of underlying redundant fatty tissue.

Radiofrequency

Radiofrequency (RF) is electromagnetic radiation in the frequency range of 3 kHz to 300 GHz. These devices induce dermal heating, collagen denaturation, and collagen remodeling.[24] Wound-healing mechanisms promote wound contraction, which ultimately enhances the appearance of mild to moderate skin laxity. One device (Thermacool, Thermage Inc, Hayward, CA) has reported efficacy in the treatment of laxity involving the lower face and neck.[26] Because RF energy is not dependent on a specific chromophore interaction, epidermal melanin is not targeted and treatment of all skin types is possible.

Kushikata and colleagues[27] reported the use of RF in a series of 85 Asian patients with skin types III and IV. Blisters occurred in 1, a burn occurred in 1, and hyperpigmentation occurred in 2 of the 85 patients. The skin types of these patients were not specified; however, in all of these cases the complications healed without permanent sequelae. Objective physician evaluation found relatively good improvement 3 months after treatment, and even better improvement at 6 months. RF treatment was concluded to be effective for skin tightening in Asian facial skin, offering safe and effective treatment of skin laxity. Although studies on RF have focused mainly on Asian skin, this modality has been widely used in African American patients with a similar safety profile.

Infrared Tightening

Titan (Cutera, Inc, Brisbane, CA, USA) is a device that uses infrared light to volumetrically heat the dermis. It is designed to thermally induce collagen contraction, with subsequent collagen remodeling and neocollagen synthesis. The epidermis is protected via pretreatment, parallel treatment, and posttreatment cooling with the sapphire tip. With this device, improvements in skin laxity and facial and neck contours have been achieved. It uses a long pulse of infrared light with a spectrum from 1100 to 1800 nm, with greatest intensity in the 1400-nm to 1500-nm range. The settings range from 32 to 40 J and are determined by patient tolerance and not by skin type. The penetration depth is 1 to 2 mm, which is best for targeting the reticular dermis.[28] Light is emitted in multisecond cycles to sufficiently heat the dermis while providing appropriate cooling of the epidermis. Like other skin-tightening devices, it is designed to thermally induce immediate collagen contraction, followed by the induction of collagen remodeling and the synthesis of new collagen. Water is the target chromophore, which allows for uniform heating of the targeted area. The procedure causes mild to moderate discomfort and mild temporary erythema. Two to 3 initial passes are performed over the entire designated treatment area, with additional passes over areas of great concern. A series of 3 to 4 treatments, 4 to 6 weeks apart, is recommended for the best results. Although an immediate tightening effect is achieved, the full effect is observed 6 months after the last treatment.[29] Liberal use of gel appears to improve patient tolerability. In all skin types, multiple sessions[3–5] are needed for best results.[30] Response rates are variable and can be influenced by patient selection.[31]

In an open-label trial in 21 Asian patients, skin tightening was observed in 86% of patients as measured by 3 independent physician observers. This improvement ranged from mild to excellent (mild 29%, moderate 38%, excellent 19%).[30,31] Variable response rates with skin-tightening technologies may be because of patient selection, energies used, and overall skin quality.[30]

Another infrared device, the SkinTyte (Sciton, Inc, Palo Alto, CA, USA) delivers infrared light in the range of 800 to 1400 nm. It uses uniform, targeted deep dermal heating to achieve skin tightening. Continuous cooling of the epidermis is achieved with thermo-electric sapphire plates.

The LuxIR and the LuxDeep IR (Palomar Medical Technologies, Inc, Burlington, MA, USA) deliver infrared light in the range of 850 to 1350 nm. The LuxDeep IR Fractional Infrared handpieces (Palomar Medical Technologies, Inc) use fractional infrared light and were designed to deliver infrared deep light extending up to 6 mm into the dermis and fat layer without damaging the epidermis. The LuxDeep IR handpiece safely delivers more effective heat to greater depths, and offers longer pulse durations. The energy is delivered through a sapphire crystal with contact cooling to prevent epidermal injury. Several treatments are required.

Clinical trials have demonstrated variable improvement in skin tightening.[32–34]

Ultrasound Tightening

In cosmetic medicine, ultrasound has been used primarily for cellulite and fat treatment, but skin tightening is its newest target. Intense ultrasound (IUS) is an energy that can propagate through tissue up to several millimeters. Ultrasound waves induce a vibration in the molecules of a target tissue during propagation, and the thermoviscous losses in the medium lead to tissue heating.[35] When the beam is directed in a firm focus of the skin tissue at a certain depth, it produces a thermal coagulative necrosis, leaving the superficial layers unaffected.

This type of intense ultrasound device has demonstrated to have the potential for correcting age-related sagging skin. Epidermal injury is minimized, and thermal energy is directed into the reticular dermis and subcutis, where immediate tissue contraction and delayed remodeling are believed to collectively cause tightening. It has been developed specifically for treating facial soft tissues and targeting the superficial musculoaponeurotic system (SMAS), a continuous fibrous network composed of collagen and elastic fibers that envelops the muscles of facial expression and extends superficially to connect with the dermis.[36,37]

One device (Ulthera P, Ulthera Inc, Mesa, AZ, USA) was introduced for use in facial rejuvenation. It is a microablation device that noninvasively treats multiple layers of tissue. This device enables visualization of target layers of subepidermal tissue immediately before the therapeutic level of ultrasonic energy is delivered. The outer epidermal layer of skin is completely spared, while deeper treatment causes collagen denaturation and wound healing.

The use of intense ultrasound (IUS) energy targeting the SMAS was studied producing thermal injury zones (TIZs) in 6 unfixed human cadaveric specimens. There were 202 exposure lines delivered bilaterally in multiple facial regions by varying combinations of power and exposure time (0.5 to 8.0 J). Subsequently, the tissue was examined grossly and histologically for evidence of thermal injury. Investigators found evidence of focused collagen denaturation and shrinkage.[38]

Alam and colleagues[39] assessed the efficacy of ultrasound skin tightening in browlifting. After evaluating 35 subjects (median age of 44 years), the investigators found that a single ultrasound treatment of the forehead produced an average brow height elevation of slightly less than 2 mm. Most subjects responded well, with only transitory mild erythema and edema as side effects. It can be concluded that IUS appears to be a safe and effective modality for facial skin tightening. In addition, this modality is safe for African American patients because melanin is not a target.

Skin tightening via nonablative energy delivery offers reduction of skin laxity with minimal downtime, and no scars or serious adverse effects.[39] All of the skin-tightening technologies discussed offer African American patients a safe alternative to surgery to treat skin laxity.

In summary, laser and light therapy can be used successfully in patients of African descent. In this patient population, it is important to choose devices that have been studied and have demonstrated safety in skin of color. Many of the lasers discussed in this article offer treatment options that have been shown to be safe and effective in dark skin. Despite this, any laser in the African American patient can cause significant complications if the appropriate settings are not used. When treating darker-skinned patients, the use of conservative settings to achieve the desired results is prudent. Following these guidelines, the clinician is most likely to achieve a favorable result with the least unwanted side effects.

LASER COMPLICATIONS IN AFRICAN AMERICAN PATIENTS

Patients with ethnic skin can have varying response to lasers and are at an increased risk of potential epidermal adverse events (AEs), including dyspigmentation, blistering, crusting, edema, and subsequent scarring. This should be taken into consideration when discussing treatment options with patients.[40]

Laser Hair Removal

Studies assessing intense pulsed light (IPL) for treatment of hirsutism in patients with darker skin types are limited. In a study of 210 subjects with skin types III to V, Bedewi[41] reported no incidence of postinflammatory dyspigmentation, burning, or scarring with IPL photoepilation. In this series, if posttreatment edema or erythema developed, a topical steroid cream and an oral anti-inflammatory agent were administered.

In 26 patients (skin types V and VI) treated with photoepilation using modified light and heat energy system for a duration of 35 milliseconds, Sadick and Krespi[42] reported that transient erythema (54%) was the most common AE reported, resolving at 6 weeks. In this study, 1 patient experienced a transient posttreatment burn with crusting and hypopigmentation in 1 treatment site, which resolved after 6 weeks. It was additionally reported that 8% experienced transient hypopigmentation that resolved after 12 weeks, and 8% experienced gradually fading hyperpigmentation that persisted at 6 and 12 weeks. No cases of blistering were reported.[42]

Other complications of hair removal that have been reported include paradoxic hypertrichosis after treatment with alexandrite (755 nm) and IPL (590–1200 nm) devices. Although the incidence ranged only from 0.6% to 5.1%,[37–40] it is suggested that individuals with darker skin types (phototypes III–V) may be at increased risk.[43,44] The exact mechanism of photostimulation remains unknown, but it is speculated that low fluences can stimulate the transformation of vellus hairs into darker terminal hairs.[43] This rare side effect of laser hair removal is less common in African American patients because of the tendency to have coarse (nonvellus) facial hair.

Persistent hypopigmentation has been observed with the alexandrite laser.[44] In one study[45] involving the long-pulsed alexandrite laser, on 150 subjects with skin phototypes IV to VI, an overall complication rate of 2.7% was reported. More severe complications, such as blistering, was reported in darker skin (phototype VI). In this study, 2 patients with skin phototype VI had AEs including blistering, hyperpigmentation, and hypopigmentation. A refrigerated gel was applied immediately before laser treatment. Also, subjects avoided the sun for 3 weeks before treatment, and were pretreated with sunscreen (SPF 15), as well as with a 2% hydroquinone/glycolic acid preparation nightly for 10 days before laser surgery. Hypopigmentation/hyperpigmentation, blistering, excoriation, crusting, ingrown hairs, and folliculitis were the main AEs reported. It was concluded that pretreatment with hydroquinone/glycolic acid and sun protection, as well as altering energy fluence, and epidermal cooling were effective in preventing hyperpigmentation. The use of topical corticosteroids, postoperatively, was considered essential in darker skin tones after treatment with the alexandrite laser.

In a study of 10 subjects (1 with skin phototype VI) treated with the super-long-pulsed 810-nm diode laser, the AEs observed included erythema, purpura, epidermal whitening, blistering, Nikolsky sign, and pain. Hyperpigmentation (11%) and hypopigmentation (9%) were noted after 6 months of treatment and hypopigmentation generally occurred in patients with darker skin and in those who had been treated under the most aggressive settings (ie, 1000-millisecond pulse duration and 115 J/cm²).[46]

Toosi and colleagues[47] analyzed the efficacy and side effects of different light sources (including the 810-nm diode, the alexandrite and the IPL [cutoff filter of 650 nm]) on the face and neck of 233 subjects with skin phototypes II to IV. As expected, a correlation between skin phototype and side-effect incidence was seen, with a higher incidence occurring in those with darker skin phototypes.

As mentioned previously, the long-pulsed Nd:YAG is the safest laser for African American patients. The Nd:YAG laser has demonstrated the lowest incidence of side effects. This is because of the minimal epidermal melanin absorption at this wavelength.[48–50] Alster and colleagues[22] found a 5% incidence of transient dyspigmentation without fibrosis or scarring in 20 patients with skin phototypes IV to VI after a series of 3 monthly long-pulsed 1064-nm Nd:YAG laser treatments. The duration of the dyschromia was approximately 4 weeks. Blistering occurred in only 1.5% of patients, suggesting that hypopigmentation and hyperpigmentation occurred independent of blister formation.

Goh[51] compared the safety and efficacy of the long-pulsed Nd:YAG laser to a noncoherent IPL system (590–1200 nm) for hair removal in 11 patients with skin phototypes IV to VI, where the Nd:YAG was applied to one half of the body and the IDL to the other. In this study, a lower rate of AEs was observed in the ND:YAG-treated patients (5/11) versus IPL-treated patients (3/11).

Tattoo Removal

Tattoos often consist of multiple pigments, and their removal may require the use of several wavelengths involving both the visible and near infrared spectrum. Tattoo treatment becomes even more difficult and unpredictable in patients with skin types IV to VI because of the presence of significant amounts of epidermal melanin that can absorb laser energy.[52] For the removal of black-and-blue tattoo pigments, as well as purple and violet pigments, the Q-switched 694-nm ruby laser is effective but risky in darker skin types.[53] Q-switched Nd:Yag lasers emit 2 wavelengths of light, 532 and 1064 nm, and remain the safest lasers in the treatment of blue and black tattoos in darker skin types.[54,55] Side effects of laser tattoo removal on darker skin can be reduced by using the minimum fluence necessary to produce immediate lesional whitening, signaling the destruction of intracellular melanosomes. When treating type VI skin with the Q-switched Nd:Yag laser, a 3-mm spot size and fluences starting between 3.4 and 3.6 J/cm² is recommended. Greater fluences resulting in pinpoint bleeding and tissue splattering are more likely to lead to transient hyperpigmentation, permanent hypopigmentation, and scarring.

Pigmented Lesions

Dermatologic conditions that result in altered skin pigmentation, such as melasma, postinflammatory hyperpigmentation, lentigines, and dermatosis papulosa nigra continue to be a primary concern among patients with darker skin tones.

IPL has been used for the treatment of melasma in patients with skin type IV. The response of melasma to irradiation with any specific laser is variable; a lack of response, worsening of the dyschromia, and recurrence are the most frequent outcomes. IPL treatment complications may result in IPL-induced melasmalike hyperpigmentation.[56] Because of the clear risk of postinflammatory hyperpigmentation observed in Asian patients,[57,58] IPL should be avoided in African American patients.

Fractional photothermolysis is currently the only laser modality approved by the Food and Drug Administration (FDA) for melasma.[59,60] Similar to IPL, it carries a risk of postinflammatory hyperpigmentation, especially in individuals who may have hyperactive melanocytes. Because of the risk of hyperpigmentation with melasma, this laser should be considered only in recalcitrant cases.

Q-switched lasers produce photomechanical effects within the epidermis and are effective for treating both freckles and lentigines. Postinflammatory hyperpigmentation is the most common side effect and tends to resolve within a few months. Reported rates of postinflammatory hyperpigmentation associated with the use of Q-switched lasers in Asian individuals have ranged from 4% to 25%.[61,62] In African American individuals, postinflammatory hyperpigmentation is likely to occur in a significantly higher proportion of patients.

Of the pigmented lesions that greatly affect darker skin phototypes, nevus of Ota is a condition that responds well to treatment with Q-switched ruby, alexandrite, and Nd:YAG lasers.[63–67] Complications, such as postinflammatory hyperpigmentation, have been observed in most patients despite pretreatment with topical hydroquinone. Postinflammatory hypopigmentation is another common side effect of Q-switched lasers in African American patients.

Skin Resurfacing and Acne Scars

Cutaneous laser resurfacing can provide an effective means for improving the appearance of diffuse dyschromia, photoinduced rhytides, and atrophic scarring in patients with darker skin phototypes.

Different studies have demonstrated that transient hyperpigmentation is the most common AE experienced after laser skin resurfacing. The incidence ranges from 68% to 100% among patients with the darkest skin types (IV).[68–71] Hypopigmentation, on the other hand, tends to be long standing, delayed in its onset, and difficult to treat. Fortunately, it is observed far less frequently than hyperpigmentation. The excimer laser, as well as topical photochemotherapy, has shown some success in repigmenting these affected areas.[61,72]

Nonablative devices are desirable therapeutic options for skin rejuvenation in those with darker phototypes. Ablative lasers have been used less often on African American individuals, because of the increased risk of transient and permanent dyspigmentation as well as scarring. Erbium:Yag and CO2 remain the gold standards for the treatment of photoaging in lighter skin types, but are not desirable in African American patients because of the increased risk of complications, including a long recovery period, scarring, and prolonged postinflammatory changes. Postinflammatory hyperpigmentation has been reported to occur in up to 68% of patients with skin type IV.[41]

In general, when compared with standard ablative therapies, fractional resurfacing is associated with a reduced side-effect profile and faster recovery times. Usually the erythema and edema tend to resolve within a few days instead of lasting weeks to months.[73]

Fractional laser photothermolysis (FP) treatment was evaluated in a retrospective study where 961 subjects with skin types I to V were treated with the 1550-nm erbium-doped laser.[11] The most common complications were acneiform eruptions (1.87%) and herpes simplex outbreaks (1.77%). These side effects were equally distributed across different ages, skin types, body locations, laser parameters, and underlying skin conditions; however, the incidence of postinflammatory hyperpigmentation augmented with increasing skin type with the incidence of hyperpigmentation in skin types III, IV, and V was noted to be 2.6%, 11.6%, and 33.0%, respectively. When treating darker skin types with FP, it is better to reduce treatment energy and treatment density to minimize the possible prolonged erythema and edema as well as hyperpigmentation.[11]

In one study, 15 subjects with acne scars and skin types IV to VI were treated using a 1550-nm erbium fractionated laser, with either 10 mJ or with 40 mJ. A significant improvement in the acne scarring and overall appearance was observed but significant postinflammatory hyperpigmentation was seen more often in those subjects with darker skin types.[74]

Vascular Lesions

For the treatment of port-wine stains, hemangiomas, and facial telangiectasias, the 585-nm pulsed dye laser (PDL) has demonstrated superiority with regard to both effectiveness and safety, despite patient skin phototype.[75–77] Although African American patients are more prone than those patients with lighter skin to develop pigmentary changes after PDL treatment, skin-cooling techniques can reduce the risk of dyspigmentation.[78]

TREATMENT OF HYPERPIGMENTATION

Hyperpigmentation is the most common side effect seen in African American patients after undergoing laser therapy. Treatment of dyschromias attributable to lasers can be complex. There are various topical agents available to treat hyperpigmentation, which interfere with the pigmentation process on different levels.

Hydroquinone

Hydroquinone (HQ) is the gold standard to treat hyperpigmentation. It is a natural, plant-derived tyrosinase inhibitor, which has been used in the United States to treat pigmentary disorders for years.[79] Despite its efficacy, safety concerns have led to regulation of HQ in Europe and Asia. In the United States, HQ is currently available over the counter in 2% concentrations and by prescription in 4% concentrations. There is an ongoing debate as to whether the FDA will further regulate HQ in the United States, partly because of reported mutagenic properties of HQ delivered systemically in animals.[80,81] No such effects have been demonstrated in humans.

For best results, a Kligman formula including a topical HQ combined with a retinoid and steroid should be used. Commercially available combination products such as Triluma (Galderma Laboratories, Fort Worth, TX, USA) and Epiquin (Skinmedica, Inc, Carlsbad, CA, USA) Micro products are useful; however, African American patients may require higher concentrations to treat hyperpigmentation that is attributable to lasers. For these patients, it is helpful to start with a compounded product that contains HQ 6% to 8%, tretinoin 0.025%, and dexamethasone 0.1%.

Localized discrete hyperpigmented patches are the most common complication of laser treatments. For this type of hyperpigmentation, patients can use a compounded HQ topically at night. A cotton-tipped applicator can be used to better localize treatment to the affected areas. This should be followed by a retinoid to the full face. For diffuse and ill-defined hyperpigmentation after laser treatment, HQ should be used sparingly. More subtle bleaching agents are effective for this type of dyschromia.

A common side effect of HQ is the hydroquinone halo, characterized by hypopigmentation around the dark macule owing to bleaching of the surrounding normal skin. As mentioned previously, use of a cotton-tipped applicator, and application of a retinoid after HQ, helps to prevent this effect.

A rare side effect of HQ is exogenous ochronosis, characterized by black macules that can progress to papules and nodules on sun-exposed areas.[82] Ochronosis was common in South Africa where long-term HQ use was prevalent. In the United States, ochronosis is observed but typically occurs with long-term continued use of HQ over decades. The risk may be reduced with sunscreen use, as the pattern of ochronosis appears to be photodistributed. Because of the risk of ochronosis, long-term continued use of HQ should be avoided. It is prudent to give "drug holidays" with HQ to maintain its efficacy over time, as clinically the efficacy of HQ appears to plateau with continued use.

Other, more common side effects of HQ include irritation and redness. When prescribing HQ it is important to recommend that patients discontinue the treatment if they notice these symptoms. Irritation from HQ is frequently caused by the HQ itself or by sodium metabisulfite, a common preservative in HQ preparations.[83] Continuing HQ despite irritation may lead to postinflammatory hyperpigmentation.

Other Therapies for Hyperpigmentation

Although none of the alternative therapies for the treatment of hyperpigmentation appear to reach the efficacy of HQ, they can be used as alternatives in patients with HQ sensitivity or during HQ drug holidays. The topical treatments that have demonstrated efficacy in vivo are discussed in the following paragraphs.

Glabridin (Glycyrrhiza glabra) is the main compound in the hydrophobic fraction of licorice extract; 0.5% glabridin has been shown to inhibit UVB-induced pigmentation and erythema in guinea pig skin.[84] Another open-label trial demonstrated improvement in the treatment of melasma.[85]

Niacinamide is a biologically active amide of vitamin B3 and exerts depigmenting effects by inhibiting the transfer of melanosomes to keratinocytes.[86] The 3.5% niacinamide/retinyl palmitate has been demonstrated to be effective in treating hyperpigmentation.

N-acetylglucosamine (NAG) is a monosaccharide derivative of glucose and a monomeric unit of chitin, which forms the outer coverings of insects and crustaceans. It inhibits the conversion of protyrosinase to tyrosinase.[87] An 8-week, double-blind, placebo-controlled, randomized, split-face clinical trial by Bissett and colleagues[88] showed that 2% NAG reduced the appearance of facial hyperpigmentation. In addition, the combination of 2% NAG with 4% niacinamide demonstrated even greater improvement.

Vitamin C (L-ascorbic-acid) reduces oxidized melanin by reducing o-dopaquinone back to dopa, thus avoiding melanin formation.[89] Because it is charged, its absorption is limited, making it difficult to traverse the stratum corneum. With iontophoresis, penetration can be increased and consequently pigmentation can be decreased significantly compared with placebo, as shown in a randomized, double-blind, placebo-controlled study.[90] Magnesium-L-ascorbyl-2-phosphate (VC-PMG) is a stable derivative of ascorbic acid. Its topical application in patients with melasma or solar lentigos demonstrated a significant lightening effect in 19 of 34 patients.[91]

Soy is a natural skin-lightening agent that acts via a novel pathway. Two natural soy-derived proteins, namely soybean trypsin inhibitor (STI) and the Bowmann-Birk inhibitor (BBI) have been shown to interfere with melanosome transfer by inhibiting protein-activated receptor 2 (PAR-2) activation. PAR-2 is a G-protein–coupled receptor, regulating the ingestion of melanosomes by keratinocytes. Inhibition of this receptor prevents transfer of melanosomes to keratinocytes and results in improved pigmentation clinically.[92–94]

Sunscreen

Sunscreen and sun avoidance is especially important when treating African American patients with lasers. Sun protection can be essential to prevent and to treat hyperpigmentation and should be emphasized to all laser patients. Newer sunscreens available in the United States now offer both long-term UVB and UVA coverage. These include formulations that contain ecamsule (Mexoryl) or avobenzone + oxybenzone (Helioplex). For patients sensitive to chemical sunscreens, physical blockers containing zinc oxide and titanium dioxide are best. Micronized formulations offer better cosmesis for patients with skin of color by minimizing the gray hue that physical sunscreens cause. Although improved, many patients still complain of this side effect of physical blockers.

Novel adjunctive therapies in treating hyperpigmentation are oral sunscreens. Polypodium leucotomos (PL) is a commercially available oral photoprotectant. In clinical studies, PL was proven to diminish sunburn cells after UVB exposure.[95] This oral therapy offers another sun-protection option to patients with pigmentary disorders.

Using a combination of hydroquinone and other natural therapies after laser treatment, dyschromias can be effectively managed. Post-laser hypopigmentation in African American patients can be more challenging to treat. Narrow-band UVB and excimer lasers can be used to reverse laser-induced hypopigmentation in African American patients.[63,72]

SUMMARY

In summary, there is an increasing demand for the use of lasers in African American patients. In this population, lasers can be used safely and effectively; however, choosing the right laser is key. Clinicians should therefore be aware of the risks when using lasers in African American patients and be prepared to manage the complications that can occur in this patient population.

REFERENCES

1. Goldberg DJ. Nonablative laser surgery for pigmented skin. Dermatol Surg 2005;31(10):1263–7.
2. merican Society for Aesthetic Surgery. 2005 Cosmetic Surgery National Data Bank statistics. Available at: www.surgery.org/download/2005stats.pdf. Accessed August 24, 2006.
3. Szabo G, Gerald AB, Patnak MA, et al. Racial differences in the fate of melanosomes in human epidermis. Nature 1969;222(5198):1081–2.
4. Montagna W, Carlisle K. The architecture of black and white facial skin. J Am Acad Dermatol 1991; 24:929–37.
5. Grimes PE. Skin and hair cosmetic issues in women of color. Dermatol Clin 2000;18(4):659–65.
6. Kim JW, Lee JO. Skin resurfacing with laser in Asians. Aesthetic Plast Surg 1997;21(2):115–7.
7. Manstein D, Herron GS, Sink RK, et al. Fractional photothermolysis: a new concept for cutaneous remodeling using microscopic patterns of thermal injury. Lasers Surg Med 2004;34:426–38.
8. Fisher GH, Geronemus RG. Short-term side effects of fractional photothermolysis. Dermatol Surg 2005; 31:1245–9.
9. Hasegawa T, Matsuka T, Mizuo Y, et al. Clinical trial of laser device called fractional photothermolysis system for acne scars. J Dermatol 2006;33(9): 623–7.
10. Lee HS, Lee JH, Ahn GY, et al. Fractional photothermolysis for the treatment of acne scars: a report of 27 Korean patients. J Dermatolog Treat 2008;19(1): 45–9.

11. Graber EM, Tanzi EL, Alster TS. Side effects and complications of fractional laser photothermolysis: experience with 961 treatments. Dermatol Surg 2008;34(3):301–5 [discussion: 305–7].

12. Kono T, Chan HH, Groff WF, et al. Prospective direct comparison study of fractional resurfacing using different fluences and densities for skin rejuvenation in Asians. Lasers Surg Med 2007;39(4):311–4.

13. Tanzi EL, Alster TS. Comparison of a 1450nm diode laser and a 1320nmNdYAG laser in the treatment of atrophic facial scars: a prospective clinical and histological study. Dermatol Surg 2004;30(2 Pt 1):152–7.

14. Lipper GM, Perez M. Nonablative acne scar reduction after a series of treatments with a short-pulsed 1,064-nm neodymium:YAG laser. Dermatol Surg 2006;32(8):998–1006.

15. Kligman AM. Solar elastosis in relation to pigmentation. In: itzpatrick TB, Pathak MA, editors. Sunlight and man. Tokyo: University of Tokyo Press; 1974. p. 157–63.

16. Gentlewave approval FDA. FDA clears GentleWaves. 2005. Cosmetic surgery–news. Available at: http://www.cosmeticsurgery-news.com/article2357.html. Accessed November 16, 2010.

17. Weiss RA, Weiss MA, Geronemus RG, et al. A novel non-thermal non-ablative full panel led photomodulation device for reversal of photoaging: digital microscopic and clinical results in various types. J Drugs Dermatol 2004;03:605–10.

18. Breadon JY, Barnes CA. Comparison of adverse events of laser and light-assisted hair removal systems in skin types IV-VI. J Drugs Dermatol 2007;6(1):40–6.

19. Nouri K, Jimenez G, Trent J. Laser hair removal in patients with Fitzpatrick Skin type VI. Cosmet Dermatol 2002;15(3):15–6.

20. Adrian RM, Shay KP. 800 nanometer diode laser hair removal in African American patients: a clinical and histologic study. J Cutan Laser Ther 2000;2(4):183–90.

21. Greppi I. Diode laser hair removal of the black patient. Lasers Surg Med 2001;28(2):150–5.

22. Alster TS, Bryan H, Williams CM. Long-pulsed Nd:YAG laser-assisted hair removal in pigmented skin: a clinical and histological evaluation. Arch Dermatol 2001;137(7):885–9.

23. Ross EV, Cooke LM, Timko AL, et al. Treatment of pseudofolliculitis barbae in skin types IV, V, and VI with a long-pulsed neodymium:yttrium aluminum garnet laser. J Am Acad Dermatol 2002;47(2):263–7.

24. Zelickson BD, Kist D, Bernstein E, et al. Histological and ultrastructural evaluation of the effects of a radio-frequency based nonablative dermal remodeling device: a pilot study. Arch Dermatol 2004;140(2):204–9.

25. Fitzpatrick R, Geronemeus R, Goldberg D, et al. Multicenter study of noninvasive radiofrequency for periorbital tissue tightening. Lasers Surg Med 2003;33:232–42.

26. Hsu TS, Kaminer MS. The use of nonablative radiofrequency technology to tighten the lower face and neck. Semin Cutan Med Surg 2003;22:115–23. 12877230.

27. Kushikata N, Negishi K, Tezuka Y, et al. Non-ablative skin tightening with radiofrequency in Asian skin. Lasers Surg Med 2005;36(2):92–7.

28. Dierickx CC. The role of deep heating for noninvasive skin rejuvenation. Lasers Surg Med 2006;38:799–807.

29. Sadick NS. Tissue tightening technology: fact or fiction. Aesthet Surg J 2008;28(2):180–8.

30. Chua SH, Ang P, Khoo LS, et al. Nonablative infrared skin tightening in Type IV to V Asian skin: a prospective clinical study. Dermatol Surg 2007;33(2):146–51.

31. Bunin LS, Carniol BJ. Cervical facial skin tightening with an infrared device. Facial Plast Surg Clin North Am 2007;15(2):179–84.

32. Dierickx C, Altshuler G, Erofeev A, et al. Skin tightening with Palomar's StarLux IR deep dermal, fractional heating. Cutaneous laser surgery. Lasers Surg Med 2007;39:15–34.

33. Weiss R. Fractional infrared light for skin tightening: six month prospective study. Cutaneous laser surgery. Lasers Surg Med 2007;39:15–34.

34. Dierickx C, Altshuler G, Childs J, et al. Dermal/hypodermal junction as a new target for deep fractional thermal treatment. Basic science/optical diagnostics. Lasers Surg Med 2007;39:1–14.

35. Kennedy Je, ter Haar GR, Cranston D. High intensity focused ultrasound: surgery of the future? Br J Radiol 2003;76:590–9.

36. Mitz V, Peyronie M. The superficial musculoaponeurotic system (SMAS) in the parotid and cheek area. Plast Reconstr Surg 1976;58:80–8.

37. Har-Shai Y, Sele E, Rubinstien I, et al. Computerized morphometric quantification of elastin and collagen in SMAS and facial skin and the possible role of fat cells in SMAS viscoelastic properties. Plast Reconstr Surg 1998;102:2466–70.

38. White WM, Makin IR, Barthe PG, et al. Selective creation of thermal injury zones in the superficial musculoaponeurotic system using intense ultrasound therapy: a new target for noninvasive facial rejuvenation. Arch Facial Plast Surg 2007;9(1):22–9.

39. Alam M, White LE, Martin N, et al. Ultrasound tightening of facial and neck skin: a rater-blinded prospective cohort study. J Am Acad Dermatol 2010;62(2):262–9.

40. Carniol PJ, Woolery-Lloyd H, Zhao AS, et al. Laser treatment for ethnic skin. Facial Plast Surg Clin North Am 2010;18(1):105–10.

41. Bedewi AF. Hair removal with intense pulsed light. Lasers Med Sci 2004;19:48–51.

42. Sadick NS, Krespi Y. Hair removal for Fitzpatrick skin types V and VI using light and heat energy technology. J Drugs Dermatol 2006;5:597–9.

43. Alajlan A, Shapiro J, Rivers JK, et al. Paradoxical hypertrichosis after laser epilation. J Am Acad Dermatol 2005;53:85–8.

44. Moreno-Arias GA, Castelo-Branco C, Ferrando J. Side-effects after IPL photodepilation. Dermatol Surg 2002;28:1131–4.

45. Garcia C, Alamoudi H, Nakib M, et al. Alexandrite laser hair removal is safe for Fitzpatrick skin types IV-VI. Dermatol Surg 2000;26:130–4.

46. Rogachefsky AS, Silapunt S, Goldberg J. Evaluation of a new super-long-pulsed 810 nm diode laser for the removal of unwanted hair: the concept of thermal damage time. Dermatol Surg 2000;28:410–4.

47. Toosi P, Sadighha A, Sharifian A, et al. A comparison study of the efficacy and side effects of different light sources in hair removal. Lasers Med Sci 2006;21(1):1–4.

48. Nanni CA, Alster TS. Laser-assisted hair removal: optimizing treatment parameters to improve clinical results. Arch Dermatol 1997;133:1546–9.

49. Tanzi EL, Alster TS. Long-pulsed 1064-nm Nd:YAG laser-assisted hair removal in all skin types. Dermatol Surg 2004;30:13–7.

50. Lanigan GW. Incidence of side effects after laser hair removal. J Am Acad Dermatol 2003;49:882–6.

51. Goh CL. Comparative study on a single treatment response to long pulse Nd:YAG lasers and intense pulse light therapy for hair removal on skin type IV to VI—Is longer wavelengths lasers preferred over shorter wavelengths lights for assisted hair removal. J Dermatolog Treat 2003;14:243–7.

52. Tanzi EL, Alster TS. Cutaneous laser surgery in darker skin phototypes. Cutis 2004;73:21–4, 27–30.

53. Zelickson BD, Mehregan DA, Zarrin AA, et al. Clinical, histologic, and ultrastructural evaluation of tattoos treated with three laser systems. Lasers Surg Med 1994;15:364–72.

54. Grevelink JM, Duke D, van Leeuwen RL, et al. Laser treatment of tattoos in darkly pigmented patients: efficacy and side effects. J Am Acad Dermatol 1996;34:653–6.

55. Jones A, Roddey P, Orengo I, et al. The Q-switched ND:YAG laser effectively treats tattoos in darkly pigmented skin. Dermatol Surg 1996;22(12):999–1001.

56. Polnikorn N. Treatment of refractory dermal Melasma with the MedLite C6 Q-switched Nd:YAG laser: two case reports. J Cosmet Laser Ther 2008;10:167–73.

57. Wang CC, Sue YM, Yang CH, et al. A comparison of Q-switched alexandrite laser and intense pulsed light for the treatment of freckles and lentigines in Asian persons: a randomized, physician-blinded, split-face comparative trial. J Am Acad Dermatol 2006;54(5):804–10.

58. Negishi K, Kushikata N, Takeuchi K, et al. Photorejuvenation by intense pulsed light with objective measurement of skin color in Japanese patients. Dermatol Surg 2006;32(11):1380–7.

59. Rokhsar CK, Fitzpatrick RE. The treatment of Melasma with fractional photothermolysis: a pilot study. Dermatol Surg 2005;31:1645–50.

60. Tannous ZS, Astner S. Utilizing fractional resurfacing in the treatment of therapy-resistant melasma. J Cosmet Laser Ther 2005;7:39–43.

61. Battle EF Jr, Soden CE Jr. The use of lasers in darker skin types. Semin Cutan Med Surg 2009;28(2):130–40.

62. Kawada A, Shiraishi H, Asai M, et al. Clinical improvement of solar lentigines and ephelides with an intense pulsed light source. Dermatol Surg 2002;28:504–8.

63. Reszko A, Sukal SA, Geronemus RG. Reversal of laser-induced hypopigmentation with a narrow-band UV-B light source in a patient with skin type VI. Dermatol Surg 2008;34(10):1423–6.

64. Chan HH, Ying SY, Ho WS, et al. An in vivo trial comparing the clinical efficacy and complications of Q-switched 755-nm alexandrite and Q-switched 1064-nm Nd:YAG lasers in the treatment of nevus of Ota. Dermatol Surg 2000;26:919–22.

65. Alster TS, Williams CM. Treatment of nevus of Ota by the Q-switched alexandrite laser. Dermatol Surg 1995;21:592–6.

66. Kono T, Nozaki M, Chan HH, et al. A retrospective study looking at the long-term complication of Q-switched ruby laser in the treatment of nevus of Ota. Lasers Surg Med 2001;29:156–9.

67. Chan HH, Leung RS, Yng SY, et al. Recurrence of nevus of Ota after successful treatment with Q-switched lasers. Arch Dermatol 2000;136:1175–6.

68. Sriprachya-Anunt S, Marchell NL, Fitzpatrick RE, et al. Facial resurfacing in patients with Fitzpatrick skin type IV. Lasers Surg Med 2002;30:86–92.

69. Tanzi EL, Alster TS. Treatment of atrophic facial scars with a dual-mode erbium:YAG laser. Dermatol Surg 2002;28:551–5.

70. Tanzi EL, Alster TS. Single-pass carbon dioxide versus multiple-pass Er:YAG laser skin resurfacing: a comparison of postoperative wound healing and side effect rates. Dermatol Surg 2003;29:80–4.

71. Tanzi EL, Alster TS. Side effects and complications of variable- pulsed erbium:YAG laser skin resurfacing: extended experience with 50 patients. Plast Reconstr Surg 2003;111:1524–9.

72. Friedman PM, Geronemus RG. Use of the 308-nm excimer laser for postresurfacing leudoderma. Arch Dermatol 2001;137:824–5.

73. Glaich AS, Rahman Z, Goldberg LH, et al. Fractional resurfacing for the treatment of hypopigmented

scars: a pilot study. Dermatol Surg 2007;33:289–94 [discussion: 293–4].

74. Mahmoud BH, Srivastava D, Janiga JJ, et al. Safety and efficacy of erbium-doped yttrium aluminum garnet fractionated laser for treatment of acne scars in type IV to VI skin. Dermatol Surg 2010;36(5):602–9.

75. Chung JH, Koh WS, Lee DY, et al. Copper vapor laser treatment of port-wine stains in brown skin. Australas J Dermatol 1997;38:15–21.

76. Chung JH, Koh WS, Young JL. Histological responses of port-wine stains in brown skin after 578-nm copper vapor laser treatment. Lasers Surg Med 1996;18:358–66.

77. Chang CJ, Nelson JS. Cryogen spray cooling and higher fluence pulsed dye laser treatment improve port-wine stain clearance while minimizing epidermal damage. Dermatol Surg 1999;25:767–72.

78. Chiu CH, Chan HH, Ho WS, et al. Prospective study of pulsed dye laser in conjunction with cryogen spray cooling for treatment of port wine stains in Chinese patients. Dermatol Surg 2003;29:909–15.

79. Penney KB, Smith CJ, Allen JC. Depigmenting action of hydroquinone depends on disruption of fundamental cell processes. J Invest Dermatol 1984;82:308.

80. Bates B. Derms react to possible FDA ban of hydroquinone: cite poor scientific reasoning, ethnic bias. Skin Allergy News 2007;38(1):1–20.

81. Nordlund JJ, Grimes PE, Ortonne JP. The safety of hydroquinone. J Eur Acad Dermatol Venereol 2006;20:781–7.

82. Lawrence N, Bligard CA, Reed R, et al. Exogenous ochronosis in the United States. J Am Acad Dermatol 1988;18:1207–11.

83. Huang Pei-Ying, Chu Chia-Yu. Allergic contact dermatitis due to sodium metabisulfite in a bleaching cream. Contact Dermatitis 2007;56(2):123–4.

84. Yokota T, Nishio H, Kubota Y, et al. The inhibitory effect of glabridin from licorice extracts on melanogenesis and inflammation. Pigment Cell Res 1998; 11(6):355–61.

85. Amer M, Metwalli M. Topical liquiritin improves melasma. Int J Dermatol 2000;39:299–301.

86. Hakozaki T, Minwalla L, Zhuang J, et al. The effect of niacinamide on reducing cutaneous pigmentation and suppression of melanosome transfer. Br J Dermatol 2002;147:20–31.

87. Bissett DL, Teresa Farmer BS, Sara McPhail BS, et al. Genomic expression changes induced by topical N-acetyl glucosamine in skin equivalent cultures in vitro. J Cosmet Dermatol 2007;6(4):232–8.

88. Bissett DL, Robinson LR, Raleigh PS, et al. Reduction in the appearance of facial hyperpigmentation by topical N-acetyl glucosamine. J Cosmet Dermatol 2007;6(1):20–6.

89. Ros JR, Rodriguez-Lopez JN, Garcia-Canovas F. Effect of L-ascorbic acid on the monophenolase activity of tyrosinase. Biochem J 1993;295:309.

90. Huh C-H, Seo K-I, Park J-Y, et al. A randomized, double-blind, placebo-controlled trail of vitamin C iontophoresis in melasma. Dermatology 2003;206:316–20.

91. Kameyama K, Sakai C, Kondoh S, et al. Inhibitory effect of magnesium L-ascorbyl-2-phosphate (VC-PMG) on melanogenesis in vitro and in vivo. J Am Acad Dermatol 1996;34:29.

92. Paine C, Sharlow E, Liebel F, et al. An alternative approach to depigmentation by soybean extracts via inhibition of the PAR-2 pathway. J Invest Dermatol 2001;116:587.

93. Hermanns JF, Petit L, Martalo O, et al. Unraveling the patterns of subclinical pheomelanin-enriched facial hyperpigmentation: effect of depigmenting agents. Dermatology 2000;201:118.

94. Babiarz-Magee L, Chen N, Seiberg M, et al. The expression and activation of protease-activated receptor-2 correlate with skin color. Pigment Cell Res 2004;17(3):241–51.

95. Middelkamp-Hup MA, Pathak MA, Parrado C, et al. Oral Polypodium leucotomos extract decreases ultraviolet-induced damage of human skin. J Am Acad Dermatol 2004;51(6):910–8.

Laser Treatment of Pigmented Lesions for Asians

Joseph K. Wong, MD, FRCS(C)

KEYWORDS

• Laser treatment • Asians • Melasma • Pigmented lesions

The term Asian refers to East Asians of the Pacific Rim who share not only a common heritage and skin type but also the same set of clinical skin problems. Pigmentation of the skin is often considered the number one esthetic skin concern in Asians. Asians idealize unblemished complexion of facial skin and are less tolerant to facial dyschromia than White.

The characteristics of the Asian skin, in general, can be described as having less wrinkles, more photoprotective effect with darker complexion than White, thicker dermal structure, and more superficial dyschromia and solar lentigines. The problems of ephelides (freckles), nevi of Ota, and melasma are common and difficult to treat.

Asian skin types have been categorized by either the Fitzpatrick grading system from grades II to IV or Fanous'[1] racial-based skin classification system that divides the globe into latitudinal zones in the temperate zones.

Problems faced in the treatment of the Asian skin are:

1. Dissimilarities between Asian populations
2. Definite anatomic traits
3. Thicker dermal layer
4. More sebaceous glands, and hence more rigorous response to exfoliation
5. Pigmentary problems
6. Prolonged erythema
7. Postinflammatory hyperpigmentation/hypopigmentation.

The study by West and Alster[2] states that an intensive preoperative regimen of tretinoin ±

hydroquinone failed to suppress postoperative melanin production, melanocytic nevi/superficial melanocytes that have been curbed by topical agents are eventually removed by the peeling process, and deeper melanocytes remain undisturbed by the preoperative treatment. For this reason, there is no evidence to support that preoperative treatment of the Asian skin with tretinoin improves postinflammatory hyperpigmentation. Treatment of Asian skin pigmentation can be divided into nonablative and ablative treatments.

NONABLATIVE THERAPY

The essence of nonablative treatment is not to affect the epidermis and target a specific chromophore in skin, for example, melanin pigments or red vascular lesions.

Common options available include:

1. Q-switched (QS) lasers
2. Intense pulsed light (IPL) therapy
3. Photodynamic therapy.

QS laser permits a short burst of intense energy that leads to a temperature gradient between the target and the neighboring tissue. Local shockwaves emitted cause tissue fragmentation and melanosomal injury and are therefore an effective nonablative treatment.

Popular QS lasers for Asians are:

1. QS neodymium:yttrium-aluminum-garnet (Nd:YAG)
2. QS ruby laser
3. QS alexandrite laser.

Department of Otolaryngology-Head & Neck Surgery, Credit Valley Hospital-Peel Regional Cancer Centre Mississauga, Ontario, Canada
E-mail address: jkhw@rogers.com

Facial Plast Surg Clin N Am 19 (2011) 417–422
doi:10.1016/j.fsc.2011.05.008
1064-7406/11/$ – see front matter © 2011 Elsevier Inc. All rights reserved.

Drawbacks of the QS laser are the following:

1. It is only good for isolated lesions.
2. Most Asians have generalized uneven facial dyschromia.

Repeated treatment may result in variation of hyperpigmentation/hypopigmentation or mottled appearance.

IPL is designed for the treatment of pigmented spots, vascular lesions, and photorejuvenation of fine wrinkles. It addresses dyschromia effectively but requires more treatment sessions. IPL is a non-coherent broadband (500–1200 nm) light device with selective cutoff filters to block specific shorter wavelengths. Pulse varies from 0.5 to 25 ms, and fluency ranges from 3 to 90 J/cm^2. IPL requires epidermal protection with a cooling gel. Ultraviolet (UV) photography may enhance the visibility of epidermal melanocytic hyperpigmentation.

Florescent pulsed light (FPL) emits a very broad spectrum: 300 to 1500 nm with the harmful UV spectrum blocked by filters. FPL transforms a substantial part of noneffective wavelengths into useful red light. The filtered wavelengths are then conducted to the target chromophores in the tissue using a sapphire crystal waveguide. The major parts of tissue structures experience a continuous pulse. The first third of the pulse with higher power heats up the target, and the remaining pulse with lower power maintains the temperature of the target tissue, thus minimizing the risk of side effects. The author's personal experience favors FPL over IPL for its gentleness toward Asian skin. The term gentleness is used here in a generic sense in that FPL tends to cause less side effects and hyperpigmentation than IPL and is a gentler and safer modality of intense light treatment with a bigger margin of safety.

Photodynamic therapy can exert 2 effects on Asian skin. Its photographic effect resembles that of a sustained IPL treatment. It is also very effective in treating active acne vulgaris. The mechanism of action is based on the skin absorbing aminolevulinic acid (ALA) and converting into protoporphyrin, a natural photosensitizer. ALA occurs naturally in the body and is involved in heme synthesis. When exposed to visible light of high intensity, protoporphyrin generates singlet oxygen, which causes cell membrane damage of target cells.

ABLATIVE THERAPY

Ablative treatment consists of:

1. Chemical peel
2. Dermabrasion
3. Lasers.

Chemical peel in Asians classically done using trichloroacetic acid (15%–35%). There are many commercial preparations available. It is effective in rejuvenation of mild to moderate rhytidosis and superficial dyschromia. However, the problem of postinflammatory pigmentation in Asian skin requires rapport and understanding between physicians and patients. The once-popular phenol peel for White is unacceptable to Asians. Not only does it cause severe postinflammatory hyperpigmentation but the permanent hypopigmentation that it may cause could be devastating for the patients. Mild gradual daily exfoliation using tretinoin or other acids is more acceptable to Asians. This can be achieved by several commercially available formulae.

Dermabrasion is mechanical abrasion of skin using a rotatory brush or diamond burr. Apart from certain type of cystic acne scars in Asians, it is not a common tool for treatment of pigmentary problems in Asian skin because of its unpredictable results and the risk of permanent scarring or hypopigmentation.

Lasers are common tools for the treatment of pigmentary problems in Asian skin. The most common ablative lasers described in the literature are:

1. CO_2 laser
2. Erbium YAG laser
3. Fractional erbium YAG laser in pixel mode
4. Fractional CO_2 laser.

CO_2 laser used as an ablative exfoliator is too aggressive for Asians because of its prolonged recovery time and the risk of scarring and permanent hypopigmentation.

Erbium YAG laser is a very effective tool for the treatment of mild to moderate dyschromia with repeated exfoliation of epidermis/dermis. It is also very effective for selected areas of deeper tissue removal. Its minimal thermal effect makes it ideal for this purpose in Asian skin with effective healing and minimal scarring. Variation of focal length (spot size) and energy level (fluency) can be altered simultaneously for the removal of skin lesions such as keratosis, melanocytic nevi, and so forth, and general exfoliation of other facial skin. However, its longer recovery time than fractional lasers limits its use for superficial lesions or isolated tissue removal.

Fractional erbium YAG laser/CO_2 laser in pixel mode is the newest form of ablative laser treatment for pigmentary problems in Asian skin. The mechanism of action is based on its effect on epidermal/dermal photothermolysis and at the same time seeks to address the limitations of both ablative resurfacing and nonablative treatments. An array of microscopic thermal wounds (microscopic treatment zones) are induced into the skin to stimulate a therapeutic response deep in the dermis. There is some promise for treatment of melasma using this therapy.

Dr Zheng,[3] a renowned dermatologist from Chengdu, China, uses the following treatment regimen for Asian dyschromia with fractional erbium YAG laser in pixel mode:

1. 7 × 7 or 9 × 9 bits
2. Pulse duration of 500 to 800, 500 to 1000, and 600 to 1200 ms
3. Each treatment requires 3 to 6 passes
4. 1 to 10 sessions
5. Duration between sessions of 2 to 6 weeks.

Postoperative care includes:

1. Immediate ice pack compress
2. Moisturizer cream 4 to 6 times daily for 7 to 10 days
3. Cold compress 30 to 60 minutes daily
4. Sun avoidance for 1 to 2 weeks
5. Tranexamic acid 250 mg orally twice a day for 3 months.

MY APPROACH TO ASIAN SKIN

The patient has to commit to a long-term treatment program and understand the risk of postinflammatory hyperpigmentation/hypopigmentation.

General Care

1. Healthy diet + vitamin C
2. No smoking
3. No excessive alcohol
4. Adequate rest
5. Exercise.

Basic Skin Care:

1. Adequate water intake
2. Sun protection with a sun protection factor of 30 for prolonged effect
3. Suitable skin cleanser: gentle pH-balanced cleanser offers proper cleansing without undue sebaceous gland stimulation
4. Toner after cleansing: it serves to further balance the skin pH and remove potential debris
5. Moisturizer: important for both dry and oily skin. Moisturizer to oily skin inhibits further autogenous production of oil.

Mild Cases

1. Microdermabrasion weekly: 1 to 2 sessions
2. Daily exfoliation systems, for example, Obagi Systems: 6 weeks
3. FPL every 3 weeks for 3 to 5 sessions

This treatment modality is best for:

1. *Mild facial dyschromia*, such as lentigines, sun-damaged skin, fine wrinkles, and ephelides (freckles). Try steps (1) to (3) for 6 weeks, and then every 3 months, repeat steps (1) and (3) for maintenance (**Figs. 1** and **2**).
2. *Mild dyschromia with acne vulgaris* with/without active inflammation:
   a. Blue light + levulan, 1 to 3 sessions monthly
   b. Acne treatment formula, for example, Clenziderm
   c. FPL: repeat step (1) 2 to 3 times if necessary. Steps (2) and (3) are for maintenance.

Moderate Cases

Moderate cases include moderate facial dyschromia, sun-damaged skin, seborrheic keratosis, actinic keratosis, melanocytic nevi, fine wrinkles, and so forth.

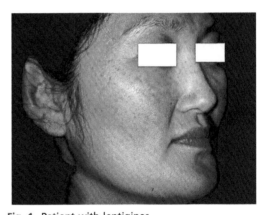

Fig. 1. Patient with lentigines.

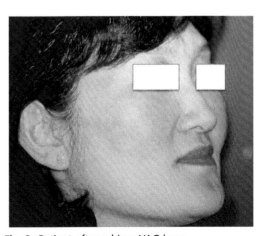

Fig. 2. Patient after erbium YAG laser.

1. Microdermabrasion weekly: 1 to 2 sessions before laser
2. Erbium YAG laser is used for individual removal of melanocytic nevi, seborrheic keratosis, actinic keratosis, and so forth with generalized resurfacing of the rest of the facial skin
3. Treatment of postinflammatory hyperpigmentation, for example, Obagi for 3 months
4. FPL is used for maintenance and repeated every 6 weeks (**Figs. 3** and **4**).

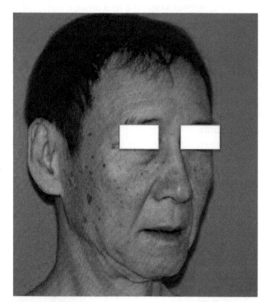

Fig. 3. Patient with sebaceous keratosis and pigmented nevi.

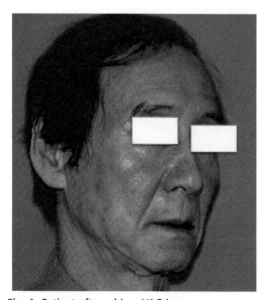

Fig. 4. Patient after erbium YAG laser.

Melasma

Melasma is a very common skin condition in Asian skin and is very difficult to treat. It is thought to be caused by stimulation of melanocytes by the female sex hormones estrogen and progesterone to produce more melanin pigments when the skin is exposed to the sun, hence the name, mask of pregnancy. There is a genetic predisposition and hence it is common in Asians. Occasionally, it is caused by overproduction of melanocytic-stimulating hormones brought on by stress, for example, thyroid disease or melasma suprarenale: Addison disease.

Severe Cases

Melasma

1. Microdermabrasion weekly, 1 to 2 sessions
2. Fractional CO_2 laser

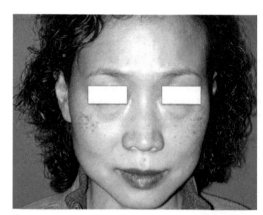

Fig. 5. Patient with melasma.

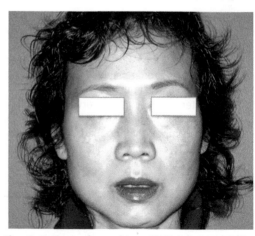

Fig. 6. Patient after erbium YAG laser resurfacing with tranexamic acid.

3. Erbium YAG laser for individual removal of melanocytic nevi, seborrheic keratosis, actinic keratosis, and so forth if necessary
4. Treatment of postinflammatory hyperpigmentation, for example, Obagi for 3 months
5. Tranexamic acid 250 mg orally twice a day for 3 months (Figs. 5–10).

TRANEXAMIC ACID

Dr Blair Ernst, a renowned hematologist from the Credit Valley Hospital-Peel Regional Cancer Center, Mississauga, Canada, has studied this topic and discovered the following facts. Tranexamic acid is mainly used in the treatment of the platelet adhesion disorder bleeding, diathesis, and in women with significant menorrhagia. Its mechanism of action is by inhibition of plasminogen activation (plasminogen→plasmin) preventing clot resorption.[4] In patients with hyperpigmentation, it has been

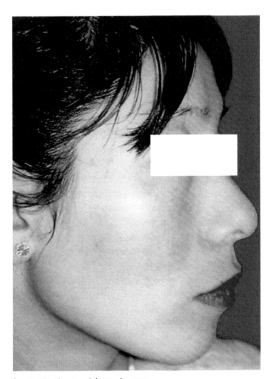

Fig. 7. Patient with melasma.

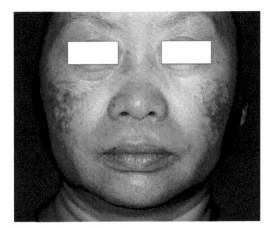

Fig. 9. Patient with melasma.

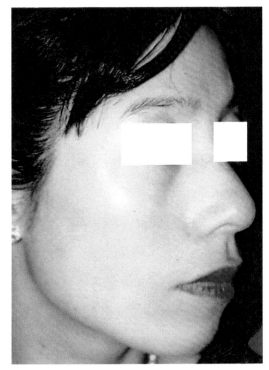

Fig. 8. Patient after fractional erbium YAG laser resurfacing with tranexamic acid.

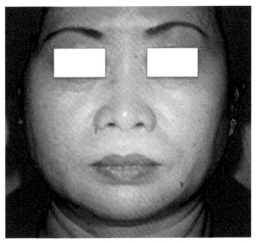

Fig. 10. Patient after fractional CO_2 laser resurfacing with tranexamic acid.

hypothesized that the same mechanism of action prevents depigmentation of keratinocytes.[5] Plasmin degrades arachidonic acid indirectly via phospholipase A_2, resulting in the production of melanogenic compounds (leukotrienes, prostaglandins, and thromboxanes).[6] Tranexamic acid inhibits this process. This has been demonstrated in UV radiation hyperpigmentation prevention in animal models[7] and ex vivo in melanocyte cultures.[5] The proposed dosage of 250 mg twice a day is far less than that used in patients with bleeding diathesis and is not associated with any significant side effects.[8]

REFERENCES

1. Fanous N. A new patient classification for laser resurfacing and peels: predicting responses, risks, and results. Aesthetic Plast Surg 2002;26:99–104.
2. West TB, Alster TS. Effect of pretreatment on the incidence of hyperpigmentation following cutaneous CO_2 laser resurfacing. Dermatol Surg 1999;25:15–7.
3. Zheng Q, He M, Li C-q, et al. The clinical application of erbium laser pixel mode. Chengdu (China): Sichuan Huamei Aesthetic Plastic Surgery Hospital; 2008. Paper serial number 1673–7040 05-0001-00.
4. Abiko, Iwamoto. Plasminogen-plasmin system. VII. Potentiation of antifibrinolytic action of a synthetic inhibitor, tranexamic acid, by alpha 2-macroglobulin antiplasmin. Biochim Biophys Acta 1970;214:411–8.
5. Maeda K, Tomita Y. Mechanism of the inhibitory effect of tranexamic acid on melanogenesis in cultured human melanocytes in the presence of keratinocyte-conditioned medium. J Health Sci 2007;53:389–96.
6. Nakano T, Fujita H, Kikuchi N, et al. Plasmin converts pro-form of group I phospholipase A2 into receptor binding, active forms. Biochem Biophys Res Commun 1994;198:10–5.
7. Li D, Shi Y, Li M, et al. Tranexamic acid can treat ultraviolet radiation-induced pigmentation in guinea pigs. Eur J Dermatol 2010;20:289–92.
8. Rapchinsky C, editor. Cyklokapron (generic: tranexamic acid), Compendium of Pharmaceuticals and Specialties. The Canadian Drug Reference for Health Professionals. Canadian Pharmacists Association. Antifibrinolytic. Pfizer; 2011. p. 717.

Index

Facial Plast Surg Clin N Am 19 (2011) 423–439
doi:10.1016/S1064-7406(11)00040-X
1064-7406/11/$ – see front matter © 2011 Elsevier Inc. All rights reserved.

Moving?